HIKE LIST

60 Hikes within 60 MILES

PITTSBURGH

INCLUDING ALLEGHENY AND SURROUNDING COUNTIES

Donna L. Ruff

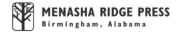
MENASHA RIDGE PRESS
Birmingham, Alabama

Copyright © 2006 Donna L. Ruff
All rights reserved
Printed in the United States of America
Published by Menasha Ridge Press
Distributed by The Globe Pequot Press
First edition, first printing

Library of Congress Cataloging-in-Publication Data

Ruff, Donna L.
   60 Hikes within 60 Miles, Pittsburgh: including Allegheny and surrounding
counties/Donna L. Ruff.—1st ed.
     p. cm.
   ISBN 10: 0-89732-591-5
   ISBN 13: 978-0-89732-591-2
   1. Hiking—Pennsylvania—Pittsburgh Region—Guidebooks. 2. Pittsburgh
Region (Pa.)—Guidebooks. I. Title. II. Title: Sixty Hikes within Sixty Miles,
Pittsburgh.

GV199.42.P42P67 2006
796.5109748'11—dc22

                                                 2006043755

Cover design by Grant M. Tatum
Text design by Karen Ocker
Author photo by Thomas E. Lobaugh
All other photos © Donna L. Ruff
Maps by Donna L. Ruff, Scott McGrew, and Steve Jones

Menasha Ridge Press
P.O. Box 43673
Birmingham, AL 35243
www.menasharidge.com

For Mum—the strongest and kindest person I have ever known

TABLE OF CONTENTS

TABLE OF CONTENTS

ACKNOWLEDGMENTS

First, I truly must simply give my thanks to God for the beautiful creation of this Earth and my fortune to have had opportunities to explore its natural wonders. I must also give a great deal of thanks to the people who work so hard to preserve our natural areas and waterways, and to build and maintain the trails that give us access to them. Whether they are volunteers, park or forest employees, or activists, all deserve credit for their hard work and cumulative effect on safeguarding and nourishing our part of the world.

A book like this takes much time, and I thank all of my loved ones, family and friends, for their understanding of my absence while I hiked, mapped, and typed. To my friends and family who have come along on various trails, thanks so much for your company, chatter, and laughter—as always, I'm privileged to know you. And to my friends who suggested trails and asked about my work, I thank you for your interest and for listening. Thanks also to my editor at Menasha Ridge Press for his insightful guidance and comments. I offer a special thanks to Bobby Nunnink for accompanying me on a number of hikes and being supportive of my efforts as the work took much of my time and energy. Finally, I'd like to thank my mother, Helen Ruff, for always encouraging me to do what I love to do.

—Donna L. Ruff

FOREWORD

Welcome to Menasha Ridge Press's *60 Hikes within 60 Miles,* a series designed to provide hikers with information needed to find and hike the very best trails surrounding cities usually underserved by good guidebooks.

Our strategy is simple: First, find a hiker who knows the area and loves to hike. And second, ask that person to spend a year hiking, mapping, photographing, and describing the most popular and very best trails around in terms of difficulty, scenery, condition, elevation change, and all other categories of information that are important to hikers. "On each hike, pretend you are a new hiker to the area and think about what any hiker would want to know," we tell each author. "Imagine their questions; be clear in your answers."

An experienced hiker and writer, author Donna Ruff has selected 60 of the best hikes in and around the Pittsburgh area. From city parks and natural reserves that highlight the area's interesting history, rivers, and diverse landscape to the more rugged mountains and forests of the Laurel Highlands, Ruff provides hikers (and walkers) with a great variety of hikes—and all within roughly 60 miles of Pittsburgh.

You'll get more out of this book if you take a moment to read the Introduction explaining how to read the trail listings. The Topographic Maps section will help you understand how useful topos will be on a hike, and will also tell you where to get them. And though this is a "where-to," not a "how-to" guide, those of you who have not hiked extensively will find the Introduction of particular value.

As much for the opportunity to free the spirit as well as to free the body, let these hikes elevate you above the urban hurry.

All the best,
The Editors at Menasha Ridge Press

ABOUT THE AUTHOR

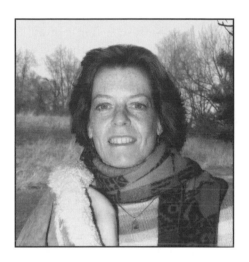

Donna Ruff was born in Pittsburgh and, although a lifetime resident of her hometown, has hiked, biked, climbed, skied, and tested her skills in mountaineering in many parts of the world. She has a special passion for hiking in southwestern Pennsylvania, not only because it is her home but because of its diverse and enchanting beauty. Ruff spent her formative years as a student at the University of Pittsburgh and was at that time beginning to explore the many trails of the area, including those of the Laurel Highlands. After numerous climbing and hiking trips here and in West Virginia, her graduation gift to herself was a climbing and hiking trip to Boulder, Colorado, sealing her fate to continually seek adventure outdoors.

A writer by trade, Ruff spends as much of her spare time as possible away from the computer and in what she calls the real world, that is, the natural world. Over the years she has been an active member of the American Youth Hostels and the Explorer's Club of Pittsburgh, where she has established valuable friendships with like-minded outdoor enthusiasts.

Her hiking and backpacking travels have taken her across the country—from Pennsylvania's "Little Grand Canyon" to Arizona's unmatchable Grand Canyon to Mount Olympus in Washington State and the redwoods of California. She has also climbed 18,470-foot El Pico de Orizabo in Mexico, and mountains in Canada, Peru, and Ecuador. Her travels have extended to many other countries and are typically planned around hiking, climbing, mountaineering, and volunteer work.

PREFACE

I was born a typical city dweller. The soles of my feet mainly tread on concrete. My first experience spending any time in the woods didn't happen until I was 17 years old and on a "retreat." Embarrassingly, our camping retreat was really an excuse for a party in a place where we weren't likely to get caught with illegal beverages, but I didn't partake enough to ruin the following day. In the morning when I opened the borrowed tent's flap and could see the beauty of the woods around me, I was taken with it. Dewdrops hung from leaves, pine needles, and blossoms. A small waterfall trickled down a rock face. The muted brown floor of the woods stood in contrast to bright red, yellow, and orange leaves, with a backdrop of many shades of green. The air smelled fresh and sweet, and the sun, as it began to burn off the fog, also warmed my shoulders and back. As the day grew warmer, the woods kept me cool. Hiking on that trip was a slow, exploratory walk, but a perfect time of discovery. Our party really did turn into a retreat—physically, mentally, and spiritually.

Since that time, I have been drawn back again and again to hiking. It has led me to trails close by, throughout Pennsylvania, then to many states, and eventually outside of the country's borders. It has allowed me to be enraptured by vistas, trees, rock formations, waterfalls, rivers, lakes, mountains, and valleys. A foray in the woods, whether in a city park or wilder terrain, allows me to relish time, a rare gift in an otherwise busy life. When else can we take a few moments to stop and notice the intricate work of a spider web or tiny blossoms emerging from the ground in spring? What is the value of the sound of songbirds, the wind whispering through pines, or the calls of animals in their natural setting over that of cars and televisions? The sight of a hawk or a deer? My experience is that there is rarely a hike or walk along a trail that fails to give something that revitalizes the soul.

Hike, in *Webster's New Universal Unabridged Dictionary,* is defined as "to take a long, vigorous walk; to tramp or march through the country, woods, etc." Ah, but it is so much more than that. Whether alone or with friends, a hike gives humans a chance to reconnect with nature. It takes us to breathtakingly beautiful places that are often unreachable by any other means. It heightens the senses, increases awareness, promotes health, relieves stress, and encourages a new appreciation for the web of life and our role in it. My hope is that this book will assist any hiker, whether a complete newbie or an experienced trekker, to enjoy the serenity that can be found all around us.

Those of us who live in Pittsburgh are fortunate to reside in an area of Pennsylvania said by some to rival parts of the western side of the United States. Our geologic makeup is what provides its diversity and beauty. The western half of the state is part of the Appalachian Plateau. Although the word plateau alludes to a flat top, it really is a geologic term that refers to the orientation of rock. Our rock lies flat and is considered a plateau by the geologist, but as any one can look around and see, our landscape is made of hills, valleys, and mountains. The hills in the Pittsburgh Plateau, which surround the city and contain many of the hikes in this book, were carved by the Allegheny and Monongahela rivers and the many drainage paths to them as they flow

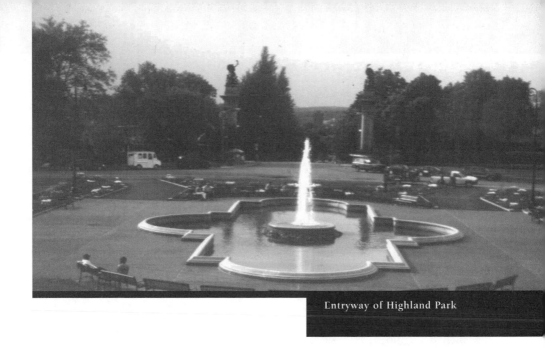

Entryway of Highland Park

west to form the Ohio. The remaining hikes in this book are in the Allegheny Mountain section of the Appalachian Plateau. Located southeast of the city are the state's highest mountains—the 3,000-foot ridges of Chestnut Ridge, Laurel Ridge, and Negro Mountain, that compose the Laurel Highlands. Pennsylvania's highest point, Mount Davis, is located on 30-mile long Negro Mountain, the easternmost of the three. At 3,213 feet, Mount Davis is the lowest high point found in any of the Appalachian Mountain states but boasts a unique ecosystem and unusual circular patterns of stone at its high point, caused by thousands of years of frost action. All of this makes for interesting, distinct, and scenic hiking.

Hikes within the city of Pittsburgh include those that incorporate some of the history of the forming of the nation, as Pittsburgh, with its three rivers, was a prized and strategic location during the American Revolution. For some Pittsburgh history, spend time with a rewarding trip to Point State Park, where you can combine an informative tour of the Fort Pitt Museum and the Fort Pitt Blockhouse with an intriguing and aesthetic walk around the Point, enjoying the view of the rivers and famous fountain. A river walk along the city's North Shore provides a moving visit to various memorials dedicated to soldiers, police officers, and our local sports heroes, and incorporates walks around the two new stadiums. The Downtown Historic Walk could be taken on a long lunch or two and integrates historic 19th-century churches, a 19th-century graveyard, grand public buildings, and the ornate theaters of the cultural district. Hikes within such city parks as Frick and Schenley allow one to combine a hike with tours of the free Frick Museum and other facilities of the Frick Art and Historical Center, or of colorful and aromatic Phipps Conservatory. For hikes that are more wooded and quiet but still within Allegheny County and very quick to reach from the city, try Hartwood Acres, Harrison Hills, Todd Sanctuary, Beechwood Farms, or the Fox Chapel Flower and Wildlife Reserve.

PREFACE

Venturing outside Allegheny County opens the way to even more spectacular natural scenery in every direction. For an adventurous hike that can easily be combined with a learning experience, head to McConnells Mill, where a tour of an old gristmill can be combined with a vigorous hike and views of Slippery Rock Creek tumbling through the gorge it has cut. In the Allegheny Mountain section, the Laurel Highlands is a famous playground for hikers, bikers, and boaters; it is lavishly adorned with natural beauty. Try a hike in the enchanting Bear Run and take a tour of nearby Frank Lloyd Wright's Fallingwater or head to Friendship Hill and tour the preserved home of Albert Gallatin, who was best known for his role as Secretary of the Treasury under Presidents Thomas Jefferson and James Madison, and afterward hike along the Monongahela. Ohiopyle has an array of hikes to choose from, with close-up views of the mighty Youghiogheny River along the Ferncliff Natural Area Loop and the sights of Cucumber Falls and the Slides—the rock formation along the Cucumber Falls to Meadow Run Loop hike. Also included in the Allegheny Mountain section are the state parks of Laurel Ridge, Laurel Hill, Laurel Summit, Kooser, and Linn Run, and the Forbes State Forest and natural areas of Roaring Run, Quebec Run, Charles F. Lewis, Lick Hollow, and Mount Davis. Each has something unique to offer—from the highest point in the state to virgin hemlocks near creek beds, walls of rhododendron to panoramic vistas.

In this book I've worked to include trails for every level of fitness and experience. Driving farther away from the city to natural areas does not mean you have to be able to hike on challenging trails, just as staying closer to the city does not limit you to short walks on easy terrain. Use the Table of Contents to assist in narrowing the geographic location of the hike and the Recommended Hikes section to assist in selecting a hike for the type of scenery or terrain you want. The latter, for example, can help with choices such as whether you want a hike that is suitable for children, is along a lake or river, is steep, or contains historical elements. Then look up the hikes and decide what grabs your interest and how much you are up for doing.

You can hike the trails using the descriptions verbatim or lengthening or shortening them to suit your own time and ability. Whichever you do, go on and get outside. Don't miss what southwestern Pennsylvania has to offer. It is all there waiting right outside your back door.

HIKING RECOMMENDATIONS

▶ BUSY HIKES

Downtown Historic Walk
Eliza Furnace Trail
Frick Park Tour Loop
Gilfillan Trail Loop
Highland Park Double Loop
Montour Trail: Cliff Mine to Five Points
Montour Trail: Panhandle Trail—
  Walkers Mill to Gregg Station

North Shore: River, Memorial, and
  Sports Walk
Schenley Park Loop
Three Rivers Heritage Trail:
  Monongahela South Shore
Twin Lakes Park:
  Loop the Lakes

▶ GOOD HIKES FOR SOLITUDE

Baker Trail: Crooked Creek Lake Area
Bear Run Nature Reserve: Southeast Loop
Blacklick Valley Natural Area:
  Parker Tract Hike
Charles F. Lewis Natural Area:
  Rager Mountain Trail Loop
Forbes State Forest: Laurel Summit—
  Spruce Flats Bog and Wildlife Area Loop
Forbes State Forest: Mount Davis
  Natural Area
Forbes State Forest: Quebec Run Wild Area
Forbes State Forest: Roaring Run
  Natural Area Loop
Friendship Hill Tour and Hike
Jennings Environmental Education Center
  Trail Loop

Keystone State Park: Stone Lodge Trail
Linn Run State Park: Grove Run Loop
McConnells Mill: Alpha Pass to Kildoo Loop
McConnells Mill: Slippery Rock
  Gorge Trail
Mingo Creek County Park Loop
Moraine State Park: North Shore Hike or
  Hike and Bike
North Park: Nature Center Loop
Ohiopyle State Park: Ferncliff
  Natural Area Loop
Raccoon Creek State Park: Lake-Forest Loop
Raccoon Creek State Park: Wildflower
  Reserve Loop
Settler's Cabin Park: Creek and Flora Hike
Todd Sanctuary Loop

▶ URBAN HIKES

Downtown Historic Walk
Eliza Furnace Trail
Highland Park Double Loop
North Shore: River, Memorial, and
  Sports Walk
Point State Park: History and
  Three Rivers Walk

Riverview Park Loop
Schenley Park Loop
Three Rivers Heritage Trail: Monongahela
  South Shore
Three Rivers Heritage Trail: Washington's
  Landing Loop

▶ GOOD HIKES FOR KIDS

Bear Run Nature Reserve:
  Southeast Loop
Beechwood Farms Nature Reserve Loop

Blacklick Valley Natural Area:
  Parker Tract Hike
Bushy Run History Loop

HIKING RECOMMENDATIONS

▶ GOOD HIKES FOR KIDS (CONTINUED)

Cedar Creek Park: Gorge Trail Loop

Downtown Historic Walk

Eliza Furnace Trail

Forbes State Forest: Laurel Summit—
  Spruce Flats Bog and Wildlife Area Loop

Forbes State Forest: Laurel Summit—
  Wolf Rocks Overlook Loop

Forbes State Forest:
  Lick Hollow Interpretive Nature Trail

Forbes State Forest:
  Mount Davis Natural Area

Fort Necessity Tour and Woods Walk

Fox Chapel Flower and Wildlife Reserve Loop

Frick Park Tour Loop

Gilfillan Trail Loop

Harrison Hills Park: Rachel Carson Trail—
  Pond and River Overlooks Hikes

Highland Park Double Loop

Jennings Environmental Education Center
  Trail Loop

Keystone State Park: Stone Lodge Trail

Kooser State Park Loop

Laurel Hill State Park: Hemlock Trail

Laurel Hill State Park: Pump House to
  Tram Road Trail

McConnells Mill: Alpha Pass to
  Kildoo Loop

Montour Trail: Cliff Mine to
  Five Points

Montour Trail: Panhandle Trail—
  Walkers Mill to Gregg Station

North Park: Braille Trail Loop

North Park: Nature Center Loop

North Shore: River, Memorial, and
  Sports Walk

Ohiopyle State Park: Ferncliff Natural
  Area Loop

Point State Park: History and
  Three Rivers Walk

Powdermill Nature Reserve Tour

Raccoon Creek State Park:
  Wildflower Reserve Loop

Riverview Park Loop

Three Rivers Heritage Trail: Monongahela
  South Shore

Three Rivers Heritage Trail: Washington's
  Landing Loop

Todd Sanctuary Loop

Townsend Park Loop

Twin Lakes Park: Loop the Lakes

▶ HISTORIC HIKES

Bushy Run History Loop

Downtown Historic Walk

Fort Necessity Tour and Woods Walk

Frick Park Tour Loop

Friendship Hill Tour and Hike

Hartwood Acres Tour

Highland Park Double Loop

McConnells Mill: Alpha Pass to Kildoo Loop

North Shore: River, Memorial, and
  Sports Walk

Point State Park: History and
  Three Rivers Walk

Schenley Park Loop

Three Rivers Heritage Trail: Washington's
  Landing Loop

▶ SCENIC HIKES

Fox Chapel Flower and Wildlife
  Reserve Loop

Harrison Hills Park: Rachel Carson Trail Pond
  and River Overlooks Hikes

HIKING RECOMMENDATIONS

▶ SCENIC HIKES (CONTINUED)

Bear Run Nature Reserve:
  Southeast Loop
Charles F. Lewis Natural Area: Rager
  Mountain Trail Loop
Forbes State Forest: Laurel Summit—
  Spruce Flats Bog and Wildlife Area Loop
Forbes State Forest: Laurel Summit—
  Wolf Rocks Overlook Loop
Forbes State Forest: Laurel Summit Loop
Forbes State Forest: Lick Hollow Pine Knob
  Overlook Trail
Forbes State Forest: Mount Davis
  Natural Area
Forbes State Forest: Quebec Run Wild Area
Forbes State Forest: Roaring Run Natural Area
  Loop
Friendship Hill Tour and Hike
Highland Park Double Loop
Kooser State Park Loop
Laurel Hill State Park: Hemlock Trail

McConnells Mill: Alpha Pass to
  Kildoo Loop
McConnells Mill: Slippery Rock Gorge Trail
Moraine State Park: North Shore Hike or Hike
  and Bike
North Shore: River, Memorial, and
  Sports Walk
Ohiopyle State Park: Cucumber Falls to
  Meadow Run Trail Loop
Ohiopyle State Park: Ferncliff Natural Area
  Loop
Ohiopyle State Park: Laurel Highlands
  Trail–Ohiopyle to First Shelter Area
Point State Park: History and Three
  Rivers Walk
Raccoon Creek State Park: Wildflower
  Reserve Loop
Three Rivers Heritage Trail: Washington's
  Landing Loop
Todd Sanctuary Loop

▶ HIKES FOR VIEWING WILDFLOWERS

Bear Run Nature Reserve: Southeast Loop
Boyce Park Log Cabin Trail Expanded Loop
Fox Chapel Flower and Wildlife
  Reserve Loop
Friendship Hill Tour and Hike
Laurel Hill State Park: Lake Trail
McConnells Mill: Slippery Rock Gorge Trail
Mingo Creek County Park Loop
Montour Trail: Cliff Mine to Five Points
Moraine State Park: North Shore Hike or
  Hike and Bike

North Park: Braille Trail Loop
North Park: Nature Center Loop
Raccoon Creek State Park:
  Lake-Forest Loop
Raccoon Creek State Park: Wildflower
  Reserve Loop
Settler's Cabin Park: Creek and Flora
  Hike
Todd Sanctuary Loop
Twin Lakes Park: Loop the Lakes

▶ HIKES WITH LAKE VIEWS

Baker Trail: Crooked Creek Lake Area
Keystone State Park: Stone Lodge Trail
Kooser State Park Loop
Moraine State Park: South Shore Trails Loop

Raccoon Creek State Park:
  Lake-Forest Loop
Schenley Park Loop
Twin Lakes Park: Loop the Lakes

HIKING RECOMMENDATIONS

▶ HIKES WITH RIVER VIEWS

Cedar Creek Park: Gorge Trail Loop
Friendship Hill Tour and Hike
Harrison Hills Park: Rachel Carson Trail—
  Pond and River Overlooks Hikes
Laurel Hill State Park: Lake Trail
McConnells Mill: Alpha Pass to
  Kildoo Loop
McConnells Mill: Slippery Rock Gorge Trail
North Shore: River, Memorial, and
  Sports Walk

Ohiopyle State Park: Ferncliff Natural
  Area Loop
Ohiopyle State Park: Laurel Highlands Trail—
  Ohiopyle to First Shelter Area
Point State Park: History and
  Three Rivers Walk
Three Rivers Heritage Trail:
  Monongahela South Shore
Three Rivers Heritage Trail:
  Washington's Landing Loop

▶ HIKES WITH WATERFALLS

Charles F. Lewis Natural Area: Rager
  Mountain Trail Loop
McConnells Mill: Alpha Pass to
  Kildoo Loop
McConnells Mill: Slippery Rock Gorge Trail

Ohiopyle State Park: Cucumber Falls to
  Meadow Run Trail Loop
Ohiopyle State Park: Ferncliff Natural Area
  Loop
Settler's Cabin Park: Creek and Flora Hike

▶ HIKES WITH STREAMS, CREEKS, AND RUNS

Bear Run Nature Reserve:
  Southeast Loop
Blacklick Valley Natural Area:
  Parker Tract Hike
Cedar Creek Park: Gorge Trail Loop
Charles F. Lewis Natural Area: Rager
  Mountain Trail Loop
Forbes State Forest: Mount Davis
  Natural Area
Forbes State Forest: Quebec Run
  Wild Area
Forbes State Forest: Roaring Run Natural Area
  Loop
Fox Chapel Flower and Wildlife
  Reserve Loop
Frick Park Tour Loop

Friendship Hill Tour and Hike
Kooser State Park Loop
Laurel Hill State Park: Hemlock Trail
Laurel Hill State Park: Pump House to
  Tram Road Trail
Linn Run State Park: Grove Run Loop
McConnells Mill: Alpha Pass to Kildoo Loop
McConnells Mill: Slippery Rock Gorge Trail
Montour Trail: Cliff Mine to Five Points
North Park: Braille Trail Loop
Ohiopyle State Park: Cucumber Falls to
  Meadow Run Trail Loop
Raccoon Creek State Park: Wildflower
  Reserve Loop
Schenley Park Loop
Todd Sanctuary Loop

▶ HIKES WITH OVERLOOKS

Baker Trail: Crooked Creek Lake Area
Charles F. Lewis Natural Area: Rager
  Mountain Trail Loop

Forbes State Forest: Laurel Summit—
  Wolf Rocks Overlook Loop

HIKING RECOMMENDATIONS

▶ HIKES WITH OVERLOOKS (CONTINUED)

Forbes State Forest: Lick Hollow Pine Knob
    Overlook Trail
Forbes State Forest: Mount Davis Natural Area
Harrison Hills Park: Rachel Carson Trail—
    Pond and River Overlooks Hikes

Laurel Ridge State Park: Laurel Highlands
    Trail—PA 653 Access to Grindle Ridge
Ohiopyle State Park: Laurel Highlands Trail—
    Ohiopyle to First Shelter Area

▶ HIKES WITH STEEP CLIMBS

Baker Trail: Crooked Creek Lake Area
Blacklick Valley Natural Area: Parker Tract
    Hike
Charles F. Lewis Natural Area: Rager
    Mountain Trail Loop
Forbes State Forest: Lick Hollow Pine Knob
    Overlook Trail
Friendship Hill Tour and Hike
Keystone State Park: Stone Lodge Trail
Kooser State Park Loop

Linn Run State Park: Grove Run Loop
McConnells Mill: Alpha Pass to
    Kildoo Loop
McConnells Mill: Slippery Rock Gorge Trail
Mingo Creek County Park Loop
Ohiopyle State Park: Laurel Highlands Trail
    Ohiopyle to First Shelter Area
Raccoon Creek State Park:
    Lake-Forest Loop
Settler's Cabin Park: Creek and Flora Hike

▶ TRAILS GOOD FOR RUNNERS

Eliza Furnace Trail
Frick Park Tour Loop
Gilfillan Trail Loop
Hartwood Acres Tour
Highland Park Double Loop
Montour Trail: Cliff Mine to Five Points
Montour Trail: Panhandle Trail—
    Walkers Mill to Gregg Station
North Shore: River, Memorial, and Sports Walk

Point State Park: History and
    Three Rivers Walk
Riverview Park Loop
Schenley Park Loop
Three Rivers Heritage Trail: Monongahela
    South Shore
Three Rivers Heritage Trail: Washington's
    Landing Loop
Twin Lakes Park: Loop the Lakes

▶ TRAILS GOOD FOR BIKES/MOUNTAIN BIKES

Boyce Park Log Cabin Trail Expanded Loop
    (mountain bikes only)
Eliza Furnace Trail
Frick Park Tour Loop (mountain bikes only)
Hartwood Acres Tour (mountain bikes only)
Mingo Creek County Park Loop
    (mountain bikes only)
Montour Trail: Cliff Mine to Five Points
Montour Trail: Panhandle Trail—

Walkers Mill to Gregg Station
Moraine State Park: North Shore Hike or
    Hike and Bike (partial)
Raccoon Creek State Park: Lake-Forest Loop
    (partial/mountain bikes only)
South Park Hike (mountain bikes only)
Three Rivers Heritage Trail: Monongahela
    South Shore
Twin Lakes Park: Loop the Lakes

HIKING RECOMMENDATIONS

▶ WHEELCHAIR-ACCESSIBLE HIKES

Downtown Historic Walk
Eliza Furnace Trail
Fort Necessity Tour and Woods Walk
  (partial)
Friendship Hill Tour and Hike (partial)
Highland Park Double Loop (partial)
McConnells Mill: Alpha Pass to Kildoo Loop
  (partial)
Mingo Creek County Park Loop (partial)
Montour Trail: Cliff Mine to
  Five Points

Montour Trail: Panhandle Trail—
  Walkers Mill to Gregg Station
North Shore: River, Memorial, and
  Sports Walk
Point State Park: History and Three
  Rivers Walk
Three Rivers Heritage Trail: Monongahela
  South Shore
Three Rivers Heritage Trail: Washington's
  Landing Loop
Twin Lakes Park: Loop the Lakes

▶ HIKES LESS THAN 1 MILE

Forbes State Forest: Lick Hollow Interpretive
  Nature Trail

North Park: Braille Trail Loop
Powdermill Nature Reserve Tour

▶ HIKES 1 TO 3 MILES

Beechwood Farms Nature Reserve Loop
Boyce Park Log Cabin Trail Expanded Loop
Bushy Run History Loop
Cedar Creek Park: Gorge Trail Loop
Downtown Historic Walk
Forbes State Forest: Laurel Summit—
  Spruce Flats Bog and Wildlife Area Loop
Fort Necessity Tour and Woods Walk
Fox Chapel Flower and Wildlife Reserve Loop
Gilfillan Trail Loop
Hartwood Acres Tour
Highland Park Double Loop
Keystone State Park: Stone Lodge Trail
Laurel Hill State Park: Hemlock Trail
Laurel Hill State Park: Pump House to
  Tram Road Trail

North Park: Nature Center Loop
North Shore: River, Memorial, and
  Sports Walk
Point State Park: History and Three Rivers
  Walk
Raccoon Creek State Park: Wildflower
  Reserve Loop
Riverview Park Loop
Schenley Park Loop
Settler's Cabin Park: Creek and
  Flora Hike
South Park Hike
Three Rivers Heritage Trail: Washington's
  Landing Loop
Todd Sanctuary Loop
Townsend Park Loop

▶ HIKES 3 TO 6 MILES

Blacklick Valley Natural Area:
  Parker Tract Hike
Charles F. Lewis Natural Area: Rager
  Mountain Trail Loop
Eliza Furnace Trail

Forbes State Forest: Laurel Summit—
  Wolf Rocks Overlook Loop
Forbes State Forest: Lick Hollow Pine Knob
  Overlook Trail
Forbes State Forest: Quebec Run Wild Area

HIKING RECOMMENDATIONS

▶ HIKES 3 TO 6 MILES (CONTINUED)

Frick Park Tour Loop

Friendship Hill Tour and Hike

Harrison Hills Park: Rachel Carson Trail—
Pond and River Overlooks Hikes

Jennings Environmental Education Center
Trail Loop

Kooser State Park Loop

Laurel Hill State Park: Lake Trail

Linn Run State Park: Grove Run Loop

McConnells Mill: Alpha Pass to Kildoo Loop

Mingo Creek County Park Loop

Montour Trail: Cliff Mine to Five Points

Montour Trail: Panhandle Trail—
Walkers Mill to Gregg Station

Moraine State Park: South Shore Trails Loop

Ohiopyle State Park: Cucumber Falls to
Meadow Run Trail Loop

Ohiopyle State Park: Ferncliff Natural Area
Loop

Raccoon Creek State Park: Lake-Forest
Loop

Twin Lakes Park: Loop the Lakes

▶ HIKES 6 OR MORE MILES

Baker Trail: Crooked Creek Lake Area

Bear Run Nature Reserve: Southeast Loop

Forbes State Forest: Laurel Summit Loop

Forbes State Forest: Mount Davis
Natural Area

Forbes State Forest: Roaring Run
Natural Area Loop

Laurel Ridge State Park: Laurel Highlands
Trail—PA 653 Access to Grindle Ridge

McConnells Mill: Slippery Rock Gorge Trail

Moraine State Park: North Shore Hike or
Hike and Bike

Ohiopyle State Park: Laurel Highlands Trail—
Ohiopyle to First Shelter Area

Three Rivers Heritage Trail: Monongahela
South Shore

60 Hikes
within **60 MILES**

PITTSBURGH

INCLUDING ALLEGHENY AND
SURROUNDING COUNTIES

INTRODUCTION

Welcome to *60 Hikes within 60 Miles: Pittsburgh*. If you're new to hiking or even if you're a seasoned trail-smith, take a few minutes to read the following introduction. We explain how this book is organized and how to use it.

▶ HIKE DESCRIPTIONS

Each hike contains eight key items: an "In Brief" description of the trail, a key at-a-glance information box, directions to the trail, a trail map, an elevation profile, GPS-acquired UTM trailhead coordinates, a trail description, and a description of nearby activities. Combined, the maps and information provide a clear method to assess each trail from the comfort of your favorite reading chair.

IN BRIEF

A "taste of the trail." Think of this section as a snapshot focused on the historical landmarks, beautiful vistas, and other sights you may encounter on the trail.

KEY-AT-A-GLANCE INFORMATION

The information in the key at-a-glance boxes gives you a quick idea of the specifics of each hike. There are 12 basic elements covered.

LENGTH The length of the trail from start to finish. There may be options to shorten or extend the hikes, but the mileage corresponds to the described hike. Consult the hike description to help decide how to customize the hike for your ability or time constraints.

CONFIGURATION A description of what the trail might look like from overhead. Trails can be loops, out-and-backs (trails on which one enters and leaves along the same path), figure eights, or balloons.

DIFFICULTY The degree of effort an "average" hiker should expect on a given hike. For simplicity, difficulty is described as "easy," "moderate," or "difficult."

SCENERY A rating of the overall environs of the hike and what to expect in terms of plant life, wildlife, streams, and historic buildings.

EXPOSURE A quick check of how much sun you can expect on your shoulders during the hike. Descriptors used include terms such as "shady," "exposed," and "sunny."

TRAFFIC Indicators of how busy the trail might be on an average day, and if you might be able to find solitude out there. Trail traffic, of course, varies from day to day and season to season.

SURFACE A description of the trail surface, be it paved, crushed limestone, rocky, dirt, or a mixture of elements.

HIKING TIME The length of time it takes to hike the trail. Most of the estimates in this book reflect an average speed of 2 miles per hour. Difficult terrain and scrambling can add significantly to the amount of time required.

ACCESS A notation of hours of service and any fees or permits needed to access the trail (if any).

MAPS Which maps are the best, or easiest, for this hike and where to get them.

INTRODUCTION

FACILITIES What to expect in terms of restrooms, water, and other amenities available at the trailhead or nearby.

SPECIAL COMMENTS These comments cover little extra details that don't fit into any of the above categories. Here you'll find information on trail-hiking options and facts, or tips on how to get the most out of your hike.

DIRECTIONS

The detailed directions along with the trail map will lead you to each trailhead. If you use GPS technology, provided UTM coordinates allow you to navigate directly to the trailhead.

TRAIL DESCRIPTIONS

The trail description is the heart of each hike. Here, the author provides a summary of the trail's essence and highlights any special traits the hike offers. Ultimately, the hike description will help you choose which hikes are best for you.

NEARBY ATTRACTIONS

Look here for information on nearby activities or points of interest.

▶ WEATHER

Despite being relatively near the Atlantic Ocean, Pittsburgh has a more continental climate, caused by prevailing winds from the western interior. The area benefits from the resulting wide temperature differences between winter and summer with four distinct seasons. Spring, summer, fall, and winter each are suitable for hiking, just with different scenery to appreciate, and different preparations for enjoyment.

Spring is a particularly delightful time to hike. During this time of year new life abounds, with wildflowers and trees blooming everywhere. Just be prepared with a jacket for chillier weather or possible rain. Pittsburgh's actual rainfall is highest from May through July. Summer brings not only heat but also increased humidity, particularly from June through August; these are great times to head to the mountains for cooler weather or choose an early morning or late afternoon for your excursion. The most important item to pack for summer months is water. Fall, with the area's abundance of deciduous trees, provides a spectacular array of color, and is my favorite time of the year to enjoy the woods. Carry a jacket and enjoy the crisp air. Winter does not come to mind for many people as a nice time to hike, but there are real benefits to getting outdoors this time of year. Snow beautifies all it touches, lining tree branches and fence posts, its white contrasting with shades of green and brown. Furthermore, trails are usually not crowded during this season, and if you get the winter blues it's a sure cure and a good time to try something new if you haven't already, such as snowshoeing or cross-country skiing. Dress in layers with a weatherproof jacket as the outermost deterrent to wind and precipitation.

INTRODUCTION

Being prepared for the weather is the easiest way to enjoy a nice hike, or is at least equal to having well-fitting shoes or boots. If you are new to hiking, it is easier than you think. Ask a friend with hiking experience or a local outdoor shop or club about proper clothing. You don't need to spend a lot of money to get good-quality clothing that's appropriate for the weather. Wicking materials assist in carrying precipitation away from your body, and wind and rain barriers for an outer layer are protective. For winter, adding a warm layer in between them takes care of most needs; you'll also need good-quality gloves and socks to protect your susceptible fingers and toes, and a hat, which retains most of your body heat (the body heat you generate with activity assists greatly in keeping you warm, too).

So go on, get out there and enjoy our beautiful areas. You'll be happier, and healthier.

AVERAGE DAILY TEMPERATURES BY MONTH

	JAN	FEB	MAR	APR	MAY	JUN
HIGH	35°	39°	50°	61°	71°	79°
LOW	20°	22°	30°	39°	49°	58°
MEAN	28°	31°	40°	50°	60°	69°

	JUL	AUG	SEP	OCT	NOV	DEC
HIGH	83°	81°	74°	63°	51°	40°
LOW	62°	61°	54°	43°	34°	25°
MEAN	73°	71°	64°	53°	43°	33°

▶ ALLOCATING TIME

Speed drops when hiking in direct proportion to the steepness of a path. Navigating obstacles such as roots and rocks, off-trail exploration of flora and fauna, photography, and rest stops also extend a hike. Give yourself plenty of time. Few people enjoy rushing through a hike, and fewer still take pleasure in hiking down a rocky path after dark. Remember, too, that your pace naturally slackens over the back half of a long trek.

▶ MAPS

The maps in this book have been produced with great care and, used with the hiking directions, will lead you to the trail and help you stay on course. However, you will find superior detail and valuable information in the United States Geological Survey's 7.5 minute series topographic maps. Topo maps are available online in many locations, including **topomaps.usgs.gov, terraserver.microsoft.com,** and **www.topo zone.com.** The downside to topos is that most of them are outdated, having been created 20 to 30 years ago. But they still provide excellent topographic detail. A

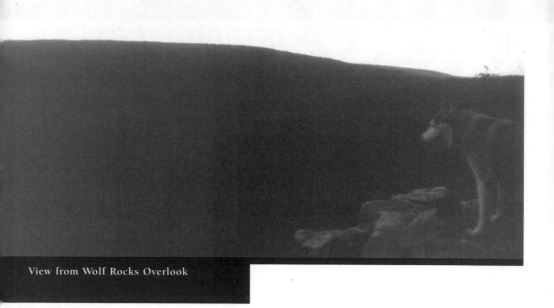

View from Wolf Rocks Overlook

fabulous new tool is Google Earth (**earth.google.com**), which allows you to zoom into a hiking area and view aerial photographs.

If you're new to hiking, you might be wondering, "What's a topographic map?" In short, a topo indicates not only linear distance but elevation as well, using contour lines. Contour lines are included across the entire map. Each line represents a particular elevation, and at the base of each topo, a contour's interval designation is given. If the contour interval is 200 feet, then the height difference between each contour line is 200 feet. Follow five contour lines up on the same map, and the elevation has increased by 1,000 feet.

Let's assume that the 7.5 minute series topo reads "Contour Interval 40 feet," that the short trail we'll be hiking is two inches in length on the map, and that it crosses five contour lines from beginning to end. What do we know? Well, because the linear scale of this series is 2,000 feet to the inch (roughly two and three-quarters inches representing one mile), we know our trail is approximately four-fifths of a mile long (two inches are 2,000 feet). But we also know we'll be climbing or descending 200 vertical feet (five contour lines are 40 feet each) over that distance. And the elevation designations written on occasional contour lines will tell us if we're heading up or down.

In addition to the online sites, outdoor shops, and bike shops, you'll find topos at major universities and some public libraries, where you might try photocopying the ones you need to avoid the cost of buying them.

GPS TRAILHEAD COORDINATES
To collect accurate map data, the author hiked each trail with a handheld GPS (Garmin GPS III) unit. Data collected was then downloaded and plotted onto a digital USGS (U.S. Geological Survey) topo map. In addition to rendering a highly

INTRODUCTION

accurate trail outline, this book also includes the GPS coordinates for each trailhead. More accurately known as UTM (Universal Transverse Mercator) coordinates, the numbers index a specific point using a grid method. The survey datum used to arrive at the coordinates is usually NAD27, but can also be NAD83 or WGS84. For readers who own a GPS unit, whether handheld or onboard a vehicle, the UTM coordinates provided on the first page of each hike may be entered into the GPS unit. Just make sure your GPS unit is set to navigate using the UTM system in conjunction with WGS84 datum. Now you can navigate directly to the trailhead.

Most trailheads, which begin in parking areas, can be reached by car. However, some hikes still require a short walk to reach the trailhead from a parking area. In those cases, a handheld unit would be necessary to continue the GPS navigation process. That said, however, readers can easily access all trailheads in this book by using the directions given, the overview map, and the trail map, which shows at least one major road leading into the area. But for those who enjoy using the latest GPS technology, the necessary data has been provided. A brief explanation of the UTM coordinates follows.

UTM COORDINATES: ZONE, EASTING, AND NORTHING

Within the UTM coordinates box on the first page of each hike, there are three numbers labeled zone, easting, and northing. Here is an example from Forbes State Forest: Mount Davis Natural Area on page 203:

> **UTM Zone (WGS84)   17S**
>
> **Easting   656847**
>
> **Northing   4406443**

The zone number (17) refers to one of the 60 longitudinal zones (vertical) of a map using the Universal Transverse Mercator (UTM) projection. Each zone is 6° wide. The zone letter (S) refers to one of the 20 latitudinal zones (horizontal) that span from 80° South to 84° North.

The easting number (656847) references in meters how far east the point is from the zero value for eastings, which runs north–south through Greenwich, England. Increasing easting coordinates on a topo map or on your GPS screen indicate you are moving east. Decreasing easting coordinates indicate you are moving west. Since lines of longitude converge at the poles, they are not parallel as lines of latitude are. This means that the distance between Full Easting Coordinates is 1,000 meters near the equator but becomes smaller as you travel farther north or south. The difference is small enough to be ignored, but only until you reach the polar regions.

In the Northern Hemisphere, the northing number (4406443) references in meters how far you are from the equator. Above the equator, northing coordinates increase by 1,000 meters between each parallel line of latitude (east–west lines). On a topo map or GPS receiver, increasing northing numbers indicate you are traveling north.

INTRODUCTION

In the Southern Hemisphere, the northing number references how far you are from a latitude line that is 10 million meters south of the equator. Below the equator, northing coordinates decrease by 1,000 meters between each line of latitude. On a topo map, decreasing northing coordinates indicate you are traveling south.

▶ TRAIL ETIQUETTE

Whether you're on a city, county, state, or national park trail, always remember that great care and resources (from Nature as well as from your tax dollars) have gone into creating these trails. Treat the trail, wildlife, and fellow hikers with respect.

- Hike on open trails only. Respect trail and road closures (ask if not sure), avoid possible trespassing on private land, and obtain all permits and authorization as required. Also, leave gates as you found them or as marked.

- Leave only footprints. Be sensitive to the ground beneath you. This also means staying on the existing trail and not blazing any new trails. Be sure to pack out what you pack in. No one likes to see the trash someone else has left behind.

- Never spook animals. An unannounced approach, a sudden movement, or a loud noise startles most animals. A surprised snake or skunk can be dangerous for you, for others, and to themselves. Give animals extra room and time to adjust to your presence.

- Plan ahead. Know your equipment, your ability, and the area in which you are hiking—and prepare accordingly. Be self-sufficient at all times; carry necessary supplies for changes in weather or other conditions. A well-executed trip is a satisfaction to you and to others.

- Be courteous to other hikers, bikers, or equestrians you meet on the trails. It is customary to yield the right of way to equestrians, hikers going uphill, and to faster hikers.

▶ WATER

"How much is enough? One bottle? Two? Three?! But think of all that extra weight!" One simple physiological fact should convince you to err on the side of excess when it comes to deciding how much water to pack: A hiker working hard in 90° heat needs approximately ten quarts of fluid every day. That's two and a half gallons—12 large water bottles or 16 small ones. So, pack along one or two bottles even for short hikes.

Serious backpackers hit the trail prepared to purify water found along the route. This method, while less dangerous than drinking it untreated, comes with risks. Purifiers with ceramic filters are the safest but are also the most expensive. Many hikers

INTRODUCTION

pack along the slightly distasteful tetraglycine-hydroperiodide tablets (sold under the names Potable Aqua, Coughlan's, and others). However, Aqua Mira, which comes in drops is tasteless. Probably the most common waterborne bug that hikers face is giardia, which may not hit until one to four weeks after ingestion. It will have you passing noxious rotten-egg gas, vomiting, shivering with chills, and living in the bathroom. But there are other parasites to worry about, including E. coli and cryptosporidium (that are harder to kill than giardia).

For most people, the pleasures of hiking make carrying water a relatively minor price to pay to remain healthy. If you're tempted to drink "found water," do so only if you understand the risks involved. Better yet, hydrate prior to your hike, carry (and drink) six to ten ounces of water for every mile you plan to hike, and hydrate after the hike.

▶ FIRST-AID KIT

A kit may contain more items than you might think. These are just the basics:

Ace bandages or Spenco joint wraps
Antibiotic ointment (Neosporin or the generic equivalent)
Aspirin or acetaminophen
Band-Aids
Benadryl or the generic equivalent, diphenhydramine (an antihistamine, in case of allergic reactions)
Butterfly-closure bandages
Emergency poncho
Epinephrine in a prefilled syringe (for those known to have severe allergic reactions to such things as bee stings)
Gauze (one roll)
Gauze compress pads (a half dozen 4 x 4 inch)

Hydrogen peroxide or iodine
Insect repellent
LED flashlight or headlamp
Matches or pocket lighter
Moleskin/Spenco "Second Skin"
Pocket knife or multi-purpose tool
Snakebite kit
Sunscreen
Tweezers (for removing ticks after placing extinguished hot match near its head)
Water-purification tablets or water filter (on longer hikes)
Whistle (more effective in signaling rescuers than your voice)

▶ HIKING WITH CHILDREN

No one is too young for a hike in the woods or through a city park. Be mindful, though. Flat, short trails are best with an infant. Toddlers who have not quite mastered walking can still tag along, riding on an adult's back in a child carrier. Use common sense to judge a child's capacity to hike a particular trail, and always rely on the possibility that the child will tire quickly and need to be carried.

When packing for the hike, remember the child's needs as well as your own. Make sure children are adequately clothed for the weather, have proper shoes, and are protected from the sun with sunscreen. Kids also dehydrate quickly, so make sure you have plenty of fluids for everyone.

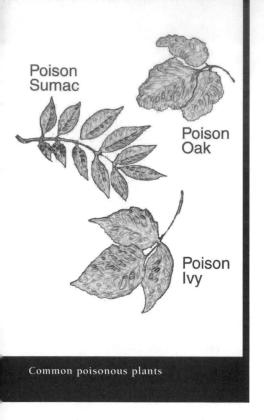

Poison
Sumac

Poison
Oak

Poison
Ivy

Common poisonous plants

A list of good hikes for children is provided in the Hiking Recommendations section earlier in this book. Keep in mind though, that if a child is used to walking and hiking and is a bit older, many other hikes may also be appropriate, but if the child is very young or not used to walking, some of the hikes listed may not be suitable or should be reduced in length.

▶ POISON IVY/OAK/SUMAC

Recognizing and avoiding contact with poison ivy, oak, and sumac are the most effective ways to prevent the painful, itchy rashes associated with these plants. Poison ivy occurs as a vine or groundcover, three leaflets to a leaf; poison oak occurs as either a vine or shrub, with three leaflets as well; and poison sumac flourishes in swampland and moist soil, each leaf containing 7 to 13 leaflets. Urushiol, the oil in the sap of these plants, is responsible for the rash.

Within 12 to 14 hours of exposure, raised lines and/or blisters will appear on the skin, accompanied by a terrible itch. Refrain from scratching because bacteria under fingernails may cause infection. Wash and dry the rash thoroughly, applying a lotion to help dry out the rash. If itching or blistering is severe, seek medical attention. And remember that oil-contaminated clothes, pets, or hiking gear can easily cause an irritating rash on you or someone else, so wash not only any exposed parts of your body but also clothes, gear, and pets if applicable.

▶ THE BUSINESS HIKER

Whether you're in the Pittsburgh area on business or are a resident, these 60 hikes offer perfect quick getaways from the busy demands of commerce. Some of the hikes are classified as urban and are easily accessible from the downtown area. Pack your lunch and take a walk for a refreshing break in the day. The Downtown Historic Walk, Point State Park, North Shore, and Three Rivers Heritage Trails are perfect escapes for the downtown-area worker.

▶ A NOTE ABOUT HUNTING

Many state parks and Forbes State Forest permit hunting in season. To learn when hunting is permitted, go to the Pennsylvania State Game Commission's Web site, **www.pgc.state .pa.us/pgc.** For specific hunting information concerning a state park or forestland, check the Pennsylvania Department of Natural Resources Web site—**www.dcnr.state.pa.us**—where you can search for hunting information under a particular park or call the contact numbers.

INTRODUCTION

▶ SNAKES

The mere mention of snakes drives fear into the hearts of some hikers. Most of the time that fear is unfounded. Just give snakes a wide berth and let them be. If you happen across a venomous variety, take extra caution when avoiding it. The best way to recognize venomous snakes is to take some time to study them before heading into the woods. As a simple rule of thumb, don't toy with any snake, especially those with triangular-shaped heads.

▶ TICKS

Ticks are frequent in southwestern Pennsylvania. But for all of the hiking that I have done over the years, I have only had one actually bite and hang on to me. Deer ticks are the most common in this area. You can use several strategies to reduce your chances of ticks getting under your skin. Some people choose to wear light-colored clothing, so ticks can be spotted before they make it to the skin. Insect repellent containing DEET is known as an effective deterrent. Most importantly, though, be sure to inspect yourself visually at the end of a hike. During your posthike shower, take a moment to do a more complete body check. For ticks that are already embedded, light a match, extinguish it, and place it near the tick's head to try and encourage it to release; then remove the tick with tweezers.

▶ MOSQUITOES

While not a common occurrence, individuals can become infected with the West Nile virus from the bite of an infected mosquito. Culex mosquitoes, the primary varieties that can transmit West Nile virus to humans, thrive in urban rather than wilderness areas. They lay their eggs in stagnant water and can breed in any standing water that remains for more than five days. Most people infected with West Nile virus have no symptoms of illness, but some may become ill, usually 3 to 15 days after being bitten.

Most at risk are the elderly and those with weakened immune systems. Though the risk of infection is relatively low, hikers should consider taking measures to prevent mosquito bites. Remedies include using insect repellent and wearing clothes that completely cover the arms and legs.

ALLEGHENY COUNTY

BEECHWOOD FARMS NATURE RESERVE LOOP

KEY AT-A-GLANCE INFORMATION

LENGTH: 1.1 miles

CONFIGURATION: Loop

DIFFICULTY: Easy

SCENERY: Native trees, flowers, and vegetation; Hart's Run; herb and Native American gardens

EXPOSURE: Mostly shaded

TRAFFIC: Light to medium; busier in spring, summer, and on weekends

TRAIL SURFACE: Dirt, grass

HIKING TIME: 1.5 hours

ACCESS: Open year-round, dawn to dusk

MAPS: Available at the Evans Nature Center or online at **www.aswp.org;** USGS Glenshaw

FACILITIES: Restrooms downstairs in Evans Nature Center

SPECIAL COMMENTS: Dogs are not permitted. Pick up a discovery book from the footpath if you wish to learn more while walking this path.

Beechwood Farms Nature Reserve Loop

UTM Zone (WGS84)   17T

Easting   592673

Northing   4488549

IN BRIEF

Beechwood Farms, at 134 acres, is one of the largest nature reserves and environmental-education centers in western Pennsylvania and is a delight to visit. It's a wonderful place to bring family members of all ages.

DESCRIPTION

The Beechwood Farm Nature Reserve is owned by the Western Pennsylvania Conservancy and leased to the Audubon Society of Western Pennsylvania, which uses it as their headquarters. The property was a part of a larger tract of land that once served as a dairy farm. The reserve itself is being allowed to return to its natural state while providing a sanctuary for humans and wildlife alike. It offers 5 miles of easy hiking trails and a host of environmental-education programs and walks.

This hike begins at the trailhead of the Spring Hollow Walk, which can be started from inside the nature center (by exiting through the back) or by walking to the left of the farmhouse and between it and the education building.

In front of the farmhouse grow many herbs, including French tarragon, chives, scotch broom, garden sage, and English thyme. Inside the farmhouse, you'll find a gift shop, bookstore, and natural history library, as well as a few chairs to sit and read or watch birds. The education building is a model of conservation. Its roof is equipped with a solar array, its furnace operates at 98-percent efficiency, its air-circulation system is designed to cool the building without the need for air-conditioning, and its toilets even operate without water. Timing

DIRECTIONS

From Pittsburgh, take PA 28 North to Exit 5B, PA 8 North. At first light, turn right onto Kittanning Road (turns into Dorseyville Road) and follow for 4.5 miles. Turn left into the parking lot.

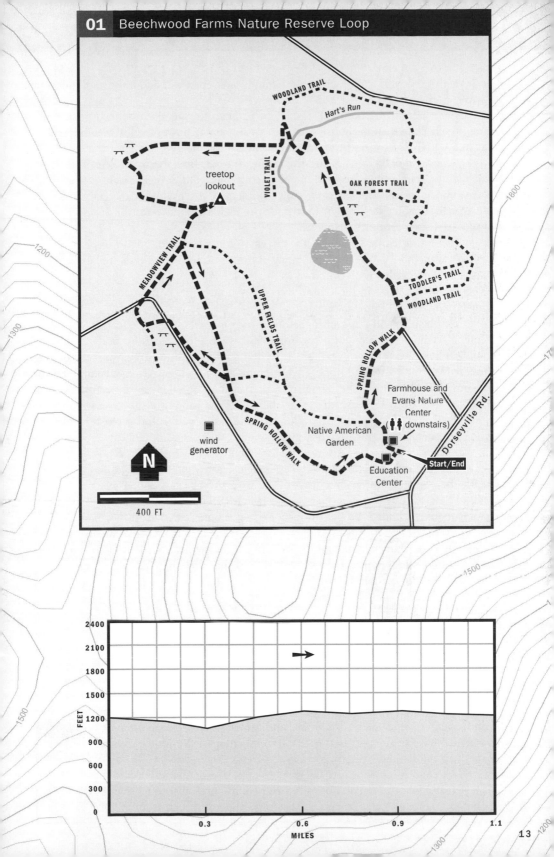

your visit with a program or when the farmhouse is open will add an extra dimension to your walk.

Once behind the building, turn right to head toward the trailhead post. Walk along the back of the farmhouse where, in spring, many flowers are sure to be blooming and a holly tree offers its shiny green leaves near the garden's split-rail fence.

Almost immediately beyond the trailhead post, find the Native American garden on the left; devil's claw, Hopi blue corn, and other vegetation harvested by Native American Indians currently grow in this area. After another 20 feet you'll find a post and a choice to turn left for the Upper Fields Trail or right for Spring Hollow Walk. Turn right for Spring Hollow.

The Spring Hollow Walk is a wide, easy, and well-maintained footpath that is perfect for the new nature explorer. Many of the trees along its length are labeled. The land surrounding this walk is known as the Native Plant Sanctuary, where plants that are common and rare in the Ohio River Valley flourish in pond meadow, hardwood forest, and stream hollow habitats.

Starting out, and if it's spring, enjoy the visual and olfactory effects of the beautifully blooming trees along the beginning of this path. Junctures for both the Woodland Trail and the Toddler's Trail are arrived at soon; continue straight for the Spring Hollow Walk at each. The pond environment on the left proves a relaxing area to explore or observe from the bench provided near it. You'll likely view some of the mallards and Canada geese that nest there. When walking again, enjoy the large pines. And just beyond, at 0.21 miles into the walk, you'll find a cluster of rustic wooden benches underneath oaks, maples, and other deciduous trees.

Mayapples also can be found in this vicinity growing in large patches under deciduous trees. These plants produce a single creamy-white, waxlike flower underneath their large, umbrella-like leaves. The fruit they bear is called an apple but is really a berry; it can be eaten but is rather tasteless. The entire remainder of the plant is poisonous. Although too poisonous for use in home remedies, it has many medicinal uses. Native Americans used the root as a strong laxative, to treat worms, and for other ailments. Currently, the root is used in cancer medications and other remedies.

Shortly, you'll bypass the Oak Forest Trail that branches off to the right; it circles back toward the farmhouse or, if you wish to take an extra jaunt, it connects to the Toddler's Trail and is only about a 20-minute walk (0.53 miles). You can retrace your steps to this point.

Continuing on the Spring Hollow Walk, you'll find an enormous tulip tree at 0.30 miles. Curving right with the path, cross Hart's Run over two small, wooden bridges. After crossing more short bridges above feeder streams, you'll reach the junction with Woodland Trail. Turn left to remain on Spring Hollow and ascend the slight incline to view many more beautiful and enormous tulip trees, a sugar gum tree, and wildflowers. The posted Violet Trail leads left. Staying on Spring Hollow, you'll come upon small, dainty violets and then cross another short series of wooden bridges. Notice the change in vegetation in this moist environment where skunk cabbage, fern, moss, and trillium thrive.

Despite some road noise, the combination of green vegetation, old trees, fallen logs (left in place to nourish both flora and fauna), and birdsong provides the feeling of being in a remote area, even on this short hike not too far from the city.

After a slight incline in the terrain, more benches, red oak trees, and a cherry tree are located at almost 0.5 miles. This is in an area where the trail is often lined with split-rail fencing. There is an old, huge chestnut oak that has been left in the middle of the trail to continue its life span. Don't miss the left turn and opportunity to walk out onto the lookout and view the treetops. Here tall, gorgeous dogwoods are in bloom and a large black oak is labeled. Enjoy the view before turning around and continuing up the trail where grass and goldenrod lead up to an old white ash.

At 0.6 miles come to an intersection with the Meadowview and Upper Fields trails and a sign indicating that there is a vista to the right. Looking for the view, we turned right and crossed the narrow, private, paved road. If you choose to do this as well, you may not find a view (we didn't) but the walk is worth taking. Looping back and to the right, there are many trees in bloom. There's also a bench to sit on and enjoy the remoteness and birdsong (we even spotted wild turkeys). After the bench, turn right at the unmarked T in the trail. Reach the unmarked private road and a post with a sign indicating the Meadowview Trail straight ahead. Go straight and reach another post. Turn right on Spring Hollow Walk and pass the turn for the vista to return to the farmhouse and nature center. Look to your right for the wind generator. At just after a mile, when you've almost reached the buildings, look at the back of the education building to see if the hawk dwelling there is visible.

▶ NEARBY ATTRACTIONS

Beechwood Farms offers many opportunities for all ages to learn in the form of hikes, programs, and tours. Visit their Web site, **www.aswp.org,** to view a calendar of activities, or call (412) 963-6100. Their gift shop, bookstore, library, education building, and the Evans Nature Center are all worth a visit if you have the time.

BOYCE PARK LOG CABIN TRAIL EXPANDED LOOP

KEY AT-A-GLANCE INFORMATION

LENGTH: 2.2 miles

CONFIGURATION: Loop

DIFFICULTY: Easy to moderate

SCENERY: Restored circa-1820 log cabin, Pierson Run, deciduous trees, flowering trees, wildflowers

EXPOSURE: Half shaded, half open

TRAFFIC: Light

TRAIL SURFACE: Dirt

HIKING TIME: 1 hour

ACCESS: Open year-round, 8 a.m. to sundown

MAPS: Available for the overall park at the administration building, call (412) 271-3110 (trails are not depicted on the park map with any detail and many are not included at all); USGS Murrysville

FACILITIES: A handicap-accessible portable toilet is in the parking lot. There are many groves and picnic shelters, a wave pool, an archery range, a model-plane field, and even downhill skiing. (See Nearby Attractions following the Description).

SPECIAL COMMENTS: Boyce Park is a large and beautiful community park. However, to enjoy the hiking here, be willing to use unmarked trails, as signage has not been a part of the park's upkeep.

Boyce Park Log Cabin Trail
Expanded Loop

UTM Zone (WGS84) 17T

Easting   606713

Northing   4479904

IN BRIEF

This hike includes both woodlands and meadows and connects many unmarked trails. As a result, the hiker passes through a variety of habitats and also sees some of the park's amenities.

DESCRIPTION

If you wish, stop at the administration building for park information; it is located on Old Frankstown Road about 0.3 miles after the turn. The Nature Center (left turn just before the administration building) features a number of displays, hosts nature programs, and offers guided tours and interpretive walks for all ages; it also has a greenhouse in which horticulture programs are conducted. (See Nearby Attractions, which follows this description.)

Boyce Park encompasses 1,096 acres and was the first of the regional parks to be dedicated in 1963. Its honoree is William D. Boyce, the locally born founder of the Boy Scouts of America. All of the picnic groves and shelters have Boy Scout–associated names. Although the park has many amenities, including the only downhill-skiing area (with lodge) in the county, about half of the land remains undeveloped, allowing for solitude, quiet hiking, cross-country skiing (trails are located near the Nature Center), and mountain biking.

DIRECTIONS

From Pittsburgh, take Interstate 376 East to Exit 14B, Plum. Follow the Orange Belt 1.4 miles and make a right on Old Frankstown Road. (Do not use the Old Frankstown Road on the left. Pass it and go over the turnpike and then turn right on Old Frankstown Road.) At 0.8 miles turn left on Spring Miller Road. At 0.3 miles Spring Miller Road turns into Pierson Run Road. The parking lot is 0.1 mile on the right just after the log cabin.

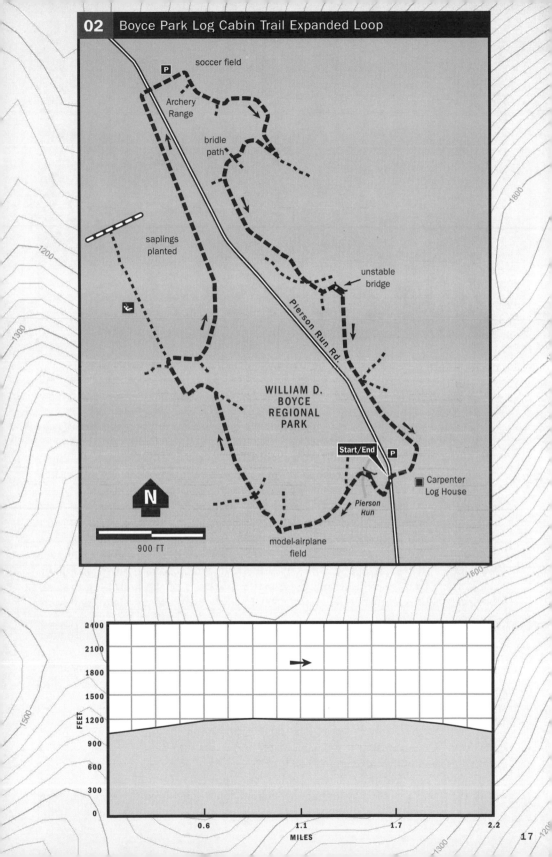

soccer field

P

Archery
Range

bridle
path

saplings
planted

Pierson Run Rd.

unstable
bridge

WILLIAM D.
BOYCE
REGIONAL
PARK

Start/End   P

Carpenter
Log House

N

900 FT

Pierson
Run

model-airplane
field

2400
2100
1800
1500
1200
900
600
300
0

FEET

0.6   1.1   1.7   2.2
MILES

17

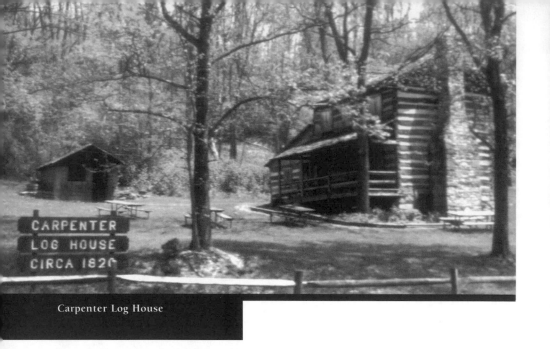

Carpenter Log House

This hike begins at the restored Carpenter Log House, erected circa 1820. (Tours of the log house are offered; see Nearby Attractions.) Cross Pierson Run Road to get to the trailhead. There is a sign for the Log House Trail, but this is the last you'll see of any marker for it. The beginning of the trail is crowded with skunk cabbage, mayapples, yellow ironweed, and wild garlic mustard. Cross the bridge over Pierson Run. Although the short bridge looks like it's about to collapse, it was quite sturdy beneath my feet. Curve left with the trail and head uphill. Growing in this area are sensitive fern (given this name because it is the first to die off at spring frost), goldenrod, red maple, sugar maple, and beech trees.

There are power pylons to your left as you come to a choice to continue straight or turn right at 0.12 miles. Go straight and up the gradual incline, heading away from Pierson Run. At the top you'll reach a model-airplane field. Make a sharp right, and walk around the fence. At 0.25 miles, pass the right turn and continue left along the path. There you'll see thistle and horse nettle, a relative of the tomato and potato families. Its fruit when ripe resembles a small yellow cherry tomato, and its flowers are star-shaped and pale with a yellow center.

At 0.33 miles you'll reach an intersection. Continue straight up the hill rather than turning left or right. Pass a white flowering dogwood, and you may find yellow violets and joe-pye weed, some more than ten feet tall. Clusters of pink flowers at the top of this so-called weed and its pagoda-like whorls of long, pointed leaves help to distinguish it from other plants; it's named for an Indian medicine man who used the hollow stalk to blow medicine into the mouths of his patients.

When the trail levels out for a bit there is unfortunately some road noise, but it begins to fade as you start to descend. Maple and sweet gum trees grow alongside the trail, and soon only birdsong prevails.

Come to a T in the trail at 0.5 miles, and turn left. The trail winds to the left and levels, and you enter a short grassy section. You'll soon arrive at a choice to turn left and go downhill, continue straight, or take a not-so-obvious path to the right.

Turn right, staying to the right of the grassy area. (If you go straight you will reach a playground with a path that leads to a dirt road.) On the way downhill, at 0.67 miles, bypass the right turn and continue downward, veering left. The trail gets wider and at 0.75 miles puts you out into a meadowlike area, which provides nice opportunities to see the bird life. You may spot a red cardinal or a field sparrow. The woods are on the right; they close in again on both sides briefly but drop off on the left as you enter a section where there are hundreds of saplings planted on the hillside. Soon you'll see Pierson Run Road paralleling the trail on the right. Walk straight until you reach the end of the saplings and the opportunity to cross Pierson Run Road.

Turn right, cross the road, and continue straight through the park gate. There is an unmarked right onto a trail and into the woods from the parking lot (well before the soccer field). Make that right (1.2 miles), and at the Y in the trail turn left (right leads to the archery range). This path is very narrow and follows Pierson Run Road. At 1.27 miles bypass a trail on the right and continue straight. Watch the trail here because it is easy to lose, as it does not appear to be heavily used and is overgrown for a short bit before it runs into a T with another trail. Turn right at the T in the trail, going downhill. Come to a Y and go right or left (they both reach the same place). At 1.5 miles, cross the unmarked bridle path and continue straight. Shortly, another trail comes in from the right; just continue straight. Mountain bikers use these trails and have a couple of jumps set up. The trail is in good condition, and the woodlands are very pretty. There are a number of large trees, including ironwood and oak, and some flowering varieties as well.

At 1.75 miles you'll come to a Y with a trail branching off to the left. Although they may lead to the same place, I took the right branch. There is also a trail paralleling this one on the right; it crosses the trail on which you are hiking at 1.8 miles. Continue straight on this rather level path. You'll pass some hawthorne growing alongside the trail and cross the water; you may want to avoid the unstable bridge. The pylons for the electrical lines come back into view, and you begin to approach the log cabin. The trail winds right and then left, and the single-track becomes grassy (this portion is isolated and in the open sun). At 2.0 miles, reach a three-way intersection and turn right. The trail goes back into the woods, is much wider, and receives a lot more use. There are some wildflowers, flowering dogwoods, and wild garlic. Use stones to cross the feeder stream once more and approach the side of the cabin grounds (you will see one of the buildings). Make a right on the road, which leads to the parking lot.

▶ NEARBY ATTRACTIONS

Tours of the log house are offered by the Allegheny Historical Foothills Society; contact them using **www.plumhistory.org.** To obtain information about programs and interpretive walks offered by the Nature Center, call (412) 733-4618. Information about renting groves or using other park attractions such as the wave pool, tennis courts, ball and soccer fields, basketball courts, model-airplane field, archery range, and downhill-skiing area and facility can be found at **www.county.allegheny.pa.us/ parks** or by contacting the park's administration building at (412) 271-3110.

DOWNTOWN HISTORIC WALK

KEY AT-A-GLANCE INFORMATION

LENGTH: 2.2 miles

CONFIGURATION: Balloon

DIFFICULTY: Easy

SCENERY: Historic landmarks, ornate building exteriors and interiors, green spaces, fountains, sculptures, and courtyards

EXPOSURE: Half shaded, half exposed

TRAFFIC: Busy

TRAIL SURFACE: Cement

HIKING TIME: 1.5 hours, not including visiting inside buildings

ACCESS: Year-round, if you wish to visit the buildings' interiors, go during the weekdays

MAPS: Maps of the streets can be purchased in many places; you can visit the city of Pittsburgh Web site, **www.city .pittsburgh.pa.us,** and search using "Walking Tours" for maps showing the locations of some buildings; USGS Pittsburgh West

FACILITIES: Eateries with restrooms are located throughout the walk

SPECIAL COMMENTS: Look at the City of Pittsburgh Web site as noted above in Maps if you wish to preview what you can see inside some of downtown Pittsburgh's most noted buildings and landmarks.

Downtown Historic Walk

UTM Zone (WGS84) 17T

Easting   584311

Northing   4477025

▶ IN BRIEF

This is a historic tour of some of Pittsburgh's most beautiful and interesting landmarks. There is far too much on this walk to describe in this space, so add more stops and sightseeing as you wish, and enjoy the city's heritage.

▶ DESCRIPTION

From the parking garage, turn right, walk to and cross Stanwix Street, and then turn left and cross the Boulevard of the Allies. Continue along Stanwix, pass Third Avenue and St. Mary's Church (A), and turn right onto Fourth Avenue. The smoked-glass and steel-framed castlelike building to the right is part of PPG Place. It was built by PPG Industries (formerly Pittsburgh Plate and Glass, founded in 1883; the present name was adopted in 1968), the first commercially successful U.S. plate and glass maker. At the end of this part of the building complex, arrive at its courtyard (B), where there are multiple vertical fountains surrounding a cement monolith showing the site dedication in 1984. The courtyard usually contains other art in the form of sculptures and, during the Three Rivers Arts Festival, large, interactive art pieces. In winter, the lobbies contain beautiful displays of international versions of St. Nicholas, as well as Christmas trees.

From the courtyard, turn around, cross

▶ DIRECTIONS

This is the heart of the city. It can be reached from the east and west via interstates 376 and 279, from the north by PA 8, and from the south by PA 51. There is street parking, but the meters are expensive. Park in the Pittsburgh *Post-Gazette* Garage on the Boulevard of the Allies (near the Fort Pitt Bridge entrance ramp, at Commonwealth Place) to begin the walk from the same spot. Or catch the bus or subway and save some money.

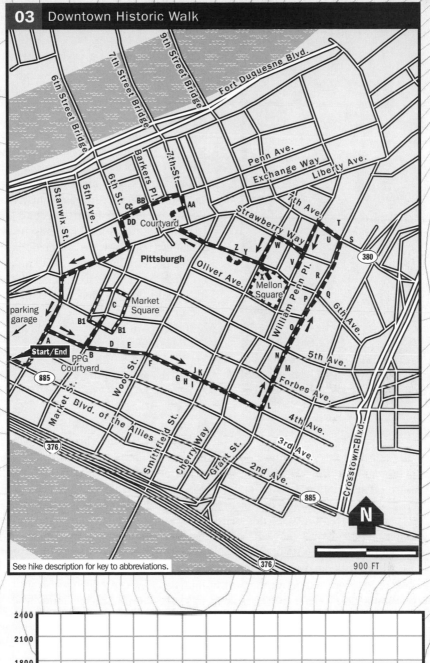

9th Street Bridge

7th Street Bridge

6th Street Bridge

Fort Duquesne Blvd.

Penn Ave.

Exchange Way

Liberty Ave.

Barkers Pl.

7th St.

Stanwix St.

5th Ave.

6th St.

CC BB AA

DD Courtyard

Pittsburgh

Strawberry Way

7th Ave.

T

380

Z Y W

V U S

Oliver Ave.

X

R

6th Ave.

parking garage

C

Market Square

Mellon Square

William Penn Pl.

Q

P

B1

B1

O

A

Start/End

B

D E

N

5th Ave.

PPG Courtyard

885

F

M

Wood St.

J K

G H I

Forbes Ave.

L

4th Ave.

Market St.

Blvd. of the Allies

Smithfield St.

Cherry Way

Grant St.

3rd Ave.

Crosstown Blvd.

376

2nd Ave.

885

N

See hike description for key to abbreviations.

376

900 FT

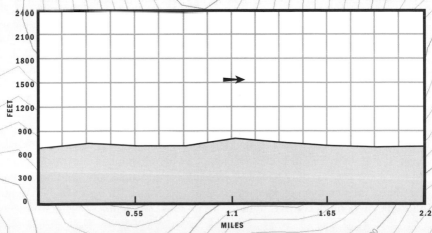

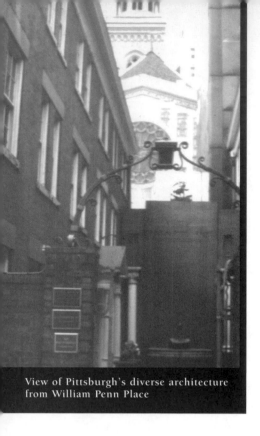

View of Pittsburgh's diverse architecture from William Penn Place

Fourth Avenue, and walk in between the other PPG buildings (B1) to Market Square (C). Here low walls, where many people sit to enjoy lunch and perhaps some music during the Mellon Jazz Festival, surround grass and trees. You'll also find the Original Oyster House, built in 1870 and still serving. This section of Forbes Avenue is composed of fitted brick with areas of cobblestone left as a reminder of the city's historic roots. Walk back out to Fourth Avenue and turn left, passing the Western Pennsylvania Conservancy (D), a historic landmark once called the Burke Building. This is the oldest office building in the city (built circa 1836), and its interior now reflects a combination of preserving the past while incorporating the best conservation materials available today.

Just beyond, the Benedum-Trees Building (E) begins a tour of what became, in the late 19th century, Pittsburgh's famous financial district, second only to Wall Street. The area's oil wells and steel mills were sources of enormous wealth that poured into banks once located here. This granite, brick, and terra-cotta building has three-story Corinthian columns and an intricately molded balcony and cornice. Inside, you'll see an elaborate lobby with marble, bronze, and plaster ornamentation. Continuing on Fourth, see the Union National Bank (F) diagonally across Wood Street, one of two Pittsburgh banks remaining from that era of prosperity. Erected in 1906, this building is rather modestly decorated for its time, though Doric columns flank the corner entry and lions' heads are above the doorways and under the roof cornice.

After crossing Wood Street, you'll see "Commonwealth Trust Company" (G) (circa 1906) inscribed above the next building's entryway. Next to it stands the Keystone Building (H) (circa 1903); look up to see keystones bearing lions' heads and an eagle with outspread wings perched atop a keystone, Pennsylvania's state symbol and the building's namesake. A couple of doors away (also across the street) is the ornate Times Building (I). Next to it stands Dollar Savings Bank, the second bank remaining from the late 19th century and the first mutual bank in Pittsburgh. This building (circa 1870) has colossal columns and life-size lions at the front steps. Stop inside for a peak at the chandelier. On your left (your side of the street) is the Engineer's Society (J) (circa 1898), and next to it the Fidelity Trust Building (K) (circa 1889).

Cross Smithfield Street and Cherry Way to reach Grant Street, which is covered in fitted brick and bisected by trees and flowers. Grant Street was named for British Major James Grant. In 1784, the street ran along the foot of Grant's Hill, which rose abruptly 80 feet above the rest of the Point. It was largely residential, and the former Pennsylvania Main Line Canal ran along it via an aqueduct from 11th Street to 7th Avenue (and on to the Monongahela River) until the 1850s and the coming of the railroad.

Cross Grant Street to reach the City County Building (L), seat of the city's government. Go inside to have a look at the beautiful barrel-vaulted corridor with its blue-and-white stenciled ceiling, which is supported by gilded columns resting on a classical marble base. Enormous arched windows provide daylight. Don't miss the elevator doors, which are cast with depictions of earlier city halls and courthouses in Pittsburgh's history.

Next you'll arrive at the County Courthouse (M). Due to a lowering of Grant Street in 1913, the entrance now opens on the original basement level, so once inside take the stairs to view the vaulted space with massive Romanesque arches and beautiful murals. When you come out, look across the street to the Frick Building (N) and notice the lions in the windows. Turn right on Grant Street, and at Fifth Avenue turn left to cross Grant again to visit the Frick Building. Its lobby is two stories high (also due to the lowering of the street), sheathed in white marble, and bordered by marble stairs. There are veined marble panels covering the ceiling and a gorgeous stained-glass window.

When finished, cross Fifth Avenue and continue along Grant Street to the Union Trust Building (O) (circa 1917), which was originally built by Henry Frick. Both the exterior and interior are designed in intricate Gothic detail. Inside, the principal corridors rise four stories with a rotunda in the middle that soars past tiers of bronze railings to a stained-glass dome. Look for the mosaics at the entrances, stained glass above the southern entry, and stenciling in the corridors. Exit at Grant Street, turn left, and cross Oliver Avenue to reach the William Penn Hotel (P) (circa 1916). This building's lobby is ornamented in a Mediterranean-Grecian classical style and has a colorfully stenciled coffered ceiling. Walk through to the William Penn Way side where you'll see the main lobby, which is larger and designed in the French classical style in white and gold and accented with glass, mirrors, and black marble at the entryways.

Return to Grant Street, turn left, cross Sixth Avenue (you'll see the USS Building and plaza [Q] across Grant Street on your right), and walk to the First Lutheran Church (R) (circa 1888). Notice the tall gabled roofs topping the stonework and 170-foot spire that are somehow complemented by the modern bronze sculpture in front. At Seventh Avenue, cross Grant Street to visit the U.S. Post Office (S) via the doorway underneath its high, arched eagle-topped doorway.

When finished, cross Grant and walk down Seventh; passing the Gulf Building (T) and the Koppers Building (U) (across the street). Turn left on William Penn Place and cross the street at Strawberry Way. Read the plaque for area history and the background of the three tiny brick row houses (V) (circa 1890) that survive here and most famously house the Pittsburgh Harvard-Yale-Princeton Club, among other organizations. Go back to Strawberry Way and turn left, and left again at Smithfield Street. Visit the Smithfield Street Church (W) (circa 1925), where you'll see 12-foot-tall stained-glass windows inside. Find more at the top of the steps in the main church as well as intricate woodwork.

Outside the church, turn left, cross Sixth Avenue, and walk up the steps to see Mellon Square (X), with its low-profile fountains, marble-wall seating, and greenery. Walk back and cross Smithfield to travel down to Sixth Avenue (on the left side) to reach Trinity Cathedral (Y) (circa 1871). Inside this English Gothic–style building are stained-glass windows, some of which date to 1872. Outside, follow the pathway through what is left of a graveyard once used by Native Americans and French,

British, and American settlers. The end of the walkway leads to the First Presbyterian Church (Z) (circa 1905). Also English Gothic in style, it houses sweeping staircases, Tiffany stained-glass windows, arched wooden roof trusses that span its length, and elaborately carved woodwork. Down at the sidewalk, go back a little to read the plaque on the wall between the buildings for interesting history about those whose remains are interred in the small cemetery.

When finished, turn left on Sixth Avenue, cross Wood Street, and then Liberty Avenue to Pittsburgh's Cultural District. Turn left, and across the street you'll see a courtyard. Walking through the courtyard and turning right leads to the Benedum Center (AA). If you walk through the courtyard and the center is open, you may be able to look at its spectacular dome and Georgian classical details. From there, walk to Penn Avenue and turn left. Across the street you'll see Cabaret at Theatre Square (BB) after the O'Reilly Theater (CC). At Sixth Street, turn left to cross Penn and visit Heinz Hall (DD) (circa 1926), an elaborately decorated music hall. When finished, continue on Sixth to Liberty (notice the public courtyard with seating, tables, and fountains) and turn right, crossing Sixth and then Fifth streets to turn left on Stanwix Street. Follow it to the Boulevard of the Allies and turn right to return to your vehicle.

▶ NEARBY ATTRACTIONS

See the Point State Park: History and Three Rivers Walk (hike 16) or the North Shore: River, Memorial, and Sports Walk (hike 15) in this book for more sites and history. There are many attractions around the city and at Point State Park throughout the year. Call the Greater Pittsburgh Convention and Visitor's Bureau at (800) 366-0093 or go to **www.visitpittsburgh.com** for more information.

ELIZA FURNACE TRAIL

IN BRIEF

The Eliza Furnace Trail is a segment of the almost complete 37-mile Three Rivers Heritage Trail, which is conveniently located and used by commuters, walkers, bikers, joggers, and skaters of all ages. This is a popular trail that offers a unique view of various city bridges, landmarks, and views of downtown.

DESCRIPTION

This Eliza Furnace Trail begins at the parking lot on Swineburne Street, following the former alignment of the once heavily traveled Baltimore and Ohio rail line. Its eastern end connects to the Panther Hollow Trail (which leads to Schenley Park), and its western end will eventually connect to Point State Park.

To begin walking on the Eliza Furnace Trail, head toward the river from the parking area and turn right. Almost immediately you'll begin to see Heritage Signs, which are found all along the Three Rivers Heritage Trail and feature interesting information about the area's history that you can learn along the way. Near this trail entrance, one sign discusses the history of the Eliza Furnace, for which the trail was obviously named. The Eliza Furnace is a type of furnace, specifically a stone blast furnace, used for smelting iron. The first was constructed in 1858, before the Civil War, by the Jones and Laughlin (J & L) Steel Company, which owned hundreds of acres of property along the Monongahela River near the current Pittsburgh Technology Center. The Eliza Furnace was named after Jones's granddaughter; its feminine name

KEY AT-A-GLANCE INFORMATION

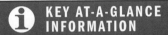

LENGTH: 5.2 miles

CONFIGURATION: Out-and-back

DIFFICULTY: Easy

SCENERY: Monongahela River, city views, urban art

EXPOSURE: Exposed

TRAFFIC: Busy

TRAIL SURFACE: Asphalt

HIKING TIME: 1.5–2 hours

ACCESS: Trail is open from dawn to dusk

MAPS: A map of this and other riverfront trails is available from Friends of the Riverfront. Contact them for maps; hiking, biking, triathlon, and volunteer mixers for all ages; volunteer and membership opportunities at (412) 488-0212 or **www.friendsoftheriverfront.org;** USGS Pittsburgh East

FACILITIES: Vending machines, water fountain, tables and seats, and bike racks are located at the First Avenue Bike and Blade Station.

SPECIAL COMMENTS: This trail is urban and noisy (next to the Parkway East). Bring a personal music player to drown out some of the noise.

DIRECTIONS

From Pittsburgh, take Second Street past Bates Street and the Hot Metal Bridge. Make a left onto Swineburne Street (there is a sign for the trail), then a right into the shuttle parking lot.

Eliza Furnace Trail

UTM Zone (WGS84)   17T

Easting   588772

Northing   4475561

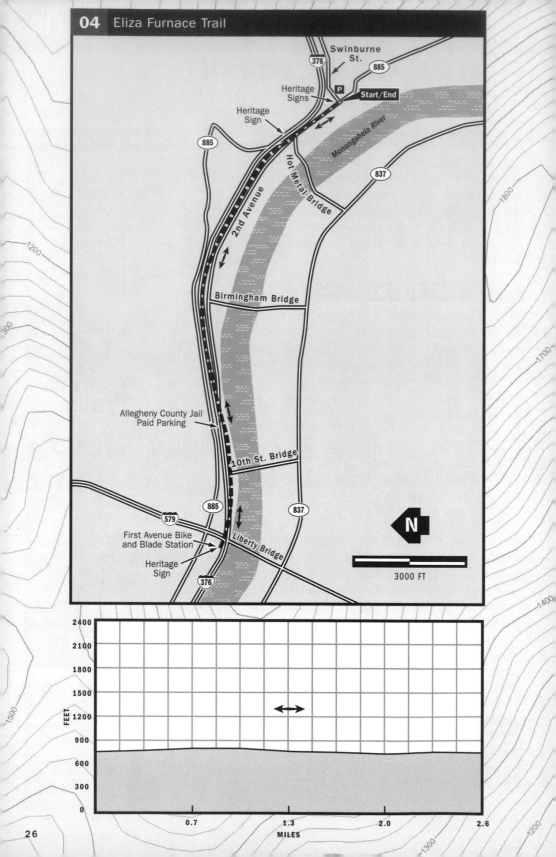

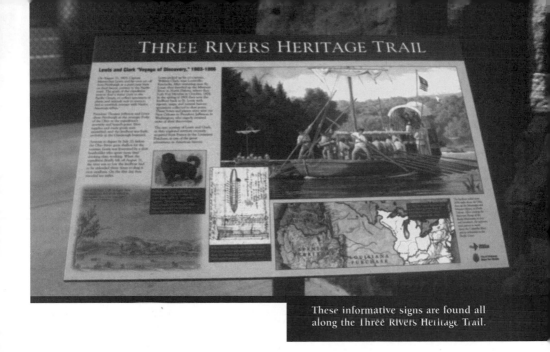

THREE RIVERS HERITAGE TRAIL

These informative signs are found all along the Three Rivers Heritage Trail.

followed the Victorian tradition of naming furnaces after women because they tended to be temperamental.

This was the first iron furnace built in Pittsburgh since 1794, and it served as a marker for Pittsburgh's future. Molten iron was transported by boat and then railcar over the Hot Metal Bridge to the city's South Side area to a Bessemer Furnace and then back again for final processing.

Continue along the asphalt trail, and you'll come to another Heritage Sign at 0.35 miles. Here, you have a good view of the recently converted Hot Metal Bridge. Plans and preparations are under way for the refurbishment of the Hot Metal Bridge to provide ramps connecting the Eliza Furnace Trail to the South Side. Adjacent to the Hot Metal Bridge stands another railroad bridge that was designed and built by J & L Steel in 1899 using steel from the company's open hearth to replace one built in 1882. Looking across the river, you'll also see the buildings of the new technology companies that now occupy—and look so much more pleasant than—the site of the former steel company. (See Nearby Attractions following this description for information on hiking and riding on that side of the river.)

Continuing the walk, look for a large mural that was still being painted on the wall during my visit. According to the artist, who was present when I was there, the mural takes graffiti to realism; at the time of this writing it depicted citizens walking in various city attire and also butterflies flying over the river. (The Sprout Fund, with the goal of painting more as the trail continues to be developed, funded this mural.)

Views of the Monongahela River, the South Side slopes, and the Birmingham Bridge span the horizon on the left. Soon, you'll pass over a small bridge above Brady Street and beneath the main span and connecting ramps of the Birmingham Bridge. Here, the noise picks up as the trail travels for a distance between busy highways.

The Eliza Furnace Trail has also been affectionately known as the Jail Trail. This is explained by the location of the Allegheny County Jail found at 1.94 miles. Parking access off Second Avenue is available in the Second Avenue parking plaza, but it's not free. Soon you will pass the Tenth Street Bridge (at 2.20 miles) and will have almost reached the end of the official Eliza Furnace Trail, near First Avenue. Once there, at 2.59 miles, you'll find the First Avenue Bike and Blade Station, owned by Golden Triangle Bike Rentals. Have some refreshments and take in the distant view of downtown Pittsburgh. Walk around and enjoy the landscaping, and you'll also find another Heritage Sign. This one clues the reader in to the Lewis and Clark Voyage of Discovery. Captain Meriwether Lewis and crew left Pittsburgh on August 31, 1803, not far from this spot. President Jefferson and Captain Lewis chose Pittsburgh, the strategic home of the "Forks of the Ohio," to be the starting point of the expedition. Credit for the financing plan for the expedition was largely due to the then U.S. Secretary of the Treasury, Albert Gallatin (see the Friendship Hill Tour and Hike, hike 52).

This is the turnaround point for the hike. When you're ready, retrace your steps to your vehicle. Alternately, see Nearby Attractions (below) for more nearby walking and touring.

▶ NEARBY ATTRACTIONS

Bikes and in-line skates can be rented at the First Avenue Bike and Blade Station. The hours are seasonal and those posted were different from those online, so call ahead at (412) 600-0675 if you wish to rent, Opportunities for eating, touring, and shopping abound in downtown Pittsburgh, as well as on the city's South Side. For more hiking close by, see other hikes in this book, including the Point State Park: History and Three Rivers Walk (hike 16), the Three Rivers Heritage Trail: Monongahela South Shore (hike 21), the North Shore: River, Memorial, and Sports Walk (hike 15), or the Downtown Historic Walk (hike 3).

FOX CHAPEL FLOWER AND WILDLIFE RESERVE LOOP

▶ IN BRIEF

This hike is within the Fox Chapel Flower and Wildlife Reserve. It is a short walk through a spectacular display of trilliums of various species and is pleasantly punctuated with the delicate Virginia bluebell. You'll also stroll along Stony Camp Run.

▶ DESCRIPTION

Walk across the road from the parking area to the trailhead. A plaque in a boulder beside Stony Camp Run commemorates Richard Boyles, the first manager of the borough of Fox Chapel; he was largely responsible for the preservation of the woodland upon which this hike travels.

Walk between the bench and boulder and down the path that crosses Stony Camp Run via well-placed, square-cut boulders. Turn right and take the stairs up to the wooden platform, which is furnished with another wooden bench. If you are here in the spring, you are certain to see hundreds of trillium.

As you travel along this pleasant path the white trillium plants are obviously dominant. But look for painted trilliums, too; their unique crimson blaze lies at the bottom of their petals and encircles their centers.

You'll notice fencing along the hillside below and to the right. This new fencing is due to an influx of a deer population that was once able to feed on the property of Teresa Heinz Kerry, wife of Senator John Kerry (D-MA). During her husband's 2004 presidential campaign, several journalists were found sneaking onto her property. To

❶ KEY AT-A-GLANCE INFORMATION

LENGTH: 1 mile

CONFIGURATION: Loop

DIFFICULTY: Easy

SCENERY: Trillium, Virginia bluebells, hardwoods, rhododendron, hemlocks, Stony Camp Run, waterfall

EXPOSURE: Mostly shaded

TRAFFIC: Light to medium

TRAIL SURFACE: Dirt

HIKING TIME: 1 hour

ACCESS: Open year-round, dawn until 1 hour after sunset

MAPS: None; USGS Glenshaw

FACILITIES: None

SPECIAL COMMENTS: Dogs are not permitted.

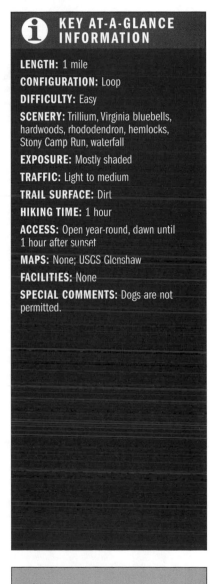

Fox Chapel Flower and Wildlife Reserve Loop

UTM Zone (WGS84)   17T

Easting   593562

Northing   4485844

▶ DIRECTIONS

From Pittsburgh, take PA 28 North to Exit 8, Fox Chapel. Take the Fox Chapel Road ramp and turn left onto Fox Chapel Road. After 1 mile, turn left at the Y onto Squaw Run Road and follow approximately 1.25 miles to parking area on the right.

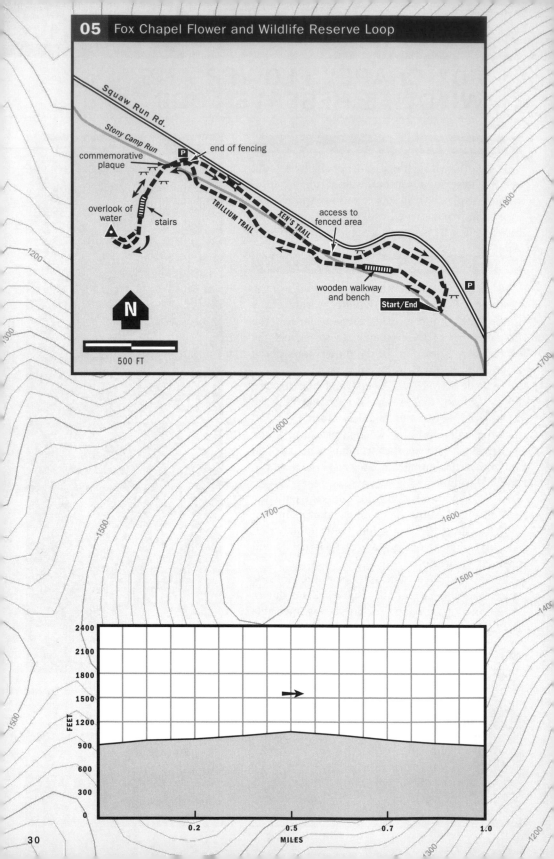

Squaw Run Rd.

Stony Camp Run

commemorative plaque

end of fencing

P

overlook of water

stairs

TRILLIUM TRAIL

XEN'S TRAIL

access to fenced area

wooden walkway and bench

Start/End

P

N

500 FT

FEET

2400
2100
1800
1500
1200
900
600
300
0

0.2   0.5   0.7   1.0

MILES

keep them at bay, she had her 100-acre property fenced off. Unfortunately, this also left a void in the food supply for local deer, which then began feeding heavily on the well-loved trillium within the reserve. To save what was left and restore the abundance of trillium once found here, Fox Chapel borough is working in conjunction with ecologists on a seven-year restoration process, as it takes this long to regenerate trillium. If I hadn't learned of this event, I would not have thought the trillium to be diminished; there is more of it here than I have ever seen together in one place before.

After a slight incline the trail levels, and you will find wooden-planked walkways and bridges in place to prevent damage and keep shoes dry. These extra touches add to the hike's pleasure. Along the first of these areas, many maple saplings are found. Afterward, you'll cross a feeder stream using the square-cut boulders. The trilliums are so eye-catching that it's easy to miss some of the other notable growth such as the many older hardwoods and garlic mustard. There's also Solomon's seal, a plant whose name comes from the leaf scars shaped like King Solomon's wax seal on its underground stem. The Iroquois tribes used to grind up the underground stem for making bread.

Periodically, if you want to see what the untouched flora will do, observe the small demonstration areas that have been fenced off against the deer since 1994. There is one down the hillside at just before 0.25 miles. Not much farther along the trail, look inside demonstration area number two, which is absolutely packed with trilliums (perhaps this is the comparison to think of before the Heinz-Kerry property was cut off). Along the trail, red trillium can be found as well. Even though this species is called red or purple trillium, as well as wake robin, some plants may be pink or salmon and less commonly yellow or whitish. If in doubt, take a whiff if you dare: this species is known for its ill scent.

Following demonstration area number two the trilliums do subside, but a beautiful display of mertensia, also known as Virginia bluebells, daintily add to the quiet splendor of this walk. These delicate nodding, trumpetlike flowers can be distinguished by their early budding; they are pink in bud and turn blue as they blossom.

The fenced-in area ends at 0.35 miles, winding through the mazelike exit. Turn left and reach a small circle of benches with another commemorative plaque set in a boulder. This one recognizes Ruth Boyles, a dedicated conservationist who encouraged environmental education and stewardship in Fox Chapel and throughout Pennsylvania. She was also essential in preserving this trail.

Walk up the obvious path, away from the road. Many more Virginia bluebells, as well as purple violets, line the trail to the left. Pass this turn or take the one on the right, which is marked by a bench underneath a large hemlock. The short trail leads down to Stony Camp Run and the base of a low-volume waterfall. Once you've finished exploring, return to the trail and follow it up a slight incline that is made more stable with stone laid at intervals; these transition into carefully placed stone stairs and finally to wooden stairs.

At the top, ferns, purple violets, and perhaps the rhythmic hammer of a woodpecker await. At almost 0.5 miles, not far from the top of the stairs, there is a choice to turn left or right. Going left, at least currently, allows one to walk a little farther until the trail just peters out. Depending on the goals of the borough, perhaps this

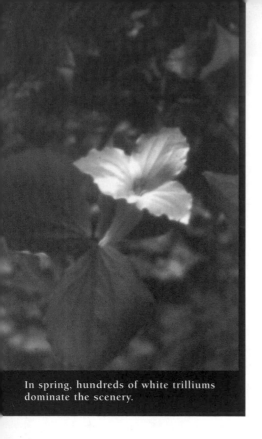
In spring, hundreds of white trilliums dominate the scenery.

portion will have been reestablished during your hike. To continue on this walk, turn right and walk out to what appears to have once been an overlook built of stone. You'll notice blocks that lay directly below, near the water at the site's base; they obviously were cut by humans. Keep children away from the edge because there is no longer a structure; it has fallen either due to landslide or malice.

Turn around and walk back to descend the stairs and retrace your steps to the edge of the fencing. Here, rather than reentering the fenced area, go left around it to follow Xen's Trail. You may see daylilies blooming and will definitely see plenty of rhododendrons. On this unprotected side of the fence, trilliums are present but in very few numbers compared with their abundance behind the fence.

This trail travels closely to Stony Camp Run and is a popular place for families to come and explore the shallow water. It's a good place to try your hand at skipping stones. Following the first wooden bridge are several large trilliums, though the large skunk cabbage may detract from their allure. At the time of my hike, a second wooden bridge was taped off, as it is in need of repair. If this is still the case, going to the right of it along the hillside isn't a bad substitute. Along this trail there are yellow violets. And at 0.75 miles you'll notice a large split sycamore.

Walk underneath the branches of several hemlocks, and you'll reach another short set of stone steps you can take. Travel through sections of large rhododendron, and pass an access into the fenced area. The final bridge of the trail leads you through more of the same scenic greenery and blooms. Just after rounding a bend toward the right, the last treat of this hike awaits.

Look up to the old pine above and on the right of the trail. Its base would likely take three people to circle and its roots have been exposed, draping over the mossy rock shelf toward the trail. Go left to cross the water, and finish the hike with Stony Camp Run to your right. The trailhead is within view shortly.

▶ NEARBY ATTRACTIONS

There are businesses along Fox Chapel Road, but if you are looking for another short hike, Beechwood Farms is a just a short drive away. To reach it, continue up Squaw Run Road and turn right on Dorseyville Road. Beechwood Farms is just a couple of miles on the left; see the Beechwood Farms Nature Reserve Loop (hike 1) for more information.

FRICK PARK TOUR LOOP

▶ IN BRIEF

The trails are prettiest in fall for leaves and in spring for wildflowers. In winter, the park can be a wonderland in the middle of the city, and is popular with local cross-country skiers when there is sufficient snow cover.

▶ DESCRIPTION

Frick Park is the largest of Pittsburgh's four major parks, boasting 600 acres of woodlands and approximately 10 miles of trails. The park originated with millionaire industrialist Henry Clay Frick. In 1908 he presented the 150-acre gift to his 17-year-old daughter, Helen, who had requested a park in which the city's children could play. The park was bequeathed to the city in 1919 along with a $2 million trust fund, which has been used to purchase additional land and maintain the park.

From the parking lot, go to the front of the Beechwood Boulevard entrance to view and walk through one of the notable French-style gatehouses; it offers a wide trail toward the Frick Environmental Center. If you are there during hours of operation, stop in to learn about the park's habitat, ecology, history, and year-round educational programs.

▶ DIRECTIONS

From Pittsburgh, take Interstate 376 East to the Swissvale–Edgewood exit. Stay left on ramps for the Edgewood exit. At the stop sign, turn right onto South Braddock Avenue. At the second light, turn left onto Forbes Avenue. At the first light, make a left onto South Dallas Avenue. Turn left at the immediate T onto Beechwood Boulevard. You will see a sign for the Frick Park Environmental Center on the left. Make the second left into the drive, following it to the parking lot.

ⓘ KEY AT-A-GLANCE INFORMATION

LENGTH: 5 miles (can be shortened approximately 1.5 miles by skipping sections as indicated in the Description)

CONFIGURATION: Modified loop

DIFFICULTY: Easy to moderate

SCENERY: Fern Hollow Creek, mixed foliage, deciduous trees, wildflowers, birds, Frick Art Museum, French-style gatehouses, wetland restoration project, educational compost displays

EXPOSURE: Mostly shaded

TRAFFIC: Light early in the day, may be heavy on the lower trail segment in afternoon, especially on weekends

TRAIL SURFACE: Varies from wide fine gravel and dirt path to narrow dirt; short section near museum is paved

HIKING TIME: 2–2.5 hours

ACCESS: Park is open year-round.

MAPS: A map of Frick Park may become available at **www.pittsburghparks.org** but currently can be purchased at the Schenley Park Visitor Center for $2; call (412) 682-7275 for details; USGS Pittsburgh East

FACILITIES: Restrooms, shelter and picnic areas, lawn bowling greens, ball fields, playgrounds, tennis courts

SPECIAL COMMENTS: The Frick Park Environmental Center is currently scheduled to be rebuilt following a devastating fire in August 2002. Contact the environmental center for information on seasonal programs and hours of operation at (412) 422-6538.

Frick Park Tour Loop

UTM Zone (WGS84)   17T

Easting   592600

Northing   4476823

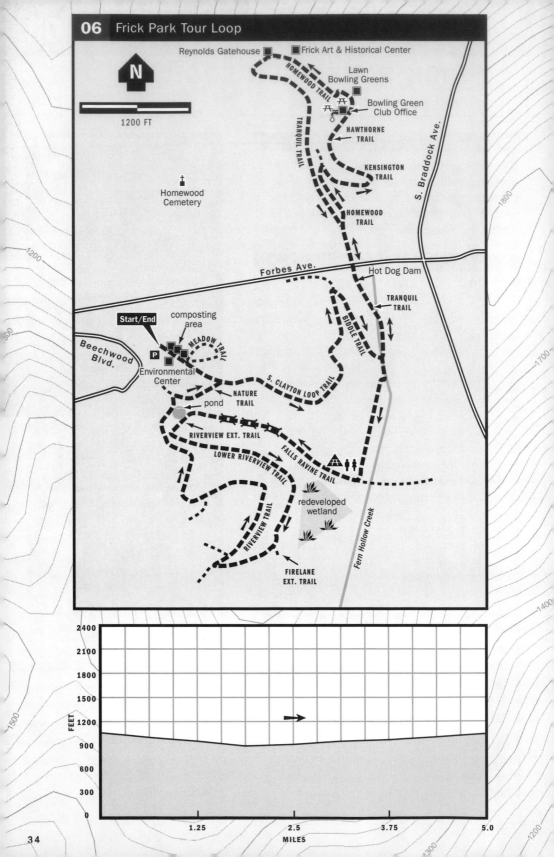

Reynolds Gatehouse ■   ■ Frick Art & Historical Center

N

1200 FT

Lawn Bowling Greens ■

Bowling Green Club Office

HOMEWOOD TRAIL

HAWTHORNE TRAIL

TRANQUIL TRAIL

KENSINGTON TRAIL

Homewood Cemetery

HOMEWOOD TRAIL

Forbes Ave.

Hot Dog Dam

TRANQUIL TRAIL

Start/End   composting area

Beechwood Blvd.

MEADOW TRAIL

Environmental Center

BIDDLE TRAIL

S. CLAYTON LOOP TRAIL

NATURE TRAIL

pond

RIVERVIEW EXT. TRAIL

FALLS RAVINE TRAIL

LOWER RIVERVIEW TRAIL

redeveloped wetland

RIVERVIEW TRAIL

Fern Hollow Creek

FIRELANE EXT. TRAIL

FEET

2400
2100
1800
1500
1200
900
600
300
0

1.25   2.5   3.75   5.0
MILES

From the environmental center, continue straight past the Woodland Area Trail on your right; you are on the unsigned South Clayton Loop. This trail is high in the park and in spring and summer you can hear the sounds of woodpeckers at work and spot scarlet tanagers, wood thrush, yellow-billed cuckoo, and many other birds flitting between the upper branches of older hardwoods. At 0.5 miles, you'll reach the intersection of South Clayton Loop, North Clayton Loop, and Biddle Trail. Make a hard right to descend down Biddle Trail, listening as the traffic noise fades into birdsong.

At the bottom you may be surprised by a red fire hydrant sprouting up from the dirt in the center of the intersecting trails. There is a sign here for Biddle Trail going straight; make a left instead onto Tranquil Trail. This section of the trail is wide and popular; Fern Hollow Creek is on the right. Soon a low wooden fence begins and you arrive at Hot Dog Dam, one of the designated legal places in the park where dogs can run free. If you have a dog, it can enjoy a dip in the water and some playtime with other canines.

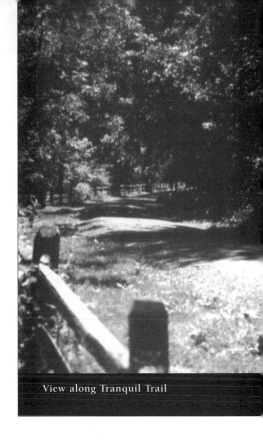

View along Tranquil Trail

At almost 1 mile, you'll arrive at the juncture with Homewood Trail; take the fork on the right. Heading uphill, the trail begins to curve left, allowing you a view of the woods and trail below on your left and a close-up of underbrush, sandstone, and shale on your right. At the T, make a right onto Kensington Trail. This brief section runs close to busy Forbes Avenue, but the trail quickly leads left, turning into Hawthorne Trail and deeper into the park again.

A small, open field passes into shade where the trail merges again with the Homewood Trail. At this point, notice on your right the only greens existing in Pennsylvania for lawn bowling, a leisure that stems from the 13th century.

Across from them is the Frick Park Bowling Green Club Office. In front of this stone building are a water fountain and, frequently, a water bowl for dogs; next to the building is a small covered shelter with a couple of picnic tables. Continue straight through a cobblestone rotunda where you may be seduced by the fragrance of calla lilies or, depending on the time of year, other bloomers. The paved path continues by an open grassy area dotted with a large variety of trees and a few tables.

Soon you'll see the Frick Art Museum across Reynolds Avenue. Part of the Frick Art & Historical Center, the museum was designed to exhibit the collection of Helen Clay Frick in an intimate atmosphere with paintings, porcelains, bronzes, and a rare collection of 17th- and 18th-century furniture. It also hosts traveling art exhibitions. If you are there during the museum's hours of operation, you may want to stop in and perhaps follow your visit with a break at its quaint cafe. Behind the museum is the remainder of the Frick Art & Historical Center grounds and buildings (see Nearby Attractions following this description).

If you've left the park for a worthwhile visit to the center, reenter through the Reynolds Gatehouse, which has been restored to its original 1935 elegance. In spring you will be greeted with flowering dogwoods and forsythia as you return to the trail. Here the trail becomes dirt again. Veer left; one of the hills of the Homewood Cemetery will be on your right.

Although there won't be a sign indicating it until later, you are back on Tranquil Trail. The dirt path is wide but quiet here; typically only the rustling sounds of chipmunks, squirrels, shrews, and deer accompany you. Pass the juncture where you originally turned uphill for the Homewood Trail, and retrace your steps past the intersection with Biddle. Walk to the left of the main trail and you'll be near Fern Hollow Creek. This area leads into an open field adjacent to the main trail and then a juncture with Falls Ravine Trail on the right. Directly in front of you is a redeveloped wetland area. Turn right on Falls Ravine Trail; a picnic shelter and restrooms are on your right. As you travel up this scenic trail, you will cross over a series of small bridges.

You'll know you've reached the top of Falls Ravine Trail when you happen upon a pond in front of you. Make a left onto the Riverview Extension Trail and then another onto the Lower Riverview Trail. This trail becomes narrow and is popular with mountain bikers. (You can skip this loop if you wish by turning right; see next paragraph.) Do not take the Firelane Extension Trail that comes up on your left; rather, turn right and continue on the Lower Riverview Trail. You will reach the top and make a right. Lower Riverview Trail turns into Riverview Trail. Continue straight on Riverview Trail. Riverview Trail becomes Riverview Extension Trail again and begins to head downward as it opens up into a much more pleasant, shaded hiking experience. After 3.5 miles, you'll be back where you made the left to hike this loop.

Continue straight and then veer right uphill (do not make the sharp right heading back down Falls Ravine Trail). Shortly you'll find yourself at the juncture with the Nature Trail. Follow it around and toward the right; the observation deck of the environmental center will be visible up the hill on your left. Make a left onto the South Clayton Loop to finish, briefly hiking out the way you came in. Before leaving, you can also hike the short, wildflower-abundant Meadow Trail loop and then take a peek at the compost area. (Contact the Frick Environmental Center for details on composting classes.)

When finished, continue back through the Beechwood Gatehouse and turn right to the parking lot.

▶ NEARBY ATTRACTIONS

Frick Art & Historical Center consists of the Frick Art Museum, Car and Carriage Museum, Café, Greenhouse Education Center, and Clayton House; all are open to the public. All facilities are free except the Clayton House (general admission, $10; seniors and students, $8; members, free; reservations suggested). Call (412) 371-0600 or visit **www.frickart.org.**

GILFILLAN TRAIL LOOP

▶ IN BRIEF

This little trail is easily accessed and easy for young children to walk. Twelve species of trees are identified by colored discs and are described in the township's map brochure. Wood chips covering the trail provide soft treading for joggers or anyone concerned about avoiding joint injuries.

▶ DESCRIPTION

In 1976, Upper Saint Clair purchased nearly 60 acres of land from the Gilfillan family to be used as a park and established the Gilfillan Trail for walking, hiking, jogging, and cross-country skiing. The trail circles through woodlands, in which some of the trees are estimated to be over 400 years old. It also travels along fields and meadows surrounding the adjacent 15-acre Gilfillan Farm, which was left to the Upper Saint Clair Historical Society in 2001 by Margaret Gilfillan.

From the parking lot, cross Orr Road and enter the trail. You can walk it either way, but turn left to follow this description. Close to this entrance, find and smell the succulent honeysuckle; crab apple trees, berry bushes, and milkweed also abound. At just 0.15 miles, walk into a section with taller trees that block the road to the left. The road noise decreases as you walk northwest, away from US 19, and cross a small bridge over a stream. You'll reach a signed entrance at 0.25 miles. From this point and the next quarter-mile

▶ DIRECTIONS

From Pittsburgh, take US 19 South through the Liberty tunnels. Starting mileage from the end of the tunnels, drive 6.2 miles and turn right onto Orr Road, across from the Upper Saint Clair Fire Station and immediately before Westminster Presbyterian Church. (Orr Road is 0.6 miles past Fort Couch Road, just past South Hills Village.) Turn left to park in the church parking lot.

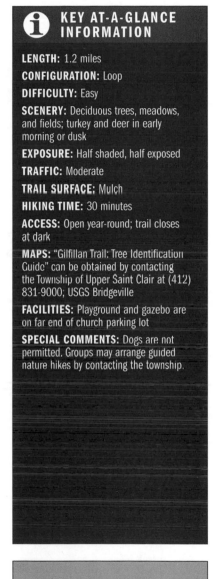

❶ KEY AT-A-GLANCE INFORMATION

LENGTH: 1.2 miles

CONFIGURATION: Loop

DIFFICULTY: Easy

SCENERY: Deciduous trees, meadows, and fields; turkey and deer in early morning or dusk

EXPOSURE: Half shaded, half exposed

TRAFFIC: Moderate

TRAIL SURFACE: Mulch

HIKING TIME: 30 minutes

ACCESS: Open year-round; trail closes at dark

MAPS: "Gilfillan Trail: Tree Identification Guide" can be obtained by contacting the Township of Upper Saint Clair at (412) 831-9000; USGS Bridgeville

FACILITIES: Playground and gazebo are on far end of church parking lot

SPECIAL COMMENTS: Dogs are not permitted. Groups may arrange guided nature hikes by contacting the township.

Gilfillan Trail Loop

UTM Zone (WGS84)   17T

Easting   579471

Northing   4466041

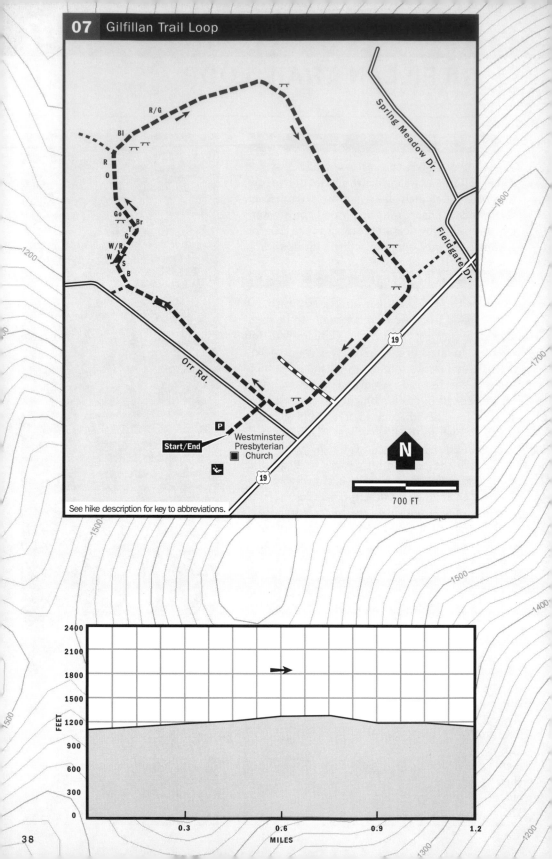

R/G

Bl

R
O

Go
Br
Y
G
W/R
S
W
B

Spring Meadow Dr.

Fieldgate Dr.

19

Orr Rd.

P

Start/End

Westminster
Presbyterian
Church

19

N

700 FT

See hike description for key to abbreviations.

1800

1200

1700

1500

1500

1400

1300

1200

FEET

2400

2100

1800

1500

1200

900

600

300

0

0.3   0.6   0.9   1.2

MILES

of trail or so, there are trees labeled with one-inch colored discs (at the bottoms of the trunks) that correspond to descriptions in the township brochure. Information about additional trees, as well as those with discs, is also provided in this description in the event that the discs are not maintained. (The discs and the township brochure were part of a Boy Scout's Eagle project.)

The first two disc-labeled trees are found before you reach the upcoming bridge on the right-hand side of the trail. The tree with the black disc (B on map) is a red maple; look for the red stem of the leaf and three pointed lobes. The tree with the silver disc (S) is a white oak; look for its distinct light-gray bark, which breaks into thick reddish scales. By the way, all of the trees named in this hike are native. Just before crossing the bridge, you'll find American basswood marked with a white disc (W); it has simple, heart-shaped leaves and often several trunks branching from one. You'll also find jewelweed. After the bridge you'll see striped maple (not labeled with a disc); this native is easy to identify even in winter due to its striped bark.

Just after the bridge, the next four types of trees are on the left side of the trail. First, look for the white and red disc (W/R) on an ironwood. This tree is a bit tough to identify without a guide. Its bark is gray and fibrous, and it spirals around the tree. Its leaves are only two to four inches long and are oval with pointed tips. Next you'll see a white ash with a green disc (G). Its bark is greenish gray with many furrows and interlacing diamond-shaped ridges. Then you'll see a sugar maple, a popular and well-known tree, marked with a yellow disc (Y). Any break or gap in a twig, branch, or trunk leaks sugary water in spring. Finally, there's an American beech, labeled with a brown disc (Br); its bark and leaves both are distinct. The bark is light gray and smooth and appears to wrap the trunk horizontally, while its leaves are narrow, pointed, and leathery dark green on top; there are some very large old ones found along this trail.

Near a bench, you'll see sassafras (on the left side of the trail and across from another American beech) marked with a gold disc (Go). This tree is easily identified by its mitten-shaped leaves, which usually have three lobes all pointing away from the stem. After this point, continue along up the slight hill. Before the hill's crest, look on the left side of the trail for a black walnut, which is labeled with an orange disc (O). The leaves of this tree are compound, meaning many leaflets grow from a stem; they are narrow and pointed. The bark is brown to black with deep pits and flat scaly ridges. These trees are easiest to identify in late summer, when their large green fruit (resembling a small tennis ball) hang from its branches and drop to the ground. Not far and also on the left, you'll see a red oak tree, appropriately labeled with a red disc (R). Like the red maple, the base of the stems of its leaves is also red.

Continue past the trail on the left that leads into the woods at 0.43 miles (unless you are in the mood for a little exploratory excursion), and you'll find some benches just after the trail levels again. The surroundings of the trail really open after passing the benches, providing a meadowlike experience. There are more sassafras trees growing in this area and black cherry trees, the latter marked with a blue disc (Bl). This is the largest member of the cherry trees, growing up to 75 feet high. In spring, their elongated, clustered white flowers are beautiful blooms, and in summer, their cherries (only one-quarter- to one-half-inch big) grow along a hanging stem, starting out green and turning dark blue or black when they are mature and ready to eat. There are quite a number of these trees along this trail.

Not much farther along, look on the left for American elm. It is one of the area's tallest native trees, growing 70 to 100 feet tall. This tree once lined almost every city street in eastern North America until Dutch elm disease arrived on infected logs from Europe in the 1920s. A bit more difficult to pick out, it produces tiny reddish-brown flowers in spring and has a flat, disc-shaped fruit called samara that turns tan when at maturity.

The trail then travels behind the yards of some residences and loops to the right. After turning the bend, find long-needled pines. By 0.79 miles, in the middle of this straight stretch, you are once again walking in a very open area where you see fields and then meadows. This would be a great spot to look for butterflies and birds. You are now walking toward US 19 again, and its noise will become a bit more noticeable. Along the way, you may be able to pick out some of the trees you've identified. After rounding the next bend, the trail parallels US 19. Look to the right through the field and perhaps see the inhabitants of some of the bird boxes placed there.

You'll cross a gravel drive at 1.12 miles. As you near the bend, there'll be silver maple; this tree is easily identified by the silver of the bottoms of its leaves, which is most obvious when the wind blows. At the bend stands a very large tulip tree. It is so named because of its large, showy flowers that resemble tulips or lilies; its leaves have a broad tip and a nearly square base. Reach the entrance you used to enter the trail just after the turn.

▶ NEARBY ATTRACTIONS

For other hikes in this area, turn to the South Park Hike (hike 20) in this book or contact the township of Upper Saint Clair's Department of Recreation and Leisure Services at (412) 831-9000, extension 256 or visit its Web site at **www.twpusc.org/ rec/parks.** There also are many establishments along US 19.

HARRISON HILLS PARK: RACHEL CARSON TRAIL—POND AND RIVER OVERLOOKS HIKES

IN BRIEF

The Pond hike has a number of side trails, but don't let it scare you off; it is easy to follow. The River Overlooks hike is very easy to follow and provides panoramic views of the Allegheny River in many spots.

DESCRIPTION

Biologist Rachel Carson (1907–1964) was born in Springdale, Pennsylvania. Her dedication to nature and the safety of all species brought her eventual world recognition and a posthumous Presidential Medal of Freedom.

POND HIKE

From the parking lot, walk past the Ox Roast picnic pavilion toward the woods, where you find the trailhead with a sign for the Rachel Carson Trail and a yellow blaze to indicate the trail's markers. The hike begins with a short downhill to cross a stream; there are plenty of rocks to keep your feet dry across it. Then a set of trail steps leads you to the top of the other side where you'll reach a T (notice that the trail blazes on the left are green). Turn right and follow more yellow blazes. Fairly quickly (0.14 miles) you'll reach a Y with a branch to the right; continue straight. At the next Y (0.20 miles), follow the double yellow blazes and veer left, ignoring a right branch once again. This trail is full of choices, and in less than 200 feet you'll encounter another one that goes to the

KEY AT-A-GLANCE INFORMATION

LENGTH: Pond hike—2.2 miles, River Overlooks hike—2.8 miles, both—5.05 miles

CONFIGURATION: Both—out-and-back

DIFFICULTY: Easy

SCENERY: Deciduous forest, ferns and mosses, pond, ducks and geese, the Allegheny River

EXPOSURE: Mostly shaded, exposed at pond

TRAFFIC: Light

TRAIL SURFACE: Dirt and grass

HIKING TIME: Pond hike—1 hour, River Overlooks hike—1.5 hours, both—2.5 hours

ACCESS: Park hours are 8 a.m.–sunset

MAPS: "A Hiker's Guide to the Rachel Carson Trail" by Steve Mentzer provides good maps, description, history, and GPS waypoints for the entire length of the 35.7-mile Rachel Carson Trail (e-mail info@rachelcarsontrail.org); USGS Freeport

FACILITIES: Restroom with pit toilets, drinking water, picnic pavilions, swings, and large playground

SPECIAL COMMENTS: Children who love playgrounds and a hike down to a pond to see the ducks or a hike along the cliffs to view the river will enjoy these hikes.

DIRECTIONS

From Pittsburgh, take PA 28 North to Exit 16, Freeport–Millerstown. Make a right onto Millerstown Road, and follow it toward Freeport for 0.6 miles. Turn right on Freeport Road and drive 0.7 miles to the left into Harrison Hills Park (there is a sign). Take the left fork and follow 0.9 miles to the Ox Roast pavilion and park.

Harrison Hills Park: Rachel Carson Trail Pond and River Overlooks Hikes

UTM Zone (WGS84)   17T

Easting   610324

Northing   4500708

41

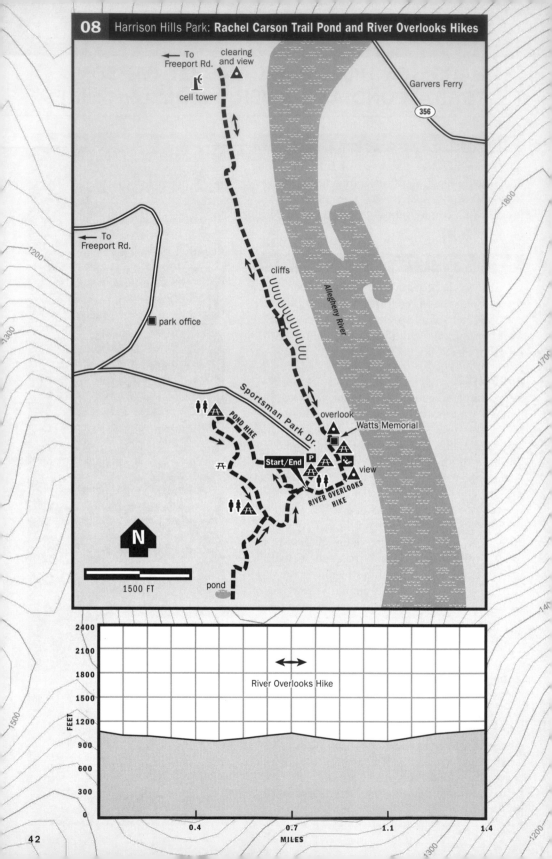

← To
Freeport Rd.

clearing
and view

cell tower

Garvers Ferry

356

← To
Freeport Rd.

cliffs

park office

Allegheny River

Sportsman Park Dr.

POND HIKE

overlook

Watts Memorial

Start/End

P

view

RIVER OVERLOOKS HIKE

N

1500 FT

pond

FEET

2400
2100
1800
1500
1200
900
600
300
0

River Overlooks Hike

0.4   0.7   1.1   1.4
MILES

1200

1300

1500

1800

1700

1400

1300

1200

left; stay straight. At the following two choices, do the same, ignoring the left branches and continuing straight.

The grasses hug the trail closely here, and the woods are thin. Step over a moss-covered log with a yellow blaze, and pass an old grill that likely once cooked dogs and burgers but now has moss growing inside. You are approaching a clearing for the new picnic area, which is equipped with a restroom and pavilion. Stay to the left of the facilities and look for the yellow-blazed tree on the left, leading back into the woods. A slight uphill grade carries you through fern and deciduous forest. Its mixture of old and young trees and lush undergrowth and moss and mayapples provides a quick escape from the hustle and bustle of busy Freeport Road just outside the perimeters of the park.

Snake through the woods on the slight uphill grade and bypass the feeder trail at 0.6 miles that leads to another picnic area. Shortly after, bypass another trail, this one from the left, which likely leads back to the beginning portion of the trail. Around 0.72 miles you'll notice another picnic area up and to your right. Keep going straight until you reach yellow double blazes on a tree at 0.77 miles, then veer left; the trail on the right appears to be another connector to the picnic area. You'll then reach a set of double-blazed (in yellow) trees, turn right heading downhill through various wildflowers.

You'll reach a gravel road at 0.92 miles; turn left on it. Follow the road briefly and veer right on the wide grassy path, following the yellow blazes. At just 0.98 miles, bear right on the trail, leaving the wide grass. Here you'll find the first conifers I saw along the trail before reaching a large field of tall grasses where purple thistle and other field flowers grow.

At the double blaze turn left; you'll immediately be immersed back into the woods and traveling downhill toward the pond, which comes into sight on the right. There are flowering trees and shrubs there in summer, and the duck and geese calls may reach you before you see them swimming about and enjoying the cool water. Daisies are along the trail and pussy willows line the pond. When you've finished lulling about the water's edge and perhaps feeding the ducks and geese, turn around and hike back.

ALLEGHENY RIVER OVERLOOKS HIKE

Note: The cliffs are steep with serious drops. Hold the hands of young children, watch pets, and warn others in your party to stay away from the edge.

If you've done the Pond Hike first, this hike begins after you've crossed the creek and come up the bank to the Rachel Carson Trail sign. Look right to see the yellow blazes located alongside the woodland at the outer edge of the grove. Turn right and follow them.

If you are doing this hike first, from the parking lot walk past the Ox Roast picnic pavilion toward the woods. There you'll find the trailhead with a sign for the Rachel Carson Trail and a yellow blaze to indicate the trail's markers. Do not go straight and cross the stream. Instead, turn left and follow the yellow blazes alongside the woodland and outer edge of the grove.

The trail begins flat and is blazed well. Be careful of the poison ivy in the area, though. Just after a slight drop in the trail, at only 0.18 miles, there is a very nice view of the Allegheny River. Continue with the cliffs to your right, and you'll come to a Y. Going right hugs the cliff's edge, but you want to choose the left branch to view the Watts Memorial. Dedicated in 1986, this plaque, which is set in a boulder, honors Michael Watts, a chemist and Pittsburgh native who worked diligently to restore clean water in western Pennsylvania and influenced environmental standards.

Just beyond the memorial, there is a formal overlook with rails, boulders, and a small monolith in its center. The view is better when there are no leaves on the trees, but even in midsummer the panoramic view is good. Leaving the overlook, continue right along the woods. Views of the Allegheny appear in various spots; stop and take them in. Bypass the four trails that diverge left, the first a grassy trail at 0.53 miles and the second at 0.62 miles (where the Rachel Carson Trail blazes actually lead left). Stay right and cross a bridge. This direction diverges then rejoins the Rachel Carson Trail and provides more views of the river, some better than any of those seen so far. If water is flowing, you'll have a chance to see some pretty runoffs. Look for the peninsula jutting out in the river as you hike along this section.

A steep descent at 1.04 miles leads to older woods with some very large trees; they are worth walking down the hill to see. More water runoffs may be trickling across the path. A brief but steep climb leads to a short roller-coaster walk down and up again, which is the direction of the remainder of the hike. Working those gluts carries you to a clearing that offers another open view of the Allegheny at 1.31 miles. If you continue beyond that, at 1.40 miles, break out of the woods and onto a gravel road. Turning right on this road leads to Freeport Road and the eastern terminus of the Rachel Carson Trail; this is a good place to turn around and retrace your hike.

▶ NEARBY ATTRACTIONS

There is a park office on the way in to the park. It was locked when I was there, but it did have a sign stating "Visitor's Welcome" and phone numbers for permits: (412) 350-2455, (724) 935-1971, and (724) 935-1766.

HARTWOOD ACRES TOUR

▶ IN BRIEF

The mansion and its grounds compose a 629-acre equestrian estate designed in the lavish style of the wealthy during the early part of the 19th century. Any visitor is impressed with the beautifully designed mansion, stable complex, and grounds.

▶ DESCRIPTION

The Hartwood Estate was initiated with a purchase of a 480-acre parcel of land on a crest overlooking the foothills of the Allegheny Mountains. The buyer was Mary Flinn Lawrence, who inherited her wealth from her father, William Flinn. She hired architect Alfred Hopkins, who captured the essence of 16th-century architecture in the Tudor style of the mansion, combining it with the desires of the Lawrences who valued the land and its similarity to the Cotswold region of England. The result is a beautiful mansion of ornamentation, detailed motifs, and stone construction surrounded by a colorful garden and meticulously kept grounds, a stately equestrian stable complex, and woodlands.

The mansion began in 1927 as a cottage in which the family could reside while the remainder of its wings were built; the magnificent home was completed in 1929. Inside, hand-carved wood paneling over stone walls and a chimney piece carved in high relief above the stone fireplace of the great room are complemented by the ornate motifs in the plaster ceiling. Detailed ceiling work is found in other rooms as well, with patterns that

KEY AT-A-GLANCE INFORMATION

LENGTH: 2.2 miles (with options for a shorter walk)

CONFIGURATION: Loop

DIFFICULTY: Easy

SCENERY: Mixed deciduous and conifer forest, garden, mansion, stables

EXPOSURE: Shaded

TRAFFIC: Moderate

TRAIL SURFACE: Dirt, pavement, and gravel

HIKING TIME: 1.5 hours (excluding tour)

ACCESS: Park closes at sunset

MAPS: Available for the overall park at the Hartwood Acres mansion (posted outside near office door) or by contacting Allegheny County Parks Department at (412) 350-7275, but there is no detail of the trails; USGS Glenshaw

FACILITIES: Restrooms are available outside the mansion, in the back, and a water fountain is located by the door entrance for tours. There is a portable toilet located near the parking lot.

SPECIAL COMMENTS: Combine your hike with a tour of the mansion by reserving ahead; call (412) 767-9200. (See Nearby Attractions following the Description below.)

▶ DIRECTIONS

From Pittsburgh, take PA 28 North to Exit 5, Etna–Butler. Follow PA 8 North 0.7 miles and turn right on Saxonburg Boulevard. Follow 4.4 miles and turn left into Hartwood Acres. Drive 0.5 miles and turn right, following the park's entrance drive to park in the mansion-area parking lot.

Hartwood Acres Tour

UTM Zone (WGS84)   17T

Easting   592303

Northing   4491385

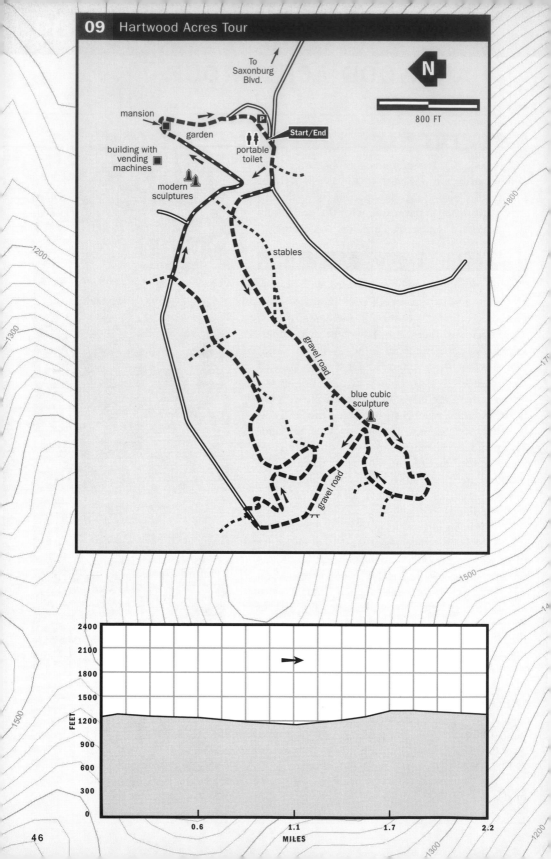

N

800 FT

To
Saxonburg
Blvd.

mansion

garden

P

Start/End

building with
vending
machines

portable
toilet

modern
sculptures

stables

gravel road

blue cubic
sculpture

gravel road

2400
2100
1800
1500
1200
900
600
300
0

FEET

0.6   1.1   1.7   2.2

MILES

provide a sense of timelessness as they reflect the equestrian life, the love of the hunt, a fondness for local wildlife, and the individual tastes of each of the Lawrences. The furnishings, including the kitchen appliances, are original and continue to complete the décor of the mansion's rooms. In 1969, Allegheny County purchased the property, including all of the buildings and furnishings as well as adjacent land, to preserve its beauty and history and to increase the park's land to its current acreage.

Begin the day with a tour of the mansion, if you have arranged it. Then start this hike from the mansion parking lot. If you have incorporated a tour of the stable complex as well, you may begin there by following the description in the second paragraph below.

From the parking lot, with the mansion to your right, walk to its end and turn right on the road. The mileage noted begins with the right turn. Walk down this scenic road, passing a trail into the woods on the left and, staying on the road, veer left at the Y. Come to an intersection and follow the gravel road; straight ahead. If you wish to walk closer to the stables (there is an option to do this later, too), take the road to the left, which passes in front of them and rejoins the gravel road. Otherwise, continue straight onto the gravel road; you can see the stables down to the left about 0.21 miles into the walk. If you wish, you can turn left from the gravel road and walk to the stables and back from here as well.

When ready to move on from the stables, continue on the gravel road until you come to a large blue cubic sculpture at 0.50 miles. Walk left off of the road, behind the sculpture, to the opening in the woods. There are no signs for the trails, but an obvious break in the woods is found by turning left at the sculpture. Note that the pipeline opening down the clearing on the right is not the opening for the trail.

Once in the woods, the trail S-curves through a mixed deciduous-and-pine woodland along an initially level dirt pathway. Oak and beech trees, along with sassafras and pines line the trail as it begins a bit of a descent. Follow the trail as it veers right, wrapping around the hillside; ignore the left branch at a Y at 0.72 miles. Do the same at the next branch, and follow the trail back up and out of the woods. Walk along the pipeline back toward the same blue cubic sculpture. Once you've reached the gravel road again, you can keep the hike short by turning right and retracing your steps along it. If you want to continue, turn left instead.

Pass a bench and arrive at a paved drive at 1.07 miles. Turn right and stay on the paved drive, ignoring the wooded trail to the left of the drive seen shortly after turning. You don't remain on the paved drive long, however (unless you wish to follow it back to the mansion rather than using the trails). Look for a quick right onto a trail leading into the woods. Turn right and follow the dirt path as it veers left back into the trees. The trail parallels the paved drive briefly. After it turns away from it, you may soon notice the enormous bur oak on the left at 1.19 miles. As the trail winds its way through the woods, two things become obvious—mountain bikers enjoy the trail as much as hikers do, and the road from which you came is not far. At 1.36 miles, pass the trail on your right that leads back to the gravel road and stay left at the Y you'll arrive at almost immediately.

The trail is easy and enjoyable. As you walk over flat boulders, try to spot fawn or deer and other wildlife; they are protected here and are sometimes visible to the observant hiker. Reach a T at 1.58 miles and turn left. There is an abundance of ferns lining the trail's edges in this area. They are beautiful but also can be a sign that the deer have eaten other vegetation and left the ferns, which they do not like, to propagate. Walk through a section where some small, embedded boulders dot the trail's surface, through another pretty section of ferns, and come to an intersection at 1.67 miles. Do not turn right or left, but continue straight. Reach the paved drive again at 1.78 miles and turn right onto it; follow it back to a triangular divider. You can either retrace your steps along the road to the parking lot from here or make a hard left to circle the mansion.

If you've chosen to circle the mansion, you'll see a few more modern sculptures off to the left. Across the open grass is a building with vending machines for beverages. The paved drive ends when the cobblestone close to the mansion begins. The back of the mansion, where the office is located, faces the cobblestone road. When the cobblestone ends, walk clockwise around the mansion in the grass to see the lovely stone veranda. This will lead past the door entrance for tours; the pathway just beyond it leads to the parking lot. You may wish to detour to the garden to the right of the pathway before returning to your car.

▶ NEARBY ATTRACTIONS

Tour fees, including stable tours, range from $5 (full-price adult ticket) to $1 (children ages 5 and younger); reservations must be made in advance by calling (412) 767-9200. Tour hours are Wednesday through Saturday, 10 a.m. to 3 p.m., and Sunday, noon to 4 p.m. All fees, including those for stable tours, and information concerning special events such as horse jumping, the celebration of lights, summer concerts, and rugby and polo matches can be found online at **www.county .allegheny.pa.us/parks** or by calling the Allegheny County Parks Department at (412) 350-7275.

HIGHLAND PARK DOUBLE LOOP

▶ IN BRIEF

You can make your trip to Highland Park an hour or a day—or anything in between. The hike incorporates many visual pleasures. If you're looking to spend some time, though, check out the park's other amenities.

▶ DESCRIPTION

Have you ever wondered how some local streets acquired their names? Most of the land upon which this park resides was originally owned by Alexander Negley (Negley Avenue) in the late 1700s. He operated a farm that was later expanded by his son, Jacob Negley. In 1837, the Negleys' land holdings were subdivided by county surveyor Robert Hiland who gave his own name to Hiland Avenue (now Highland Avenue). The city of Pittsburgh annexed areas in 1868, and the current site made it ideal for the city's drinking-water reservoir, which began operation in 1879 and quickly became a destination for residents. In 1893, after exhaustive efforts by Pittsburgh Director of Public Works Edward Bigelow (Bigelow Boulevard), Highland Park officially opened.

Today, Highland Park continues to be one of Pittsburgh's most popular outdoor destinations. Its 380 acres attract walkers, joggers, bicyclists,

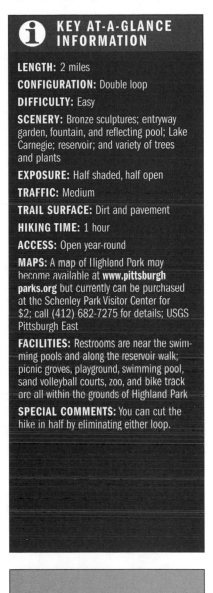

▶ KEY AT-A-GLANCE INFORMATION

LENGTH: 2 miles

CONFIGURATION: Double loop

DIFFICULTY: Easy

SCENERY: Bronze sculptures; entryway garden, fountain, and reflecting pool; Lake Carnegie; reservoir; and variety of trees and plants

EXPOSURE: Half shaded, half open

TRAFFIC: Medium

TRAIL SURFACE: Dirt and pavement

HIKING TIME: 1 hour

ACCESS: Open year-round

MAPS: A map of Highland Park may become available at **www.pittsburgh parks.org** but currently can be purchased at the Schenley Park Visitor Center for $2; call (412) 682-7275 for details; USGS Pittsburgh East

FACILITIES: Restrooms are near the swimming pools and along the reservoir walk; picnic groves, playground, swimming pool, sand volleyball courts, zoo, and bike track are all within the grounds of Highland Park

SPECIAL COMMENTS: You can cut the hike in half by eliminating either loop.

▶ DIRECTIONS

From Pittsburgh, take Interstate 376 East to Exit 9, Edgewood–Swissvale; use the left ramp following Edgewood signs. Again, stay left following Braddock Avenue signs. Turn right at the stop sign onto South Braddock Avenue, and continue straight through the first and second lights. At the third light turn left onto Penn Avenue. Follow Penn Avenue to Highland Avenue. Turn right onto Highland Avenue and follow it 1.8 miles to the entrance of Highland Park. Drive between the columns and turn right onto Reservoir Drive and park.

Highland Park Double Loop

UTM Zone (WGS84) 17T

Easting 591954

Northing 4481465

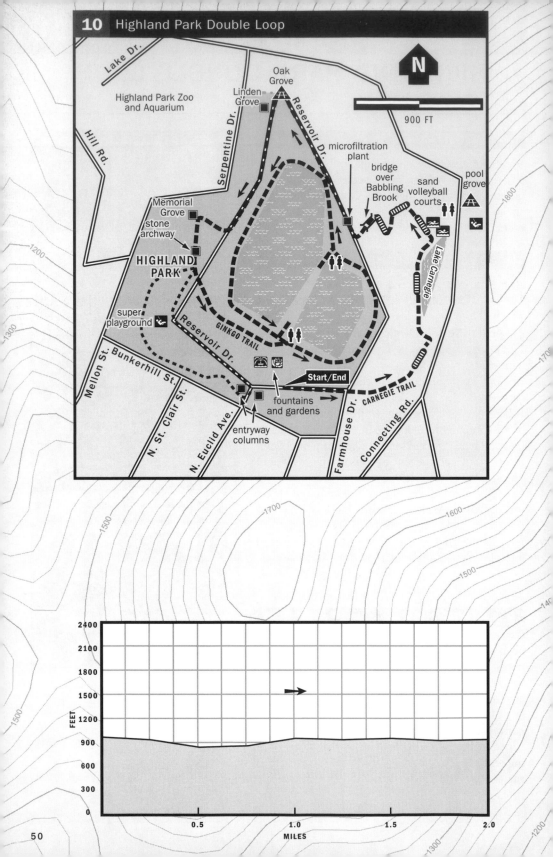

Lake Dr.

Highland Park Zoo
and Aquarium

Hill Rd.

Oak
Grove

Linden
Grove

Serpentine Dr.

Reservoir Dr.

N

900 FT

microfiltration
plant

bridge
over
Babbling
Brook

sand
volleyball
courts

pool
grove

Memorial
Grove
stone
archway

HIGHLAND
PARK

Lake Carnegie

super
playground

Reservoir Dr.

GINKGO TRAIL

Start/End

Carnegie Trail

fountains
and gardens

Mellon St.

Bunkerhill St.

N. St. Clair St.

N. Euclid Ave.

entryway
columns

Farmhouse Dr.

Connecting Rd.

-1200

-1300

-1500

-1700

-1600

-1500

-1400

-1300

-1200

-1800

-1700

FEET

2400

2100

1800

1500

1200

900

600

300

0

0.5   1.0   1.5   2.0

MILES

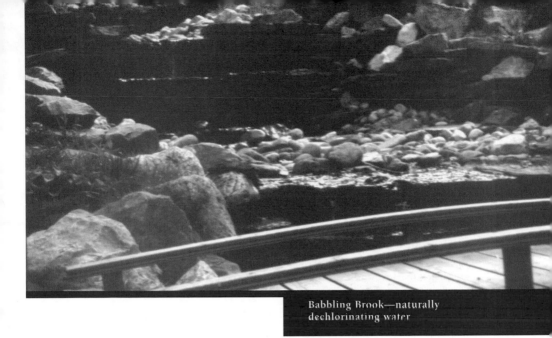

Babbling Brook—naturally
dechlorinating water

swimmers, anglers, and visitors to the Pittsburgh Zoo and Aquarium.

Once you park your car on Reservoir Road, walk over to the columns to view the exquisite detail of the bronze sculptures by Giuseppe Moretti. You can visit the entryway gardens, fountain, and reflecting pool now or later. This entryway, including the walkways, benches, and lighting, was part of a project to restore the entrance to its original grandeur as recently as 2003.

Walk to your right on Reservoir Drive, with the fountain and gardens on your left. Swamp white oak and a variety of other deciduous trees line the sidewalk. Cross Farmhouse Drive (the 140-year-old Negley farmhouse is down this road and has been used as a park office). Immense Norway spruces, with their weeping branches, line the path briefly. This may be the most common spruce in the state, and it produces the largest cones of all spruces. Just beyond them, turn right down the unmarked, wide cement path before Oak Grove. This is Carnegie Trail; follow the path and stone stairs down to Lake Carnegie. Turn left to walk on the western side of the lake. In the 1870s, Andrew Carnegie partially financed the creation of this lake, which was used as a halfway station for water being pumped out of the Allegheny River. Lake Carnegie was established for recreation when this former lower reservoir became obsolete. In 1932, the lake was halved in size to make room for the park's swimming pools (coming up), but is still used for fishing in summer.

Enjoy the view and scent of honeysuckle until you reach stairs that lead to the lake. Follow them down and out onto the cement pad if you'd like or sit and relax on one of the benches. Ducks, geese, and fish make this area their home. Back along the path, you'll find daisy fleabane, identifiable by its numerous thin rays.

As the end of the lake draws near and the pools come into view, continue walking on the path; the surface changes to gravel. Birds and chipmunks seem to frequent the area, so you may spot a few. Walk past the pool building; there are restrooms on the other side. This pool is the city's only long-course pool and occupies 13,600 square feet. There is also a 3,000-square-foot wading pool for toddlers. Nearby are sand volleyball courts.

Just beyond this point (0.4 miles), turn left and ascend the stairs (continuing straight leads to Lake Drive). Cross over an unmarked path (called Sycamore Trail) and veer slightly right to ascend another set of steps. The stone on the left cascading down the hillside is Babbling Brook. Water may not be flowing in this lower section, but it should be above. The watercourse comes from a new microfiltration plant that has proved an international model. As the water runs down the rocks and leaves within the brook, it is naturally dechlorinated before reaching Lake Carnegie.

Cross the small arched bridge that fords the brook. Either turn left to walk along the fine gravel path, up a set of steps, and right along the grove, or take the steps closer to the brook. Both lead to Reservoir Drive. You can cut the hike short here by taking the stairs across the road by the microfiltration plant up to the reservoir or make a right on Reservoir Drive to continue.

Pass by the unfinished trail that veers off to the right at 0.68 miles. According to the park map, this trail is finished, but it wasn't yet during my visit. Walking along Reservoir Drive, continue past Oak and Linden groves. Along the way find a tree of heaven, oaks, maples, and chokecherry. At 1 mile, you'll notice another set of stairs leading up to the reservoir. Shortly after, turn right down the steps and path to Memorial Grove. The memorial you'll find is dedicated to Alexander Negley; both he and his wife are buried here. Turn left and walk along the asphalt path; you'll see wildflowers growing in this area.

Go up the steps and through the stone archway. This trail is called Ginkgo Trail, and at least 16 ginkgo trees grow along it. Veer left with the trail to go to the entryway gardens and the reservoir. Turning right leads to what's called the super playground, built in just five days by community volunteers.

When you reach the wall in front of the stairway there is a plaque showing that the reservoir is a historic landmark. Take the stairs up and begin your walk around the water. It's likely that there will be a mix of other walkers and joggers enjoying it as well. The water is quite soothing, especially if you are fortunate enough to be here on a beautiful spring or summer evening. A quarter of the way around is a restroom on the right and a walkway leading between the water pools. There are a number of blooming trees along this three-quarter-mile walkway, as well as benches on which you can sit and watch the world go by for awhile. After encircling the reservoir, there are many choices for additional activity or relaxation.

▶ NEARBY ATTRACTIONS

For shelter permits, call the Department of Public Works at (412) 255-2370; for more information visit **www.city.pittsburgh.pa.us.** For swimming, call the city's aquatic-information line at (412) 594-4645; during the summer, contact the pool at (412) 665-3637. Contact the Pittsburgh Zoo at (800) 474-4966 or visit **www.pittsburgh zoo.com.** For information about events and activities at the Washington Boulevard Bike Track, contact the Allegheny Cycling Association at **www.acaracing.com** or the Pittsburgh Masters Velo Club at (412) 521-2207.

MONTOUR TRAIL: CLIFF MINE TO FIVE POINTS

▶ IN BRIEF

Currently, multiple sections of the Montour Trail totaling more than 40 miles are completed. The trail is ideal for all forms of nonmotorized use: bicycling, walking, running, cross-country skiing, and nature appreciation. In certain sections horseback riding is also permitted, but not on the improved trail surface.

▶ DESCRIPTION

This segment of the Montour Trail begins at the Cliff Mine Trailhead and ends at the Enlow (Five Points) access.

Enter the Cliff Mine Trailhead heading west. Here you immediately spot lady slipper, which is prominent in different intervals on the trail. You quickly arrive at a road crossing at 0.2 miles; it is the only one along this segment. Watch for cars making the curve at high speeds on your left. At 0.46 miles, you'll see an interpretive sign that explains the efforts of the Montour Run Watershed Association to stabilize the stream banks along Montour Run. Carbonate rock linings have been installed in the banks in 12 locations to offset the erosive effects of increased storm-water runoff. The Montour Run Watershed Association also planted vegetation along the banks to hold the soil in place and to create more shade along the run to assist in habitat development for fish and other aquatic life. Walk down to the water running on your left at this point, if you wish, before continuing on to reach a lookout from a

ⓘ KEY AT-A-GLANCE INFORMATION

LENGTH: 3.8 miles (can be lengthened by walking farther on the Montour Trail)

CONFIGURATION: Out-and-back

DIFFICULTY: Easy

SCENERY: Montour Run, wildflowers, wetlands, former railroad tunnel, and interpretive signs

EXPOSURE: Mostly sunny

TRAFFIC: Heavy use on weekends

TRAIL SURFACE: Wide, paved path covered with crushed limestone

HIKING TIME: 1–1.5 hours

ACCESS: Trailhead never closed

MAPS: A map of the Montour Trail, access points, walking bypasses of uncompleted sections, and information on trail developments and events can be found at **www.montourtrail.org** or by calling (412) 831-2030; USGS Oakdale

FACILITIES: Portable toilets, drinking fountain

SPECIAL COMMENTS: The Montour Trail is a result of the nationwide Rails-to-Trails program and was honored with the designation of a National Recreation Trail in 2004. When completed, the trail will ultimately extend 47 miles from Coraopolis to Clairton. The Montour Trail is also part of the Great Allegheny Passage, a 152-mile bicycle and walking trail that will eventually connect Pittsburgh with the C & O Canal in Cumberland, Maryland.

▶ DIRECTIONS

From Pittsburgh, take Interstate 279 South to PA 60 toward the airport. Take Exit 2, Montour Run Road. Bear right at the end of the ramp. Turn left onto Cliff Mine Road and follow 0.6 miles to the parking area where Cliff Mine Road, Steubenville Pike, and Enlow Road intersect.

Montour Trail: Cliff Mine to Five Points

UTM Zone (WGS84)   17T

Easting   567883

Northing   4478175

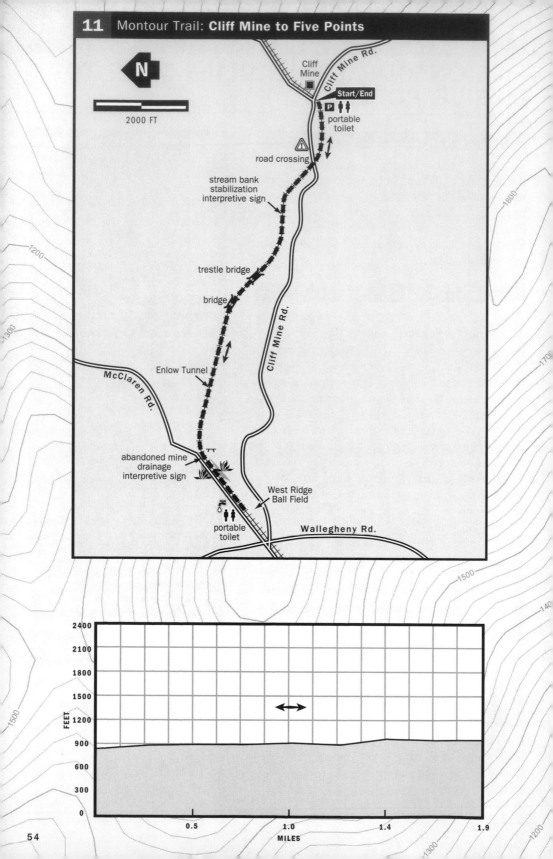

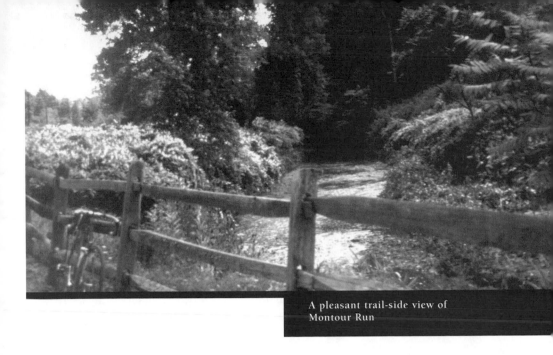

A pleasant trail-side view of
Montour Run

bridge over the water. The run curves left, out of site until the next bridge crossing.

You will cross an old railroad trestle before coming upon another of the many small bridges that dot this trail over the meandering Montour Run. At a little more than 1 mile you reach the entrance of the lighted Enlow Tunnel. This remnant of the Montour Railroad offers a very pleasant reprieve from the heat of the sun. As you emerge from the tunnel look up to the right where you'll see the rock walls through which the tunnel was blasted in the 1920s, 50 years into the construction of the Montour Railroad.

About 60 feet up the trail on the left is a bench, the only one between the beginning and end of this segment. A wetland begins to come into view at about 1.6 miles. There is an interpretive sign that gives information on the abandoned-mine drainage that's causing metal pollution within the Montour Run watershed. If you notice an orange or rust color in the streambed bottom, the metal pollution is coming from iron; if white, it's from aluminum. The wetlands here assist in mitigating the effects of the abandoned Cliff Mine drainage by trapping the metals. They also offer a beautiful display of large cattails and grasses to the passerby. Along the trail you will also enjoy wild mustard, daisies, Queen Ann's lace, and purple thistle.

The Enlow (Five Points) turnaround is made obvious with a small parking area on the right, the West Ridge Ball Field on the left, and a portable toilet. There is a drinking fountain near the ball field's backstop.

▶ NEARBY ATTRACTIONS

For a large selection of restaurants, drive to the Robinson Town shopping area; there are a couple of other choices close by. At the Enlow (Five Points) access is a service station across the street with vending machines containing snacks and beverages. Schmidt's Tavern is a half mile from the Cliff Mine access, and the Settle Inn (located in Imperial) is at 297 Mahoney Road.

MONTOUR TRAIL: PANHANDLE TRAIL—WALKERS MILL TO GREGG STATION

KEY AT-A-GLANCE INFORMATION

LENGTH: 4.8 miles

CONFIGURATION: Out-and-back

DIFFICULTY: Easy

SCENERY: Rock quarry, quarry windmill, landscaped flowerbeds, butterfly garden

EXPOSURE: Sunny but shaded areas throughout

TRAFFIC: Moderate

TRAIL SURFACE: Packed, crushed stone

HIKING TIME: 1 to 2 hours

ACCESS: Trailhead never closes

MAPS: A map of the Montour Trail, access points, walking bypasses of uncompleted sections, and information on trail developments and events can be found at **www.montourtrail.org** or by calling (412) 831-2030; USGS Oakdale

FACILITIES: Portable toilets at Walkers Mill and Gregg Station access points, numerous picnic pavilions, grills

SPECIAL COMMENTS: The Panhandle Trail, Pennsylvania's 100th rail-trail, will eventually span 29 miles from Walkers Mill in Collier Township through the northern sector of Washington County to Weirton, West Virginia, along the former Conrail line known as the Panhandle Railroad. Contact the Panhandle Trail Association to obtain the most recent trail development information at **www.panhandletrail.org.**

Montour Trail: Panhandle Trail—
Walkers Mill to Gregg Station

UTM Zone (WGS84)   17T

Easting   573711

Northing   4472132

IN BRIEF

The Panhandle Trail is chock-full of interesting diversions, and is a great place for family hiking and picnicking. The trail is suitable for hikers, joggers, or bikers of every age and ability level. It is also easy to navigate with a stroller or wheelchair.

DESCRIPTION

When you enter the trailhead you will be immediately impressed with the quality of this trail, and you will not be disappointed during the entire hike. Only a few feet away from the trailhead on the right, stop and take in the butterfly garden, which is adorned with colorful butterfly houses interspersed with orange, white, yellow, and purple colors from daylilies, black-eyed Susans, hostas, and other flowering beauties. If you pause here you will find that the garden is doing its job, as there will be several species of butterflies enjoying it. Within sight, about 30 feet farther along the trail, is a welcoming picnic pavilion equipped with a grill that is roomy enough for a family or two. If you are traveling with a family, this is a great place to picnic either before or after using the trial. There is also a portable toilet at the trailhead.

As you continue walking or biking, you will soon cross what will be a series of bridges that allow you to traverse Robinson Run without getting your feet wet. At just about 600 feet from the trailhead, there is an access path to Cliff Cave, which is posted against trespassing and is under camera surveillance but can be explored

DIRECTIONS

From Pittsburgh, take Interstate 279 South (Parkway West) and merge onto I-79 South. Take Exit 57 toward Carnegie and merge right from the ramp onto Noblestown Road. At 1.6 miles turn left onto Walkers Mill Road. Drive about two blocks; there are signs for the trailhead and parking.

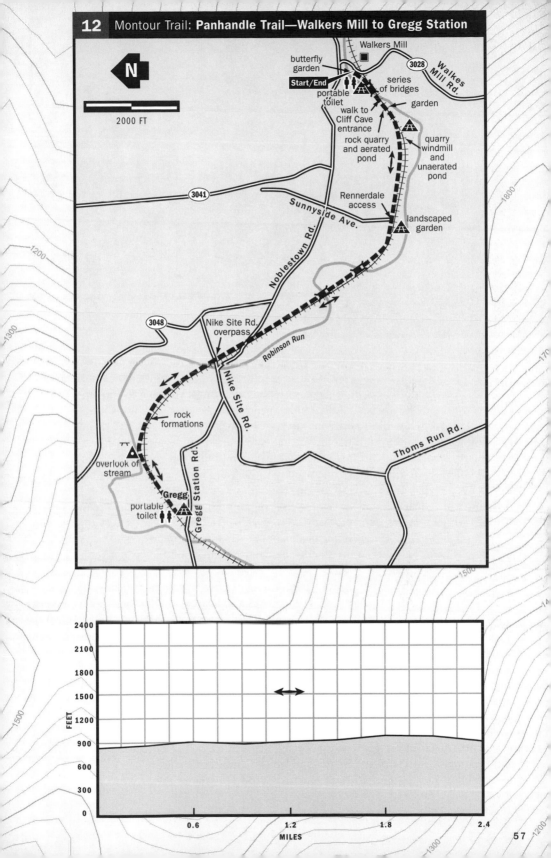

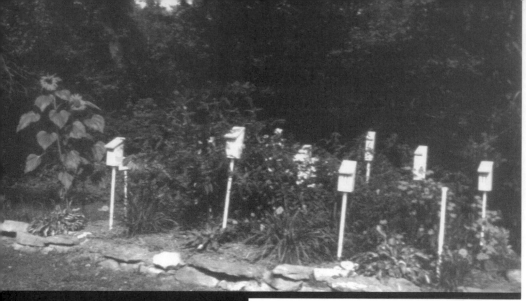
Butterfly garden near trailhead

with permission. See Nearby Attractions following this description for information.

Another 300 feet from the path to the cave brings you to a rock quarry, framed on both sides with beautifully landscaped small gardens; you'll also see a 10- to 15-foot-tall white birdhouse for martins. The rock wall of the quarry stands at least 100 feet tall, and toward the top are lights that are used during special events. At the quarry's base is a pond that is aerated by a windmill; stop and look in the pond for bubbles. If wind is crossing the windmill, the bubbles are a testament to the oxygen being pumped in through an underground pipe to assist fish life by reducing summer and winter fish kill and increasing fish appetite for spawning; it also reduces algae growth, eliminates odor problems, improves water clarity, and reduces organic bottom sediments. Take note of the quality of the water in this pond so that you may compare it with the water in the smaller, unaerated quarry pond located a short distance farther up the trail.

Directly in front of the rock quarry is a large fire ring formed with—what else?—rocks. The fire ring is surrounded by benches and a large boulder for fireside comfort. This area is used for various events; see the Web site (**www.panhandletrail.org**) to obtain event news and dates. Across from the quarry are another picnic pavilion and a garden that even has tomato plants. A lucky hiker or biker may find a sweet ripe tomato to snack on along the way.

Shortly you'll find yourself at the quarry windmill on the left-hand side of the trail, and next to it the smaller, unaerated pond. After reading the informative sign and walking on, you'll see Robinson Run on your left before you reach the Rennerdale access on the right (at approximately 0.6 miles). Across from it, you can't miss yet another landscaped garden and covered picnic area. You also likely will have noticed by now the numerous hummingbird houses and plastic jugs hanging from the trees on both sides of the trail; several more martin houses dot the way as well.

Both slightly before and after 1 mile, you will cross two bridges over Robinson Run as it weaves its way through the land. As you continue on from this area the landscaping ends, but the trailside abounds with wildflowers of every color. You'll walk under the Nike Site Road overpass at about 1.5 miles, where you can look up on the nearby hillside to see the former installation of the Nike missile launch sites of the 1950s. You'll pass between rock formations that rise up on both sides of the trail before reaching an open, scenic overlook of Robinson Run and a bench to rest on if you wish to indulge.

You'll arrive at Gregg Station at 2.35 miles, which is the turnaround point. There is another picnic pavilion here as well as a portable toilet. If you wish you can travel farther and turn around later.

▶ **NEARBY ATTRACTIONS**

Call the Collier Township office at (412) 279-2525 to prearrange permission to explore the cave at Cliff Mine. The closest restaurant is Doug's Family Restaurant, located two blocks from the Walkers Mill access.

NORTH PARK: BRAILLE TRAIL LOOP

 KEY AT-A-GLANCE INFORMATION

LENGTH: 0.5 miles

CONFIGURATION: Loop

DIFFICULTY: Easy

SCENERY: Wildflowers, deciduous forest, lush undergrowth

EXPOSURE: Shaded

TRAFFIC: Light

TRAIL SURFACE: Dirt

HIKING TIME: 20 minutes

ACCESS: Open year-round, sunrise–midnight

MAPS: Available for the overall park and (more detailed) for the trails near the Latodami Nature Center at the park office (see Directions), (724) 935-1766; USGS Emsworth

FACILITIES: Portable toilets are located at the Latodami Nature Center just a short way farther on Brown Road, on the right.

SPECIAL COMMENTS: All ages and abilities can enjoy this short walk in the woods.

North Park: Braille Trail Loop

UTM Zone (WGS84)   17T

Easting   581937

Northing   4496984

▶ IN BRIEF

This trail represents a wonderful concept. To the right of the trail along its entire length is a guiding wire covered in soft black tubing, which enables the visually handicapped to experience the trail more independently.

▶ DESCRIPTION

I was surprised and happy to find a trail that was constructed in such a way that the visually impaired could more easily enjoy a walk in the woods. The trail, originally constructed in 1970 to be self-guided, included posts along the way with interpretive signs both in print and in Braille. Unfortunately, I saw only one sign remaining in either format. The trail was rebuilt in 1987 for use by all, but the signage has not been restored. For this I was saddened because its existence is important. However, even though most of the signage is gone, the trail remains wide and easy, and the guiding rail along it still makes it better than many for someone with visual difficulty or impairment.

To begin the hike, walk left on the loop with the guiding rail on the right; the trail is meant to be hiked clockwise. In the spring, find gray-headed coneflowers and colorful phlox in the beginning of the hike. Here, the surrounding

▶ DIRECTIONS

From Pittsburgh, take PA 28 North to Exit 5, Etna–Butler. Follow PA 8 North 7.3 miles, and make a left onto Wildwood Road (Yellow Belt). Follow 2.7 miles and turn right onto Babcock Boulevard. Drive 0.2 miles and turn left on Pearce Mill Road. To visit the park office, turn left at 1.4 miles; otherwise drive 2.1 miles and turn left on Kummer Road. Veer right at the Y for Brown Road, drive 0.2 miles, and turn left at the small parking area.

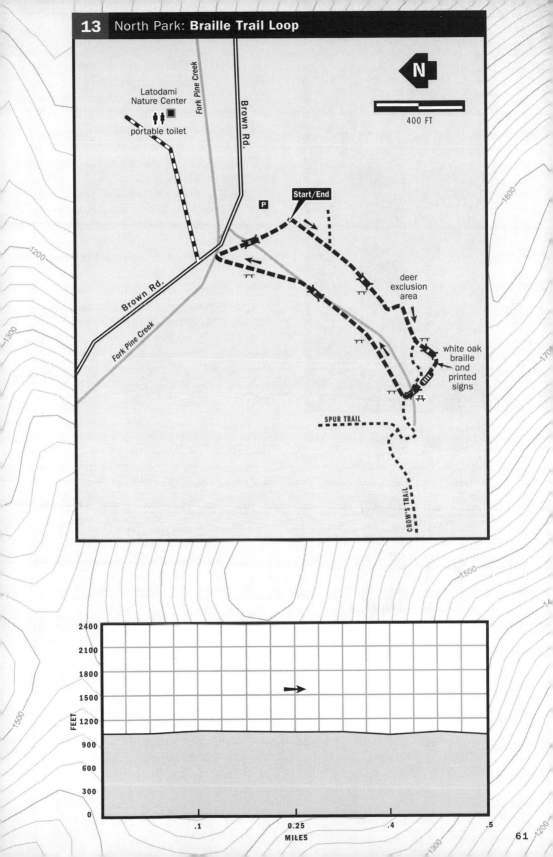

N

400 FT

Latodami
Nature Center

portable toilet

Fork Pine Creek

Brown Rd.

P

Start/End

deer
exclusion
area

Brown Rd.

Fork Pine Creek

white oak
braille
and
printed
signs

SPUR TRAIL

CROW'S TRAIL

FEET

2400
2100
1800
1500
1200
900
600
300
0

.1   0.25   .4   .5
MILES

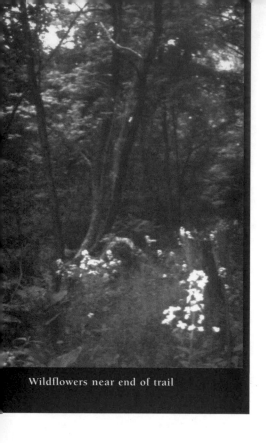

Wildflowers near end of trail

woodlands appear to be very young and consist of deciduous trees. There also are many birdhouses, a nice addition because the sound of birds calling and singing allows more immersion into nature. You may hear or see swifts, swallows, finches, woodpeckers, and warblers. I was fortunate enough to see a scarlet tanager.

You'll quickly arrive at a post marked with a deer hoof and a mushroom at the edge of a path that leads back and left. There is no indication on the map of what these markings are, but they are found on a legend board at the nature center.

Continue straight, and you'll find yourself among some much older and larger trees including red oak. The forest floor is covered with wildflowers, ferns, moss, and mayapples. Cross over a small feeder stream, and pass a bench. The water is feeding into Fork Pine Creek, also known as Grom Run, and the moisture it provides is a perfect breeding ground for the skunk cabbage along this section.

At 0.12 miles, turn left to see if you notice a difference between the white-tailed deer exclusion area and the unprotected woods. There is some information posted about which flora might be better able to survive without the grazing deer and its habitat. Look for bloodroot, ginseng, wild leeks, trout lily, false Solomon's seal, and Indian strawberry among them.

Upon returning to the main trail, you'll find that it begins to travel closer to the water. There is a choice at 0.16 miles to head right or straight. Walk straight ahead (turning right rejoins this trail but cuts out a small portion). There is a nice sitting bench just prior to a bridge. Cross the bridge, walk up the slight incline, and stop at the post with the last remaining printed page and braille plate; both give information about the enormous white oak standing to the right of the post.

White oaks are one of the most important trees of this area. From the time this land was settled, this species has provided lumber for furniture, buildings, whiskey barrels, crates, and much more. Also, white oak is one of the best woods from which charcoal is made. In autumn you'll find its acorns on the ground, an important food source for turkeys, squirrels, grouse, deer, and other wildlife. They can be consumed by humans, too, but should be boiled in several changes of water to leech out the bitter and slightly toxic tannins.

Continue and walk down a short set of shallow trail steps. Pass the trail coming up from the right. (This is the shortcut mentioned previously.) Almost immediately you'll arrive at two long benches that line each side of the trail. There is also a picnic bench on the other end of the benches. This is indeed a beautiful spot to relax and enjoy, being located next to the trickling water run. When ready, cross the bridge over the creek and at 0.23 miles arrive at a junction with Spur Trail. According to the more detailed map or the trails near the nature center, the Spur Trail heads east and then loops north and west again and reconnects with this trail. It also provides a connection to Crow's Trail, which is a one-way trail to McKinney Road. Take the Spur Trail loop if you like, or continue right for this hike.

You'll see wild geranium, false Solomon's seal, and lilies, and another bench on the left of the trail. Walking on a slight decline, you'll find another bench on the right of the trail, in addition to flowering trees and a variety of wildflowers. At the other end of another small bridge are beautiful stands of fireweed. After the last bench you are very near the end of the trail. In this area you'll find gorgeous displays of phlox before crossing the last and largest of the trail bridges to return to the parking area.

▶ NEARBY ATTRACTIONS

For more hiking, leave the parking lot, turn left on Brown Road and then right up the dirt road leading to the Latodami Nature Center. See the North Park Nature Center Loop (hike 14). Information about renting groves or using other park attractions such as the pool, tennis courts, golf course, boat house (boat rentals available), and ice-skating facility is available at **www.county.allegheny.pa.us/parks** or by contacting the park office at (724) 935-1766.

NORTH PARK: NATURE CENTER LOOP

KEY AT-A-GLANCE INFORMATION

LENGTH: 1.7 miles

CONFIGURATION: Loop with optional out-and-back

DIFFICULTY: Easy

SCENERY: Latodomi Nature Center, meadow with lots of birds and wildflowers, deciduous forest

EXPOSURE: Half shaded, half open

TRAFFIC: Light

TRAIL SURFACE: Grass and dirt

HIKING TIME: 1 hour

ACCESS: Open year-round, sunrise–midnight

MAPS: Available for the overall park and (more detailed) for the trails near the Latodomi Nature Center at the park office (see Directions), (724) 935-1766; USGS Emsworth

FACILITIES: Portable toilets are located at the Latodomi Nature Center

SPECIAL COMMENTS: The symbols on some of the posts along the trail are found on a board at the nature center but are not marked on the park map.

North Park: Nature Center Loop

UTM Zone (WGS84)   17T

Easting   582086

Northing   4497132

IN BRIEF

If you enjoy birds and wildflowers, you'll love this hike. An uphill jaunt carries you to an open meadow complete with an observation blind. Bring your binoculars.

DESCRIPTION

The Latodomi Nature Center is open only for special programs: many are offered both in the field and inside the center, and outings take place elsewhere in the park. (If you are interested, see Nearby Attractions following this description for contact information.) The surroundings of the nature center include a butterfly house, planted flowers, and a picnic shelter. On the side of the nature center are vibrant colorful paintings of the various butterflies of the area including the Titus swallowtail, fritillary, checkered white, spicebush swallow, spring azure, pink lady, and silver-spotted skipper. There is also a pond you can reach by taking a 10- to 15-minute walk on the Pond Trail below the nature center.

To begin this hike, walk from the parking lot through the picnic shelter and turn left at the post marked with bird, wagon-wheel, and fox-head symbols. Almost immediately after you begin walking uphill, you will reach another post, this one with arrows pointing right and straight ahead.

DIRECTIONS

From Pittsburgh, take PA 28 North to Exit 5, Etna–Butler. Follow PA 8 North 7.3 miles and turn left onto Wildwood Road (Yellow Belt). Follow 2.7 miles and turn right onto Babcock Boulevard. Drive 0.2 miles and turn left on Pearce Mill Road. To visit the park office, turn left at 1.4 miles; otherwise drive 2.1 miles and turn left on Kummer Road. Veer right at the Y for Brown Road, drive 0.3 miles, turn right, and drive up the dirt road to the parking area.

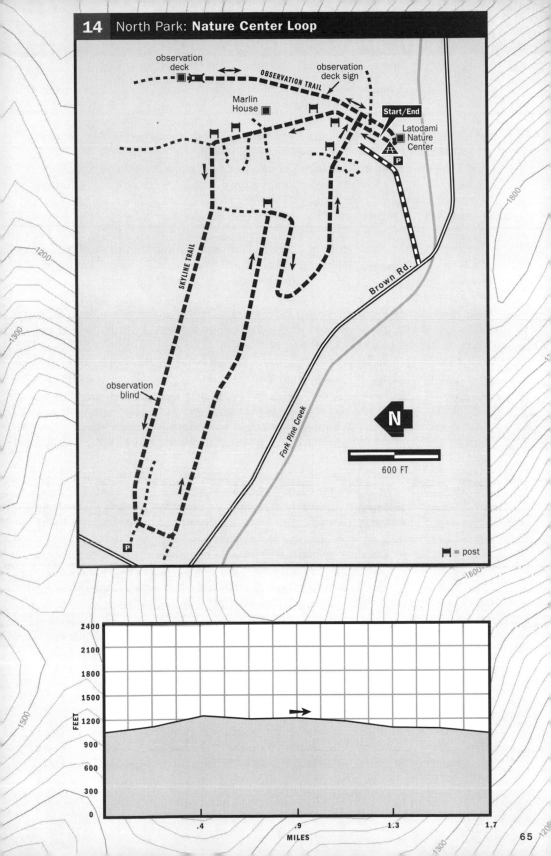

observation
deck

OBSERVATION TRAIL

observation
deck sign

Marlin
House

Start/End

Latodami
Nature
Center

P

SKYLINE TRAIL

observation
blind

Brown Rd.

Fork Pine Creek

N

600 FT

P

= post

Continue straight and upward—and into the beginning of your reward for continuing uphill. This leads to a clearing with a marlin house and choices for turning straight, left, or right. Take the middle trail straight ahead for a walk through the ecotone between the lower deciduous forest and the meadow ecosystems.

If you're lucky, the yellow irises I saw growing in this middle section will be in bloom. Yellow iris, an escapee from European gardens and a beautiful visual treat, is typically the only type of iris to be found growing wild. Continue straight, passing two posts, following the bird symbol. Through this open area will be a few unmarked choices to cut to the left; continue straight, also passing the choice to go left at the fox-head symbol posted at 0.16 miles.

At 0.20 miles you'll arrive at a post with arrows pointing left and back the way you came; there's also a choice to go straight here. Turn left and begin entering the meadow. You'll pass some black cherry trees (hopefully in bloom) on the left of the trail as you arrive at 0.26 miles and another choice, this one for an unmarked left or straight ahead path onto the posted Skyline Trail. Go straight for a wonderful walk through this wide-open meadow. The plentiful birds, open sky, wildflowers, and flowering trees make a great combination.

Flowers seen right away include daisy fleabane and several species of dandelions and thistle. There are many, many bird boxes placed throughout (a big thanks to the volunteers who built them). Birds are everywhere in the meadow—chirping, singing, and calling—and the open fields offer great views of them. Some you may see are tree swallows, bluebirds, golden- and blue-winged warblers, and yellow-breasted and common yellow chat. Find the observation blind at 0.46 miles and sit a spell if you wish to admire them.

Beyond the observation blind, the hike continues straight. Find honeysuckle and oxeye daisies, named for their large depressed yellow disc centers. At 0.59 miles you'll see a gate a little farther ahead that leads to an entrance from Reynolds Road and a choice to turn left. Turn left, then bypass a second sharp left. Walk to the far end of the field, turning left once more at 0.63 miles.

Along this section you may find black mustard (a yellow four-petal flower on a tall stalk) and phlox. Along the woods on the right is a mixture of deciduous and conifer trees. At almost 1 mile are more black cherry trees and a post near them indicating a right or left turn; turn right. Here you'll begin to head downhill and back into deciduous forest; maples and young tulip trees are among the species you'll see. The trail turns sharply left, taking you into a U-turn; Brown Road becomes visible to the right. The forest here is very young and the understory thin. You'll see the beautiful fringe tree here. When it is in bloom, its flowers look like groups of small white fireworks.

At 1.23 miles, ignore the right turn on the grassy path, and walk straight onto a narrow path into the woods. There is a post here with the bird symbol. These woods hug the trail, and you have a much different experience walking through them than the meadow and wide trails hiked thus far. Quickly reaching an intersection with an unmarked trail, continue straight and come to another post with the bird symbol. You'll see familiar surroundings and the marlin house; bear right downhill. You can either continue down and return to your car, or turn left when you reach the bottom of the fielded area to hike out to an observation deck.

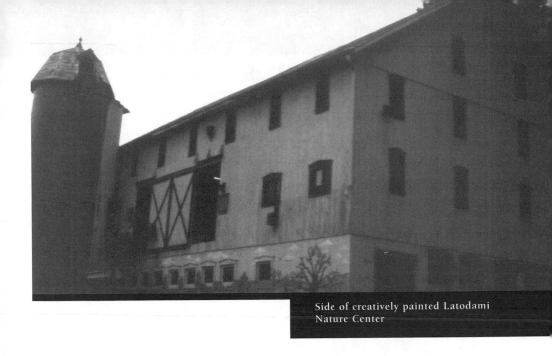

Side of creatively painted Latodami
Nature Center

I turned left and hiked out to the observation deck. This short out-and-back is
included in this hike, but the best part of the hiking is done. Note that the Observation Trail doesn't appear to be well maintained. If you are going out to the observation deck, after turning left and walking about 100 feet or so you'll see a
right-pointing wooden sign with "Observation Deck" carved into it. Once you reach
it, take the narrow dirt trail back; in spring it is dotted with purple violets, mayapples, and phlox. This forested area also has much larger deciduous trees. Cross a
small bridge and reach the observation deck at 1.48 miles. You can continue to hike
on this trail if you'd like; it connects with other trails to loop or can be done as an
out-and-back. I chose this as my turnaround. When finished, hike back out and to
the parking lot the way you came in.

▶ NEARBY ATTRACTIONS

For information about the many programs and outings offered at the Latodami Nature
Center, call (724) 935-2170 or go to **www.county.allegheny.pa.us/parks/calendar/
latodami.asp** for their calendar of activities. For more hiking, leave the parking lot,
turn left on Brown Road and then right into the small parking lot. See the North Park:
Braille Trail Loop (hike 13) write-up in this book for this hike and additional information on other park facilities.

NORTH SHORE: RIVER, MEMORIAL, AND SPORTS WALK

KEY AT-A-GLANCE INFORMATION

LENGTH: 2.2 miles

CONFIGURATION: Loop

DIFFICULTY: Easy

SCENERY: Allegheny River; Korean War, Vietnam War, and Allegheny County Law Enforcement Officers memorials; baseball and football statues and player flags; PNC Park; Heinz Field; 150-foot-high fountain at rivers' confluence across Allegheny; and views of the three rivers and opposite shores, including the Pittsburgh skyline

EXPOSURE: Exposed

TRAFFIC: Moderate

TRAIL SURFACE: Paved walk

HIKING TIME: 2 hours

ACCESS: Year-round

MAPS: None this specific. A map of the Three Rivers Heritage Trail (which is updated as the trail is developed) is available from Friends of the Riverfront by calling (412) 488-0212 or in PDF format at **www.friendsoftheriverfront.org;** USGS Pittsburgh West

FACILITIES: Bike racks and emergency phones are found along the river; eating establishments at PNC Park

SPECIAL COMMENTS: This walk is wheelchair accessible and very scenic.

North Shore:
River, Memorial, and Sports Walk

UTM Zone (WGS84)   17T

Easting   584245

Northing   4477958

IN BRIEF

If you haven't been to the renovated North Shore, visited the memorials, and enjoyed the views and the statues at the new stadiums, you shouldn't miss this walk.

DESCRIPTION

From the parking lot, go to the corner of General Robinson Street and Mazerowski Way and cross the street toward PNC Park. Immediately on the opposite corner find a large statue of Honus Wagner, considered by many to be Major League Baseball's greatest all-around player. The former shortstop (until 1917) and then manager of the Pittsburgh Pirates, Wagner retired with more hits, runs, doubles, triples, games, and steals than any other National League player. He was also admired when he had his valued baseball card recalled because he objected to it being included with tobacco, not wanting to set a poor example for children. Continuing along the side of the baseball stadium, you'll see vertical flags with the photos and names of some of baseball's great players, including Roberto Clemente, Dave Parker, Mannie Sanguillen, and many more.

Turn left, following the circular walk past the gate for right field and continue on it, passing the stairs and ramp down to the river. Turn left and travel briefly on the uppermost walk and turn left, beginning down the ramp for easiest access to the Korean War Memorial. (Note that if you are not in or pushing a wheelchair you can cross the street to the uppermost walk and turn left down the ramp.)

Quickly arrive at the first memorial—a plaque set in marble dedicated to all Korean War

DIRECTIONS

From Pittsburgh, cross the Sixth Street Bridge and turn left onto General Robinson Street. Park in the General Robinson Parking Lot, across from PNC Park.

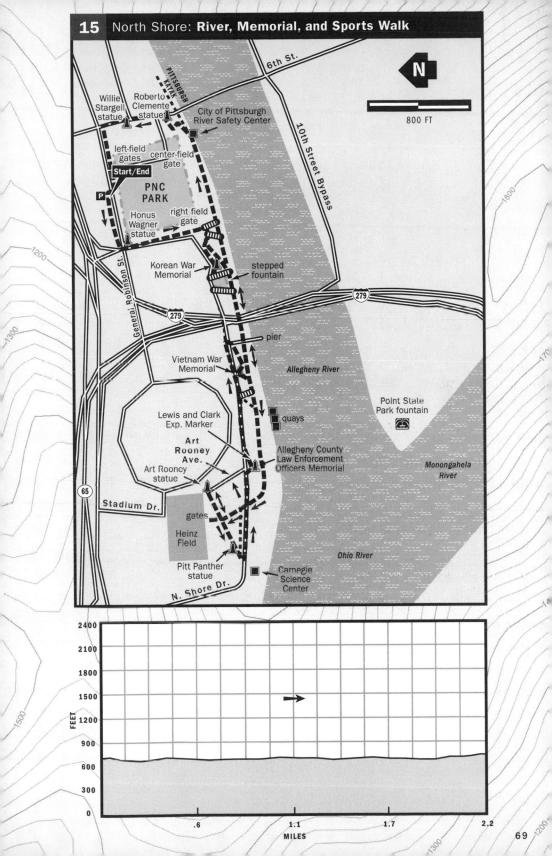

N

800 FT

6th St.

PITTSBURGH KAYAK

Willie Stargell statue

Roberto Clemente statue

City of Pittsburgh River Safety Center

left-field gates

center-field gate

Start/End

P

PNC PARK

Honus Wagner statue

right field gate

10th Street Bypass

Korean War Memorial

stepped fountain

279

General Robinson St.

279

pier

Vietnam War Memorial

Allegheny River

quays

Point State Park fountain

Lewis and Clark Exp. Marker

Art Rooney Ave.

Art Rooney statue

Allegheny County Law Enforcement Officers Memorial

Monongahela River

65

Stadium Dr.

gates

Heinz Field

Pitt Panther statue

Ohio River

Carnegie Science Center

N. Shore Dr.

FEET

2400
2100
1800
1500
1200
900
600
300
0

.6   1.1   1.7   2.2
MILES

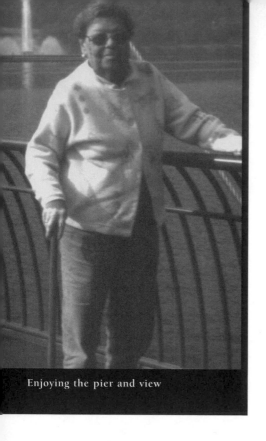

Enjoying the pier and view

veterans. Farther down the path, which is lined with pines and flowering bushes, you'll find four large marble slabs with plaques chronologically showing all of the major dates and events of the Korean War, which lasted from 1950 to 1953. Amazingly, U.S. involvement in this conflict began and ended on the same dates of each year, July 27. The memorial continues with more plaques honoring those who served, were taken prisoner, are missing in action, or died. A large and beautifully designed marble amphitheater-shaped memorial with sketches of North and South Korea showing the 38th parallel is on the left. The end of the memorial and ramp leads to a T with steps alongside an interactive stepped fountain. There is no wheelchair access down or up here; if you have wheels, turn around and go back up the ramp, turn right at the esplanade, and right again on the ramp down to the river. Otherwise, you can walk down the steps.

Whichever way you go, make a right. Near the stepped fountain you'll see a sign about the history of the first World Series, played in 1903, in which the National League champion Pittsburgh Pirates lost to American League champion Boston Americans. Games four through seven of the nine-game series were played in Pittsburgh's home to baseball at the time, Exposition Park. (In favor of the Pittsburgh Pirates, they did win the last game played in Exposition Park in 1909 against the Chicago Cubs.) Walk under the Fort Duquesne Bridge and the new Fort Duquesne Flyover, a bike and walker's bridge to Point State Park and downtown Pittsburgh. Shortly after, at 0.50 miles, take a walk out onto the pier that juts out over the Allegheny River. The pier and most of the river walk provide spectacular views of the fountain, rivers, surrounding shores, and downtown Pittsburgh.

The Vietnam War Memorial is within sight just beyond the pier. You can walk straight up the stairs across from the pier, or use the ramp located just a little farther down the shore to the right of a double set of steps. Either way, be sure to see this very moving "Welcome Home" memorial. The life-size bronze statues beneath the large canopy (in the shape of a hibiscus flower, a symbol of rebirth) have unbelievably real expressions—happiness, uncertainty, concern, and wonder come to life in their faces. They are surrounded by the word "Peace" in many languages, and a plaque depicts a poem written by T. J. McGarvey, president of the Pittsburgh–Allegheny County Vietnam Veterans Monument Committee, on which the late John Heinz also served.

Use the ramp to walk back down to the river. As you walk along, you'll notice many docking quays along the river where people can access the North Shore and its attractions by boat. Across the shore, the Duquesne Incline and Mount Washington are in clear site. When you reach the point where the wall curves right, follow it to take a look at Heinz Stadium and its grounds. The wheelchair ramp is not obvious but is designed so that it zigzags between the two large sets of steps in front of Heinz Field. Go to the set of steps on the left to begin up the ramp or take the stairs. At the top you can go up to the gate for a look inside. Then turn, and with the stadium at your back, go left to see the larger-than-life statue of the late Art Rooney, the much loved and admired former owner of the Pittsburgh Steelers. Remember: He never met a player he didn't like.

Follow the walk back, recrossing the front of the stadium to find another large statue, this one a panther representing the Pitt Panthers, who now share Heinz Field with the Pittsburgh Steelers. Continue straight after the statue and come to North Shore Drive. Make a left, walking past the many large cement flower-filled planters. You are above the walkway near the river and will cross a bridge. Make a right at Art Rooney Avenue to cross North Shore Drive and reach the Allegheny County Law Enforcement Officers Memorial, which describes the risks law-enforcement officers take daily while serving the public and is dedicated to those who have fallen. A bronze statue of an officer, plaques, and emblems mark the site and, appropriately for Pittsburgh, cobblestones are included within its grounds. Crossing Art Rooney Avenue on this side of North Shore Avenue, also find a small marker dedicated to the Lewis and Clark Expedition.

Shortly after, you'll see a brick path lined with benches that leads back down to the river; North Shore Drive continues straight. Veer right down the path that leads to the esplanade above the walkway next to the river. You can use the steps or ramp here to reach riverside, or turn left and make a right down the ramp just beyond the Vietnam War Memorial (the latter is the choice depicted on the map that accompanies this hike description). Once on the lower riverside walkway, follow it back past the stepped fountain and the ramp used to come down from the west side of PNC Park. Reach a Three Rivers Heritage Trail information board about the turf sports of the past, when Pittsburgh and Allegheny (now the North Side) were separate cities that rivaled each other. Continuing straight, notice that this portion of the walk, near PNC Park, has diamond shapes included in the sidewalk's design. When you reach the City of Pittsburgh River Safety Center, leave the shore by turning left up the ramp (or steps) to travel along the eastern side of PNC Park.

At the top, you'll see an enormous statue of Roberto Clemente, perhaps Pittsburgh's most loved player in history; he died in 1972 in a plane crash off the coast of San Juan, Puerto Rico (his home country), on his way back from a humanitarian trip. Take the time to walk around it and see that first, second, and third "plates" placed here contain hallowed ground—dirt brought from the three stadiums in which he most played: Santurce Field of Carolina, Puerto Rico, and Forbes Field and Three Rivers Stadium of Pittsburgh. Continuing along PNC Park, you'll see more flags commemorating treasured players. As you pass the eateries that line the sidewalk you'll see a large bronze statue of Willie Stargell, another great player in the history of the Pittsburgh Pirates. Turn left onto General Robinson Street at the corner and walk along this side of PNC Park to view more memorable players depicted on flags. Cross the street to the parking lot when you have finished.

▶ NEARBY ATTRACTIONS

For more river walking, follow the River Trail to the Point and use the description for the Point State Park: History and Three Rivers Walk (hike 16) in this book. There are many eating establishments at PNC Park and attractions around the city throughout the year. Go to **www.visitpittsburgh.com** for more information.

POINT STATE PARK: HISTORY AND THREE RIVERS WALK

KEY AT-A-GLANCE INFORMATION

LENGTH: 1 mile

CONFIGURATION: Loop

DIFFICULTY: Easy

SCENERY: Fort Pitt blockhouse and museum, memorials, 150-foot-high fountain at rivers' confluence, views of the three rivers and opposite shores

EXPOSURE: Half shaded, half exposed

TRAFFIC: Moderate

TRAIL SURFACE: Paved walk

HIKING TIME: 1 hour, not including tours

ACCESS: Park hours are 7 a.m.–11 p.m.; Fort Pitt Museum open Tuesdays–Saturdays, 9 a.m.–5 p.m., and Sundays, 12–5 p.m.; Fort Pitt Blockhouse open Tuesdays–Saturdays, 9:30 a.m.–4 p.m., and Sundays 12–4 p.m. Museum fee charged for ages 12 and older; no fee for blockhouse

MAPS: Point State Park map is available at the Fort Pitt Museum; it can also be obtained from the Pennsylvania Department of Conservation and Natural Resources Web site, **www.dcnr.state.pa.us,** or by calling (412) 471-0235; USGS Pittsburgh West

FACILITIES: Restrooms at the Fort Pitt Museum and northern side of the fountain; drinking fountains throughout park, and beverage vending machines on southern side of fountain

SPECIAL COMMENTS: The park is wheelchair accessible except a couple of steps down to access the inside of the blockhouse. There is only one wheelchair access ramp to the side of the fountain and rivers.

Point State Park:
History and Three Rivers Walk

UTM Zone (WGS84)   17T

Easting   584217

Northing   4477201

IN BRIEF

A few hours spent in Point State Park are rewarding both historically and aesthetically. If you are feeling a need to learn about the history of the city or want to pump up your pride, this is the best place to start.

DESCRIPTION

Enter the park at the corner of Commonwealth Place and Liberty Avenue along the wide brick path. Almost as soon as the park is entered, landmarks and memorial plaques describing the Point's rich history begin—the first is reached in just 243 feet.

As this first plaque states, the moatlike channel shows the restored Music Bastion. (Today, many children can be found playing there during free summer concerts.) A bastion is a projecting part of a fortification. Fort Pitt had five in a pentagonal arrangement; of these, three have been restored. Looking beyond the plaque, view the rampart walls and the curtain wall, in which a drawbridge was once located. It was originally intended that the fort be surrounded by a moat, but it was usually dry due to low water levels.

Fort Pitt was constructed by the British between 1759 and 1761, after an army of 6,000 British soldiers led by Brigadier General John Forbes came to attack Fort Duquesne, which was

DIRECTIONS

Point State Park is in the heart of the city. It can be reached from the east and west via interstates 376 and 279, from the north by PA 8, and from the south by PA 51. There is street parking, but the meters are expensive. Park in the Pittsburgh *Post-Gazette* Garage for easy access to the park entrance at Commonwealth Place and Liberty (near the Fort Pitt Bridge entrance ramp, across from the Hilton Hotel).

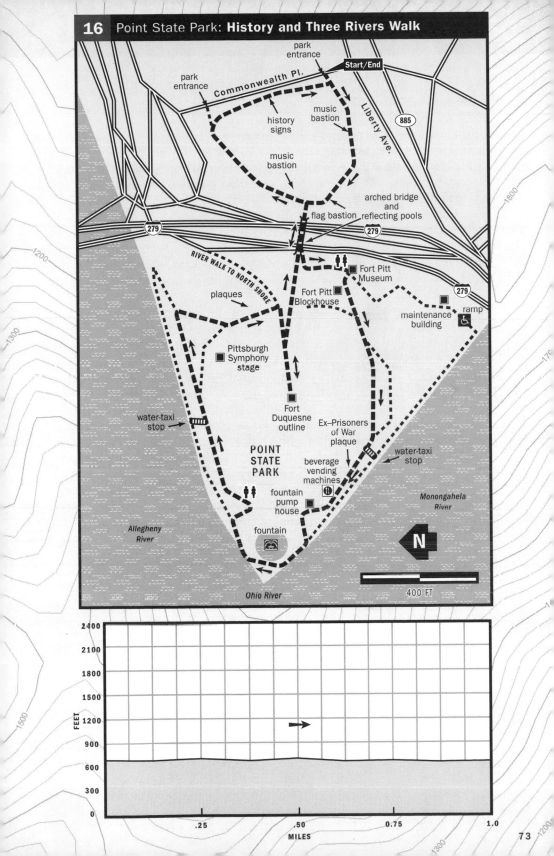

park entrance

park entrance

Start/End

Commonwealth Pl.

history signs

music bastion

music bastion

Liberty Ave.

885

arched bridge and reflecting pools

flag bastion

279

279

RIVER WALK TO NORTH SHORE

plaques

Fort Pitt Museum

Fort Pitt Blockhouse

279

maintenance building

ramp

Pittsburgh Symphony stage

Fort Duquesne outline

Ex-Prisoners of War plaque

water-taxi stop

POINT STATE PARK

beverage vending machines

water-taxi stop

Monongahela River

fountain pump house

Allegheny River

fountain

N

Ohio River

400 FT

built by the French and occupied by them until 1758. During the struggle between the British and French for control of the Ohio Valley, known as the French and Indian War, the "Forks of the Ohio" was viewed as a prized command. For the French, the Ohio River represented the only way to connect their colonies in New France (present-day Canada) to their colonies in Louisiana. For the English, control of the Ohio River meant the expansion of their colonial power beyond the Appalachian Mountains. Native Americans, caught between the two most powerful nations of Europe, were trying to preserve their land and culture.

Continuing on, you arrive at the Flag Bastion found on the left side of the path, just before veering right to cross over the arched bridge beneath the overpass and over a reflecting pool that can be lit from the sides. At the end of the bridge, turn left and walk toward the Fort Pitt Museum. A plaque located to the right of the museum's doorways, beyond the cannons, explains that the museum in housed in the Monongahela Bastion.

Inside, find a beautiful floor mosaic of the Arms of William Pitt, Earl of Chatham, who selected Brigadier General John Forbes to lead the attack against Fort Duquesne and for whom the city was named. When paying the admission, ask when the next discussion will take place around the 16-foot-wide circular well (visible from the entrance) that surrounds a model of Fort Pitt, the Point, and the surrounding area. Learn about the history of the Point from the time of early French expeditions into the region to the beginning of Pittsburgh's industrial age, and you'll better associate present-day landmarks with their history. Exploring the first floor, view the inside of a fur trader's cabin and a soldier's barracks in full-size replicas. Upstairs follow the many dioramas, exhibits, and films clockwise for a rich learning experience about the intense struggle for control of the Forks of the Ohio.

After exiting the museum, walk over to the Fort Pitt Blockhouse and through its wrought-iron gate. (There is not a ramp down the couple of steps to the doorway.) Along the short path inside the gate are commemorative plaques and a sundial. Inside, you'll find a very informative volunteer and displays of artifacts.

Here's a brief history of the blockhouse: In the 1700s, the undammed rivers ran high and low, periodically flooding and eroding the western and riverside walls of Fort Pitt, which were built of dirt and sod. In 1763 during Pontiac's War (see the Bushy Run History Loop hike [hike 24] for more information), Native Americans took advantage of this situation by walking through the dry moat and attacking the fort's weakest walls. To guard against more invasions of this type, Colonel Henry Bouquet had a blockhouse (also known as redoubt) built at each of the structure's five corners in 1764. The Fort Pitt Blockhouse is the only one remaining, and it stands as the oldest building in Pittsburgh and one of the oldest in western Pennsylvania. After Fort Pitt was abandoned in 1792, this blockhouse was used as a kitchen, slum tenement, candy store, and saloon before being purchased and restored by the Pittsburgh Chapter of the Daughters of the American Revolution in 1894.

When you walk outside again, turn right on the path and notice the ginkgo trees, which were planted in 1908. These almost century-old trees are known for their tolerance of pollution and poor environmental conditions, allowing them to survive the many industrial uses of the Point before its development into a state park. (Note that if you want wheelchair access to the fountain you must use the ramp behind the Fort Pitt Museum, near the maintenance building. However, on the opposite side, assistance is required to get a wheelchair back up so you may wish to stay on this level or go down and come back using this same ramp.) On this walkway, go around the bend to find a plaque marking the end of Forbes Road at Fort Duquesne. The pleasant environment of trees, flowers, views, and benches to rest on makes it difficult to imagine the Point when it was occupied by warehouses, freight yards, rail lines, industrial workers, and was considered the backwash of the city.

In just a short distance the path splits, and you can choose to walk closer to the river using the path on the left or stay in between the planted areas; the paths meet very quickly at just 0.3 miles. Across the Monongahela River, the heart of Station Square and the many ships and boats used for cruises and tours along the river come into view. Mount Washington and the incline up to it are also visible. Not long after the paths meet, there is a set of steps that lead down to the water's edge and one of the water-taxi stops. Shortly after, arrive at a plaque about the first ceremony at the Point to honor imprisoned, fallen, and missing soldiers.

This path leads around the corner of the pump house, where there is a spectacular view of the 150-foot columnar fountain. Three peacock fountains surround it and represent the meeting of the Allegheny River, which drains southwestern Pennsylvania and parts of West Virginia, Maryland, and Virginia; and the Monongahela River, which drains northwestern Pennsylvania and New York. These great rivers meet here to form the Ohio River, which flows to the mouth of the Mississippi River in New Orleans to reach the Gulf of Mexico. Enjoy time at this beautiful spot. The 200-foot circular basin around the fountain provides ample room to sit or walk along its wide rim and take in the sites. As you round its perimeter, the renovated North Shore—home of the new stadiums, Carnegie Science Center, and many memorials—can be seen across the Allegheny.

You can choose to walk down immediately next to the river or on this path above. Stone bleachers and stairs along the Allegheny provide access. If you are on the lower walkway with a wheelchair, access back up is found past the water-taxi stop with assistance only; otherwise, you must turn and go back around to the ramp by which you came down to the river. On this upper walkway, when you are near the back of the Pittsburgh Symphony Stage, turn right at 0.62 miles to walk back toward the entrance and find plaques for David L. Lawrence and the Forks of the Ohio. Just beyond these, make a right and walk out onto the grass to better view the outline of the former site of Fort Duquesne.

When you're ready to leave, recross the arched bridge and turn left on the other side to exit the park farther north. When you reach Commonwealth Place, turn right and walk past the remaining informative signs that commemorate the succession of forts built here. Another is dedicated to David L. Lawrence, who was born at the Point and was a driving force in the renaissance and the creating of Point State Park.

▶ NEARBY ATTRACTIONS

For more river walking, follow the River Walk to the North Shore and use the description for the North Shore: River, Memorial, and Sports Walk (hike 15) in this book. There are many attractions around the city and at the Point throughout the year. Call the Greater Pittsburgh Convention and Visitor's Bureau at (800) 366-0093 or go to **www.visitpittsburgh.com** for more information.

RIVERVIEW PARK LOOP

 ## KEY AT-A-GLANCE INFORMATION

LENGTH: 2.4 miles

CONFIGURATION: Balloon

DIFFICULTY: Easy

SCENERY: Cherry and apple blossom trees, many old deciduous trees, Allegheny Observatory

EXPOSURE: Mostly shaded

TRAFFIC: Light to medium

TRAIL SURFACE: Dirt and briefly pavement

HIKING TIME: 1.5 hours

ACCESS: Open year-round

MAPS: A map of Riverview Park may become available at **www.pittsburgh parks.org** but currently can be purchased at the Schenley Park Visitor Center for $2; call (412) 682-7275 for details; USGS Pittsburgh West

FACILITIES: Restrooms are inside the visitor's center and at the activities building

SPECIAL COMMENTS: The trails are open to horses and their riders; they are much less frequently seen than hikers, but be aware—especially if you are with a dog.

Riverview Park Loop

UTM Zone (WGS84)   17T

Easting   583019

Northing   4481760

IN BRIEF

The hillside in front of the Allegheny Observatory, where the hike begins, is especially beautiful in early spring (late March through mid-April or so) when many of the trees planted here are in spectacular bloom. Plan your hike for April through October on a late Thursday or Friday afternoon, and couple it with a tour of the observatory in the evening. See Nearby Attractions at the end of this description.

DESCRIPTION

Riverview Park was known as Watson Farms in the era of 1894, when the city of Allegheny purchased 200 acres of land from Samuel Watson. The former dairy farm and grazing land became a prized park with an amphitheater, merry-go-round, and small zoo that even had an elk paddock. These attractions do not exist today, but the park has grown to 287 acres and has added hiking and equestrian trails, playgrounds, special-event facilities and pavilions, and a pool.

One of the most important attractions of the park is the Allegheny Observatory. Dating to 1912, it is designated a historical landmark and is one of the world's major astronomical institutions. Its predecessor, the city's first observatory, was built in 1859 on Perrysville Avenue by prominent city businessmen who had formed the

DIRECTIONS

From Pittsburgh, take Interstate 279 North to the Perrysville Avenue exit. Turn right at the end of the ramp onto Perrysville Avenue. At 1.5 miles, turn right on Riverview Avenue. In 0.2 miles, turn right on Riverview Drive. Drive to the top (about 0.2 miles) and park. When leaving, turn right on Perrysville Avenue and left (almost immediately) on Venture Street to reach I-279. (This street is one way and cannot be used to reach the park.)

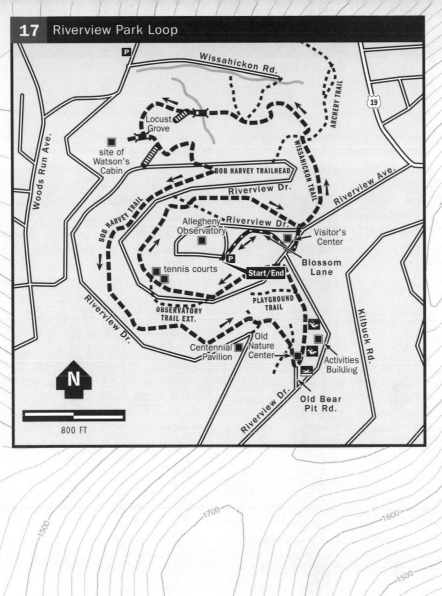

Wissahickon Rd.

ARCHERY TRAIL

19

Locust Grove

site of Watson's Cabin

BOB HARVEY TRAILHEAD

Riverview Dr.

WISSAHICKON TRAIL

Riverview Ave.

BOB HARVEY TRAIL

Allegheny Observatory

Riverview Dr.

Visitor's Center

Blossom Lane

tennis courts

Riverview Dr.

OBSERVATORY TRAIL EXT.

PLAYGROUND TRAIL

Centennial Pavilion

Old Nature Center

Activities Building

Kilbuck Rd.

Riverview Dr.

Old Bear Pit Rd.

Start/End

P

N

800 FT

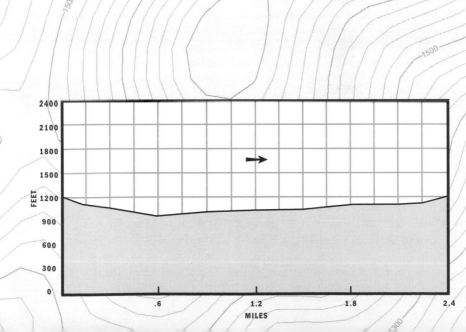

Allegheny Telescope Association. Waning interest and funds caused the group to turn it over to the Western University of Pittsburgh (now the University of Pittsburgh) in 1867; it was then that the observatory was used for truly scientific purposes. With improved equipment made possible by Pittsburgh industrial leader William Thaw, Professor Samuel P. Langley was able to observe the position of the stars as they crossed the celestial meridian and provide accurate time to industrial subscribers, including the Pennsylvania Railroad, thus providing money for financing research and maintaining the building. It was also from this observatory that James Keeler provided visual evidence of the particulate matter of Saturn's rings and the velocity of their travel around the planet. Recognition of the shortcomings of the old observatory sparked the project that resulted in the prominent Allegheny Observatory that resides within Riverview Park today. The new Allegheny Observatory houses a 30-inch Thaw telescope, the primary instrument used by the University of Pittsburgh for research. The observatory is open to the public by appointment (see Nearby Attractions following this description).

The hike begins at this historic site in front of the Allegheny Observatory. With your back to the observatory and the open hillside in front of you, walk left to the beginning of Blossom Lane, so named because of the many cherry and apple blossoms to be enjoyed in early spring. Blossom Lane is not marked at the top but is the only paved pathway down the hillside; there is a sign at the bottom. The end of the path leads to the stone entryway of the park. Walk to its center and make a sharp left to walk down the stairway. Cross Riverview Drive, walk up the stone stairs and along the slate sidewalk, which leads to the attractive stone visitor's center and meeting place. (The visitor's center is not marked, and its hours of operation are not posted.)

Walk past the visitor's center to the Wissahickon Trail behind it. Turn right on the wide trail. There are blooming trees at the top and old oaks and maples along the beginning. At 0.32 miles you'll come to a four-way intersection with the unmarked Archery Trail. Veer left (not a sharp left) and downhill to continue on Wissahickon Trail, which becomes narrower and runs alongside drainage. Along this portion of the trail enjoy the mayapples. Check for blossoms underneath their large umbrella-like leaves. There is also wild garlic mustard, a nonnative biennial (it does not flower until its second year). Because it is both nonnative and hardy, this plant competes with natives for nutrients and space. For some insects, such as the West Virginia butterfly, this can cause problems by pushing out natives they use.

In this area there are Ohio buckeye, silver maple, and English oak trees. After rounding the bend toward the left, pass the two trails near 0.5 miles that join in succession from the right; these lead to Old Wissahickon Road, a dirt road that leads to the main park road and a small parking area. Continue down and cross a bridge over a creek. The stairs up the hillside lead to Locust Grove. You can take these or stay on the trail traveling right around the grove. Following the trail as it wraps around the grove, enjoy more of the many older trees found in this park. A large old beech is among them, and I always hear the sound of woodpeckers here.

On the other side of Locust Grove is a bridge to the right that crosses over the feeder stream. The bridge goes to the site of Watson's Cabin; two buildings are on the site, but both are currently in a deteriorated state and are closed to use. Do not cross the bridge; rather, head slightly left through Locust Grove and up the cement stairs.

Turn left on Riverview Drive, where there are bike and walking paths, one on each side of the road. Cross the one-way road to the Bob Harvey Trailhead; it is easily seen and is signed. Turn right and head uphill. The trail quickly levels out to a rolling stroll along a wide path through old, long-established trees, including white ash, sugar maples, American bladder nut, and a variety of oaks. There is a right turn down some stairs to a grove. There are no picnic tables in this grove, but if you are interested in a break there are some in the grove coming up on the left. The stairs to that also lead up to the main park road.

You may spot deer walking through this section. They are abundant throughout the park, and there is evidence here on some of the trees showing that the bucks have been rubbing their antlers on them. At 1.36 miles you can look down the hill and across the road to the site of the former swimming pool (there is a new Olympic-sized pool located elsewhere in the park). The stairs now lead to the blue-topped Centennial Pavilion. Pass the log and dirt stairs on the left and then the single-track dirt trail that drops down to the road on the right. At 1.5 miles you'll come to a four-way intersection close to Old Bear Pit Road behind the former nature center, which, sadly, is not currently in operation. Turn right to walk up to the old road and then make a quick left in front of the nature center, where a white-flowered dogwood blooms in the spring. Continue up the slightly graded road. The activities building is up the hill on the right; two large playgrounds and a number of picnic and sitting benches surround it. Along this old cement road, you'll see ginkgo trees and slippery elm; its fruit (samara) are the scattered brown discs all around it.

Pass Playground Trail on the left (this trail follows below the road and then crosses it later to Observatory Trail). Cross the road and go up the five cement stairs to Observatory Trail. The path is dirt and stays left of the hillside. The observatory quickly comes into view. Enjoy the large old trees that line this trail, which include an enormous red oak.

If you wish, you can cut the hike short by walking up the hill to your car. I stayed straight on the trail, dropping behind and below the observatory. At 1.8 miles, the unsigned Observatory Trail Extension drops down to the left. Continue straight and you'll see where the extension comes up to meet the main trail again across from two tennis courts. Follow the trail back into the woods. Here is the first time on the hike I spotted a few wildflowers, including some yellow ones that appear to be members of the Saint-John's-wort family.

At the next four-way intersection, go straight to follow the path back to the visitor's center. (Left leads down to the road and right cuts up toward the observatory.) There is a brief but noticeable uphill climb to the back of the visitor's center. Round the corner of the visitor's center, turning right on the slate sidewalk. Retrace your steps across the road, up the stairs to the park entryway, and along Blossom Trail to your car.

▶ NEARBY ATTRACTIONS

Tours of the Allegheny Observatory are offered from April to October free of charge; **www.pitt.edu/~aobsvtry.** For shelter permits, call the Department of Public Works at (412) 255-2370; for more information visit **www.city.pittsburgh.pa.us.** For swimming, call the city's aquatic-information line at (412) 594-4645; during summer contact the pool at (412) 323-7223.

SCHENLEY PARK LOOP

KEY AT-A-GLANCE INFORMATION

LENGTH: 1.7 miles

CONFIGURATION: Modified loop

DIFFICULTY: Easy

SCENERY: Panther Hollow Lake, ducks, Panther Hollow Run, wetland-restoration project, mixed foliage, deciduous trees, wildflowers, birds, Phipps Conservatory and Botanical Gardens

EXPOSURE: Mostly shaded

TRAFFIC: Light on the lower trail, busier on the upper trail

TRAIL SURFACE: Varies from dirt and flat rocks next to the run to very wide packed-sand trail above

HIKING TIME: 1 hour

ACCESS: Park is open year-round.

MAPS: A map of Schenley Park may become available at **www.pittsburgh parks.org** but currently can be purchased at the Schenley Park Visitor Center for $2; call (412) 682-7275 for details; USGS Pittsburgh East

FACILITIES: Restrooms and cafe in visitor's center, picnic shelters, and playgrounds

SPECIAL COMMENTS: The trail at Panther Hollow Run narrows in a couple of spots and may be slippery. It can easily be avoided by taking the upper trail as described as an alternative. Hiking down by the water though is a fascination for children and fun for dogs.

Schenley Park Loop

UTM Zone (WGS84)   17T

Easting   589367

Northing   4476935

IN BRIEF

Schenley Park is Pittsburgh's flagship park and should not be missed. It has a pleasant environment, historical value, and aesthetics that reflect its roots and the care devoted to it through time. In addition to hiking, the park offers biking and running on most trails, and facilities and fields for tennis, soccer, baseball, roller hockey, and ice skating; there is also a golf course (and golf programs for kids) and a disc golf course. For nostalgia, visit the Neil Log House, one of the last three existing 18th-century buildings in Pittsburgh.

DESCRIPTION

Mount Airy Tract became the object of desire between developers and Edward Bigelow, director of Pittsburgh's Department of Public Works in 1889. Bigelow felt strongly about the preservation of the land for recreation and athletics. When he heard developers were sending lawyers to London to pursue its purchase from Mary Schenley (originally Mary Elizabeth Croghan of Pittsburgh), he sent his own via train and steamer to reach her first (beating the others by two days). Schenley agreed to donate 300 acres of land, with the option to purchase 120 more if the park were named after her and never sold. The city agreed and purchased the remaining property immediately.

Bigelow did not disappoint Pittsburghers in the park's development. He hired William Falconer, who was trained at London's Kew Gardens,

DIRECTIONS

From Pittsburgh, take the Boulevard of the Allies; go through two traffic lights and over the Anderson Bridge.

At the second exit into Schenley Park, turn right. (This takes you under the Anderson Bridge and over the Panther Hollow Bridge.) At the fork, bear left. The visitor's center is across from Phipps Conservatory. Park at an open parking meter.

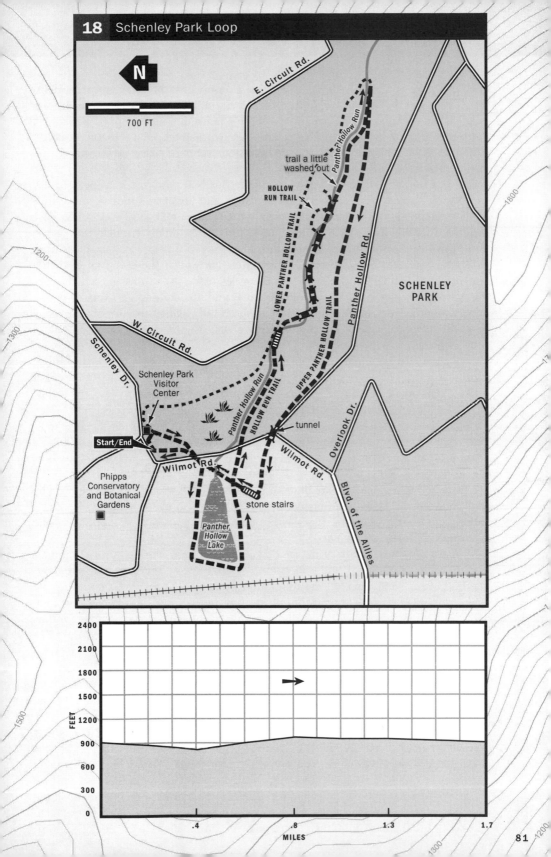

to lead the design and building of Phipps Conservatory and Botanical Gardens, which was built in 1893. Bigelow also saw to the fulfillment of athletic needs, and today Schenley Park remains one of Pittsburgh's finest and most popular parks with 456 acres set aside for hiking, biking, running, ice skating, tennis, soccer, baseball, golf, quiet contemplation, and social and cultural events (see Nearby Attractions following this description).

For a full morning or afternoon, combine this hike with lunch at the Schenley Park Visitor Center, a tour of Phipps Conservatory and Botanical Gardens, and a drive or walk around Schenley Park to the Westinghouse Memorial and Pond. If you have children, they will love a visit to one of the park's playgrounds as well.

This hike begins directly behind the Schenley Park Visitor Center (across from Phipps Conservatory). Walk around the center and down the stone stairs. You'll notice that "WPA 1939" is chiseled in the sides of most of the stairs and bridges throughout Schenley Park. Through President Franklin D. Roosevelt's Works Progress Administration program, Schenley Park was improved, giving those setting the stone over which we walk today the ability to enjoy at least some relief during the hard years of the Great Depression.

Continue down the second pair of steps, a ramp, and over the small bridge; turn right to walk through some of Schenley Park's continued work. A restoration of native plants and wetland is in progress and may be noticeable because of the yellow plastic tied around various small trees and bushes. While following the path, enjoy the open scenery of trees, wetland, Panther Hollow Run, and the bridges that span it.

Turn right to walk around Panther Hollow Lake, which was dug in 1909 for boating; a boathouse once sat on its shores. Water enthusiasts turned out in numbers to rent the boats and enjoy the lake. The boathouse was demolished in 1979 or 1980, but plans to build a new one are under discussion. Today, the lake is still enjoyed by anglers and is populated with many ducks. Children also like to play on its shores, and although there are two bridges within view, when you reach the far side of the lake, the area is relatively quiet.

As you follow the turn of the far side of the lake, take the trail up to the right, away from the lake's shore, and walk past the steps on the right, continuing straight. The trail opens wide here and the restoration project continues. Walk straight, past where you originally turned right to walk around the lake, and continue on the wide path until reaching a slight incline that leads up to the main Lower Panther Hollow Trail (there are no signs). At a little more than a half mile, before reaching the main trail, look right and you'll see a short pair of stone stairs that lead down to Panther Hollow Run (this trail is currently being restored); there are many small WPA bridges and a path following the run. If you wish to hike on easier terrain (with no mud and very wide) then go up to the main trail. The run stays within view and the hike can also be followed from there.

If you choose to hike down in Panther Hollow Run, enjoy a pleasant and mostly quiet and enjoyable walk in solitude, over the many small, charming, arched bridges constructed by the WPA. There are a couple of places where the trail narrows and you must step carefully or cross the small run using the many flat rocks, but it is worth it if you like to avoid popular trails and feel a bit more removed. As the hike along the water ends, there will be a choice of two turns. For each turn right—the first begins to take you up to the main trail; the second puts you on the main trail, making a U-turn

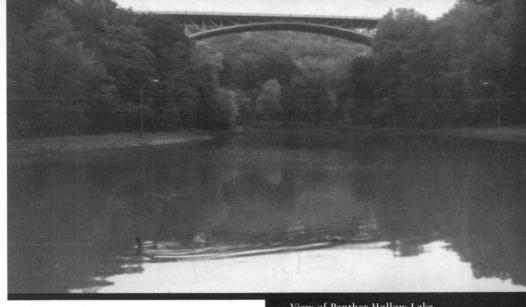

View of Panther Hollow Lake

and avoiding going up to Panther Hollow Road. You should then be hiking on the wide main Upper Panther Hollow Trail (packed sand and no sign), with Panther Hollow Road above and left and Panther Hollow Run now below and to the right. (Note that if you took the main Lower Panther Hollow Trail rather than the Hollow Run Trail along the water, simply continue turning right, cross a larger bridge and make a U-turn onto the Upper Panther Hollow Trail, also avoiding going up to the road.)

Although you're hiking closer to the road now, the trail remains below it and therefore a low noise level is maintained. As you hike along, you'll notice the restoration project's plants and trees. Where the trail and road begin to meet and, if the leaves are down, the University of Pittsburgh's Cathedral of Learning and Phipps Conservatory come into view. Stay on the path and follow it through a tunnel under Panther Hollow Bridge, where the lake will soon come back into view. Take a set of stone stairs (watch your step in places) down toward the lake. Reaching the trail, make another right (or go straight down the short wooden stairs to be directly at lakeside) and follow the same trail you took leaving the lake. This time, make a left to go over the bridges back into the wetland-restoration area and return rather than going straight. Follow both sets of stairs back to the visitor's center.

▶ NEARBY ATTRACTIONS

Schenley Park offers many recreational and cultural amenities. Phipps Conservatory and Botanical Gardens has both regular and special displays and makes a beautiful tour; visit **www.phipps.conservatory.org** or call (412) 622-6914 for more information. The park also hosts popular public events, such as the Vintage Grand Prix, Race for the Cure, and movies on Flagstaff Hill in the summertime; go to **www .pittsburghparks.org** and select "Events." To visit the Neil Log House, learn about disc golf and the course, swimming pool, Schenley Oval (tennis, track, and soccer), skating/hockey rink, or the golf courses, visit **www.pittsburghparks.org** and select "Parks," then "Schenley Park," then "Where to go."

SETTLER'S CABIN PARK: CREEK AND FLORA HIKE

 KEY AT-A-GLANCE INFORMATION

LENGTH: 1.6 miles

CONFIGURATION: Out-and-back

DIFFICULTY: Moderate

SCENERY: Creek with small waterfall, wildflowers, mixed deciduous and conifer forest

EXPOSURE: Shaded

TRAFFIC: Light

TRAIL SURFACE: Dirt

HIKING TIME: 40 minutes

ACCESS: Open year-round, sunrise–midnight

MAPS: Available for the overall park at the park office or by calling the Allegheny County Parks Department at (412) 350-7275 (the trails are not depicted in detail on the county park map); USGS Oakdale

FACILITIES: Restrooms within picnic grove near trailhead

SPECIAL COMMENTS: Wear shoes with good treads to avoid slipping on wet clay or rocks.

Settler's Cabin Park:
Creek and Flora Hike

UTM Zone (WGS84)   17T

Easting   571614

Northing   4475028

IN BRIEF

This short hike is a nice way to take in a variety of flora, enjoy a small waterfall, and get a little exercise on some hills without spending much time.

DESCRIPTION

From the parking lot, walk left, along a gravel road toward swings and a picnic shelter. Find the trailhead by keeping the picnic shelter to your left and passing the swings on your right. Veer slightly right, to the southwest, and look for an opening in the woods. There is no sign or trail name.

Maple and crab apple trees are found at the beginning of the trail. Be careful of the undergrowth because some of it is thorny. At the T, reached at 0.17 miles, turn right. It quickly becomes apparent that mountain bikers are likely the most frequent visitors to this trail. There are tracks and a few jumps set up. As in a number of the county parks, the mountain bikers are also likely the ones who do the most trail maintenance. Shortly after, at 0.23 miles, there is a choice to turn left and head south or go straight and continue west; turn left. If you are hiking in spring or summer, keep your eyes open for uncommon wildflowers. Perhaps you will have better luck than I did identifying them.

The gradual descent you've been making since the trailhead becomes a bit more noticeable.

DIRECTIONS

From Pittsburgh, take Interstate 376 West to US 22–30 West. Take the first exit, Tonidale, and turn left at the stop sign. Following the PA 22–30 East signs, curve left in just 0.1 mile. Make the first right onto Bayer Road and drive 1.3 miles to Papoose Drive. Make a right onto Papoose Drive and follow it for 0.5 miles to the T. Turn left on Teepee Drive and follow for 0.5 miles. Make a right and park in the lot below Arrowhead Grove.

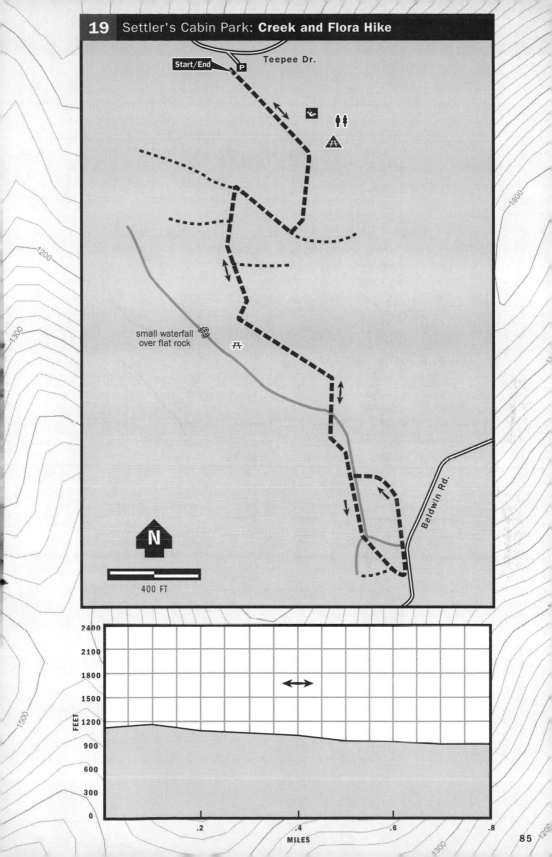

Teepee Dr.

Start/End

P

small waterfall
over flat rock

Baldwin Rd.

N

400 FT

FEET

2400
2100
1800
1500
1200
900
600
300
0

.2   .4   .6   .8

MILES

Berry trees, daisy fleabane, and yarrow can be found along this section. At 0.26 miles, pass the trail on the right and continue south, veering left. Find rhododendron and oxeye daisies as you carefully make your way through this muddy area and find yourself among pines and spruces mixed with the deciduous trees. Continue straight past the left at 0.29 miles. If the ground is wet, watch your step; the soil is mainly clay and is very slippery in damp conditions.

Take a right turn downhill at 0.33 miles, and the next right as well. You are heading toward water and may hear it running by now. Come to a vantage point where you can see a creek with water flowing over the smooth surface of a large flat rock, creating a small waterfall over its edge; if you want, you can go down a small steep trail to enjoy it at a picnic bench or put your feet in. Look around near your feet up and on the hillside, too; again, you'll see some unusual wildflowers.

If you've gone down to visit the creek, climb back up the narrow trail and turn right, using the trail you walked on to overlook the water, to rejoin the main trail. If you've stayed on the hillside, just continue along the spur trail and follow it back up to the main trail. As you continue on the main trail, the creek remains visible on your right. The area appears to be popular for deer, and you may see their tracks in this red clay section of the trail.

The trail becomes much wider, and its surface briefly changes to flat rock at 0.4 miles. Once the trail surface changes to dirt again and shelved rock appears above the trail on the left, look for the trees with shaggy bark on the younger sections of the trunk and then up to the older sections that have peeled and are entirely smooth. After this, the trail winds to the right and becomes very narrow; continue downhill to its low point to cross the creek at 0.47 miles.

The creek is now on your left, and you snake a bit with its path until you cross it again at 0.58 miles. Here you can decide to turn around and retrace your steps to avoid going uphill and then making a steep descent to rejoin it later, or you can continue up the hill toward the left.

If you decide to go up, climb the hillside; at the top you'll reach Baldwin Road. Turn left, following the path that parallels the road; do not cross the road. Walk over a water runoff. Not long after a small diameter pipe can be seen along the left side of the trail; notice the enormous oak tree on the left (before the pipe crosses the trail and travels along its right side). Shortly after, at 0.7 miles, the trail veers left and downhill. Almost halfway down, you can veer to the right to make the descent a little easier. At the bottom, cross the creek at 0.8 miles and retrace your steps.

▶ NEARBY ATTRACTIONS

Information about renting groves or using other park attractions such as the wave pool, tennis courts, and picnic shelters and groves can be found at **www.county .allegheny.pa.us/parks** or by contacting the park office at (412) 787-2750.

SOUTH PARK HIKE

▶ IN BRIEF

There are many activities and facilities in South Park, but if a walk in the woods is a part of your visit, this little hike will help. Plan to come on a Sunday to visit the Oliver Miller Homestead (April through December), and stop by the game preserve to see the buffalo while you're in the park.

▶ DESCRIPTION

Begin the hike by walking to the left corner of the parking lot to enter the trail, which is not signed but is marked with white rectangular blazes and easy to find. Follow the trail back into the woods until you reach a junction at 210 feet and turn right. In less than another few hundred feet another trail connects this one to the parking lot as well; trees to be seen in this area include American beech and Shumard oak, a species not very common in Pennsylvania. At 0.21 miles, pass another trail coming in from the right (it appears to lead to the road), as well as the next two trails from the left, the second of which just loops to rejoin the main trail.

You'll notice that the trail is popular with mountain bikers, which is part of the reason there are so many branching trails and also part of the reason the trails are maintained. There is a right turn (marked with yellow triangular blazes) onto a mountain bike path at 0.27 miles; continue straight to another junction where there is a

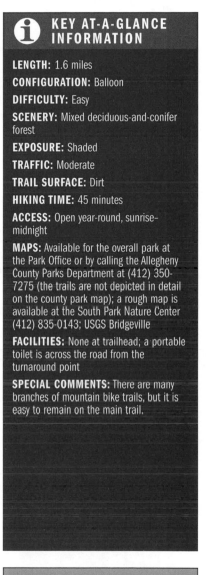

KEY AT-A-GLANCE INFORMATION

LENGTH: 1.6 miles

CONFIGURATION: Balloon

DIFFICULTY: Easy

SCENERY: Mixed deciduous-and-conifer forest

EXPOSURE: Shaded

TRAFFIC: Moderate

TRAIL SURFACE: Dirt

HIKING TIME: 45 minutes

ACCESS: Open year-round, sunrise-midnight

MAPS: Available for the overall park at the Park Office or by calling the Allegheny County Parks Department at (412) 350-7275 (the trails are not depicted in detail on the county park map); a rough map is available at the South Park Nature Center (412) 835-0143; USGS Bridgeville

FACILITIES: None at trailhead; a portable toilet is across the road from the turnaround point

SPECIAL COMMENTS: There are many branches of mountain bike trails, but it is easy to remain on the main trail.

▶ DIRECTIONS

From Pittsburgh, take PA 51 South to PA 88 South. Follow it 4.7 miles to the entrance of South Park; this entrance is Corrigan Drive. Follow Corrigan Drive 0.4 miles. Turn left onto Hundred Acres Drive; follow it 1.3 miles and turn right (just past West Virginia Grove). At the stop sign (almost immediate), turn right onto East Park Drive and make a quick left into the small parking area.

South Park Hike

UTM Zone (WGS84)   17T

Easting   584320

Northing   4464667

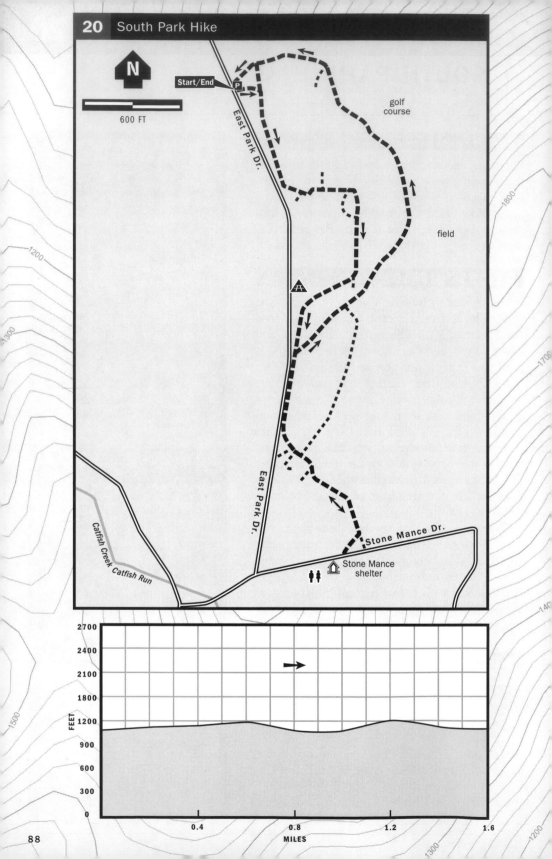

choice to veer toward the left or turn right with the main trail. Turn right to stay with the white-blazed main trail and pass the junction where the mountain-bike trail rejoins the main. Here, you'll notice that the trail is now marked with both the white and yellow blazes. The trails share the path only until 0.38 miles, where the mountain bike trail continues straight and you turn right with the hiking trail.

The trail veers right and runs closer to the road. Not long after passing a picnic shelter on your right, arrive at a choice to veer right or turn left. Veer right to continue hiking. You will hike out and back on this next portion to return to this point (left returns to the parking lot if you wish to reduce the length of the hike). Walk through a section where pitch pines are growing, staying on the main trail and passing the Y at 0.57 miles. Almost immediately, you'll arrive at a junction of a network of trails. Continue straight even though there is a white blaze on the trail heading left and uphill; there is also a white blaze straight along the trail that's not visible from this point. Pass another trail feeding in from the right, and walk over a culvert to reach a junction. Turning right keeps you on the main trail, although the path straight ahead leads to the same road, Stone Mance Drive, just a little farther up.

If you are in need, there is a portable toilet across Stone Mance Drive, not far from the Stone Mance shelter; this is the turnaround point. Retrace your steps to return to the second Y juncture with the white-blazed trail at 1.03 miles. (The first will lead to the same place if you take it instead.) After veering right, begin a slow, steady incline. There is a field to the right, followed by a golf course. The trail meanders away from and back toward the golf course after you reach its plateau and begin to head downhill.

After the trail veers left at 1.45 miles, pass the last of the mountain bike trails branching off to the left and reach the junction where you originally turned right to enter the loop from the parking lot. Walk straight to reach your vehicle.

▶ NEARBY ATTRACTIONS

If you wish to hike more, you can cross the road to find similar trails. If you want to see other parts of the park, you can visit the buffalo at the park's game preserve (off Sesqui Drive) or walk the paved trail around the park. Information about renting groves or using other park attractions such as the Oliver Miller Homestead, wave pool, tennis courts, golf courses, BMX track, model-airplane field, and ice-skating rink, among many others, can be found by contacting the park office at (724) 935-1766. Visit **www.county.allegheny.pa.us/parks** to find additional details about the facilities and events, such as the summer concert series. The South Park Nature Center hosts many programs; visit the above Web site for a calendar of events, or call (412) 835-0143.

THREE RIVERS HERITAGE TRAIL: MONONGAHELA SOUTH SHORE

 KEY AT-A-GLANCE INFORMATION

LENGTH: 6.6 miles (can be shortened by turning around sooner or lengthened by continuing past parking area on way back for an additional 1.5-mile out-and-back)

CONFIGURATION: Out-and-back

DIFFICULTY: Easy

SCENERY: Monongahela River, ducks and geese, Steelers and Panthers University of Pittsburgh Medical Center Sports Complex facility and mural (in lobby), Steelworkers Monument

EXPOSURE: Mostly sunny

TRAFFIC: Light, but well used on weekdays

TRAIL SURFACE: Wide and mostly paved with crushed gravel path alongside for joggers

HIKING TIME: 1–1.5 hours

ACCESS: Park is open year-round

MAPS: A map of this and other riverfront trails is available from Friends of the Riverfront. Contact them for maps, hiking, biking, triathlon, volunteer mixers for all ages, and volunteer and membership opportunities at (412) 488-0212 or **www.friendsof theriverfront.org;** USGS Pittsburgh East

FACILITIES: Portable toilets, picnic tables, boat launch, and pay phone

SPECIAL COMMENTS: This is a popular trail used by South Side workers and residents. It's a fun way to get out for a walk along the river and combine it with some city touring in the unique South Side, where old Pittsburgh and trendy shops come together for a unique experience.

Three Rivers Heritage Trail:
Monongahela South Shore

UTM Zone (WGS84)   17T

Easting   587116

Northing   4476173

▶ **IN BRIEF**

This trail segment is part of the almost complete 37-mile Three Rivers Heritage Trail, which is used by hikers, bikers, and skaters of all ages.

▶ **DESCRIPTION**

This segment of the Three Rivers Heritage Trail is in the South Side Riverfront Park, where you can vary your hike by feeding the ducks and geese, riding a bike, or jogging and ending with a jaunt into the South Side commercial district (see Nearby Attractions following this description).

The trail segment begins from the upper parking lot (note: do not confuse the shorter sidewalk along the river with the trail). Turn right as you face the river and then follow the trail southward underneath the Birmingham Bridge. The trail breaks with a left fork onto gravel that quickly rejoins the paved trail, leaving you with the option to take either path. At approximately 0.75 miles, cross Hot Metal Street and notice the Steelworkers Monument, which is part of the city of Pittsburgh's South Side Works Public Art Project. The industrial art here also includes a steel bench and slag mounds, remnants of the city's heritage. Continue on until 0.9 miles, where you may wish to walk down the gravel path to the riverfront. You're likely to find out what the catches of the day have been (or hear a few good fish tales) from the anglers who frequent this spot. The deviation offers a good view of the river and large boulders to sit and contemplate on or just enjoy the breezes that typically come off the water.

▶ **DIRECTIONS**

From Pittsburgh, take the Boulevard of the Allies (PA 885) to the Tenth Street Bridge. Turn right to cross the bridge and get to the South Side. Turn left onto East Carson Street (PA 837) to 18th Street. Make a left onto 18th Street and follow it to South Side Riverfront Park.

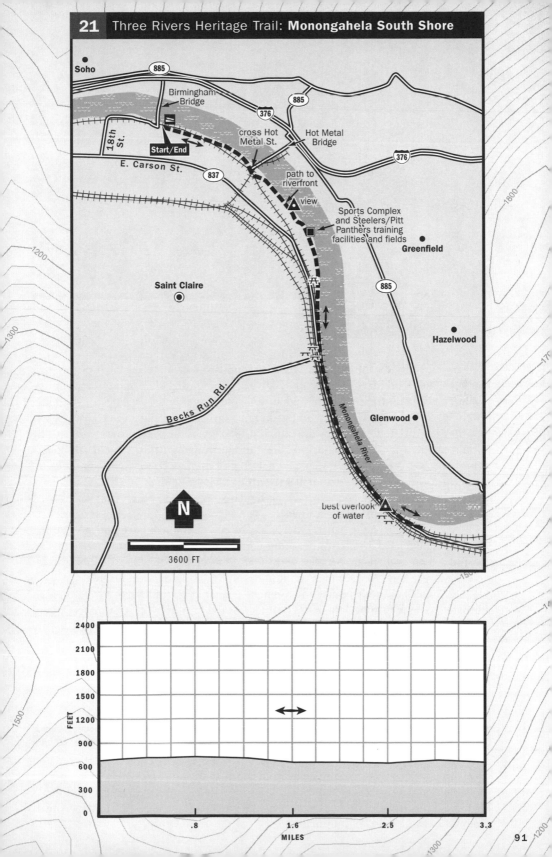

Soho

885

Birmingham
Bridge

885

376

18th
St.

Start/End

cross Hot
Metal St.

Hot Metal
Bridge

376

E. Carson St.

837

path to
riverfront

view

Sports Complex
and Steelers/Pitt
Panthers training
facilities and fields

Greenfield

885

Saint Claire

Hazelwood

Becks Run Rd.

Glenwood

Monongahela River

best overlook
of water

N

3600 FT

2400

2100

1800

1500

FEET 1200

900

600

300

0

.8   1.6   2.5   3.3

MILES

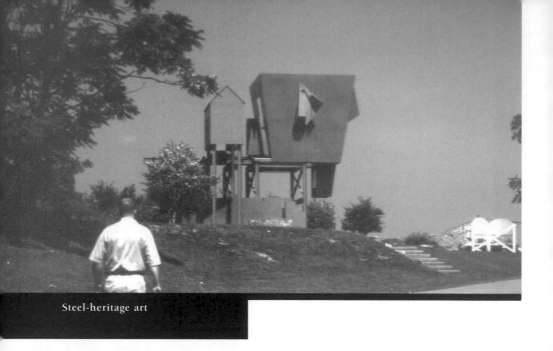

Steel-heritage art

At 1.1 miles, beautiful landscaping surrounds the area. To the right of the path you'll see the University of Pittsburgh Medical Center (UPMC) Sports Performance Complex, which encompasses the indoor and outdoor training facilities of the Pittsburgh Steelers and the University of Pittsburgh Panthers, as well as the UPMC Center for Sports Medicine. If you enjoy art, stop in the lobby of the center to view the 10- by 60-foot mural. The Steelers' and Panthers' outdoor training fields immediately follow the center; each has viewing towers and lighting for evening sessions. The entire complex, developed as part of Pittsburgh's riverfront revitalization, is one-half mile in size and sits on the site of the long-closed Ling-Temco-Vought (LTV) South Side Works Steel Mill. (Note: LTV purchased the former Jones and Laughlin [J&L] Steel Company.)

At 1.5 miles a picnic bench is available; although you will have noticed that the landscaping ended 0.2 miles prior to this, this is not a great stop for picnicking. At 1.6 and 1.8 miles there are benches with small roofs facing the river; you can stop for a pleasant rest here. At 1.9 miles you'll find another trail down to the river.

At 2 miles the trail's quiet environment is altered by traffic noise from a parallel road. You may turn back here or continue for the best overlook of the river found on this segment of the trail at 3 miles. I recommend turning around at approximately 2 miles, passing back through the lot where you parked, and taking the brief (additional 1.5-mile out-and-back) but scenic walk north along the trail. Here you will find shade in the overhanging trees, clear views of the Pittsburgh skyline, and interpretive signs highlighting the city's history in the steel- and glass-making industries, railroad lines, its canal system, and its many immigrant workers.

▶ NEARBY ATTRACTIONS

The South Side is packed with interesting new- and used-book stores, offbeat and specialized retail stores carrying items from beads to furniture, restaurants known for their international specialties and quaint atmospheres, clubs with music and dancing, and stairs to the slopes for spectacular views of the city. Visit **www.south sidepgh.com** for loads of information.

THREE RIVERS HERITAGE TRAIL: WASHINGTON'S LANDING LOOP

▶ IN BRIEF

This island is exemplary of successful remediation. Its close proximity to downtown Pittsburgh, flat terrain, and consistent views of the Allegheny River make it convenient and enjoyable for walkers and joggers of all ages.

▶ DESCRIPTION

Anyone who isn't familiar with the history of the remediation and development work that turned the former Herr's Island into the new Washington's Landing may have a difficult time believing that this beautiful, serene haven was once an environmental nightmare. Condemned as a contaminated brownfield site in the 1970s, this 42-acre island on the Allegheny River was once home to oil refining and storage, tube works, soap works, stockyards and a rendering plant, scrap-metal recycling, hotels, and worker lodging houses. The most descriptive quote I've read tells the story: "Odors from the island's animal-rendering plant were foul enough to make a fellow just about swear off breathing" (O'Neill, 1986).

Fortunately, these sentiments are left in the past. In their place is an admiration from community and city dwellers for the walking and jogging path that encircles the island, its landscaping, magnificent view of the river and downtown skyline, and many other amenities. In addition to the path, which is part of the Three Rivers Heritage

▶ KEY AT-A-GLANCE INFORMATION

LENGTH: 1.2 miles

CONFIGURATION: Loop

DIFFICULTY: Easy

SCENERY: Allegheny River, praiseworthy landscaping, rock sculpture, history signage

EXPOSURE: Sunny with areas of shade

TRAFFIC: Medium to busy

TRAIL SURFACE: Packed, fine stone

HIKING TIME: 45 minutes

ACCESS: Open year-round

MAPS: A map of this and other riverfront trails is available from Friends of the Riverfront. Contact them for maps, hiking, biking, triathlon, volunteer mixers for all ages, and volunteer and membership opportunities at (412) 488-0212 or **www.friendsof theriverfront.org**; USGS Pittsburgh East

FACILITIES: There is a portable toilet in the parking lot; Troll's restaurant has a restroom for customers only; vending machines for beverages are located at the marina.

SPECIAL COMMENTS: You may extend the hike by making a right at the marina, walking out and back to the trail bridge, and then walking the path as described on the following pages.

▶ DIRECTIONS

From downtown Pittsburgh, take Interstate 579 North (Veteran's Bridge) and merge onto PA 28 North. Follow 1.3 miles and turn right onto the 31st Street Bridge. Make an immediate right (0.1 mile) onto River Avenue. Make the immediate left (0.1 mile) onto the 13th Street Bridge, which becomes Waterfront Drive. Turn left to enter the parking area under the 31st Street Bridge.

Three Rivers Heritage Trail: Washington's Landing Loop

UTM Zone (WGS84) **17T**

Easting **586663**

Northing **4479779**

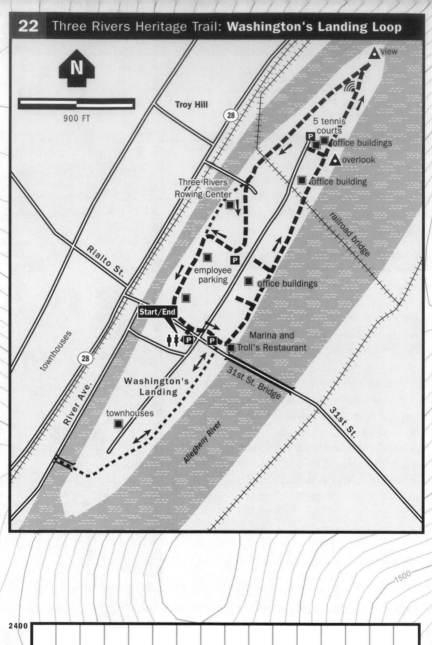

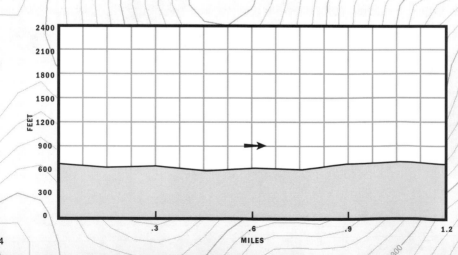

Trail, the island is also home to a seven-acre residential development of 93 town-houses, a public park, tennis courts, a fitness and rowing center, a 150-slip marina with dry dock, and low-profile office buildings.

To begin the hike, cross the street and turn left on the sidewalk. Just as you reach the first office building, make a right onto the crushed-stone path. You'll walk by maples and through the woody berry trees that press close to the path, reminiscent of an arbor, to reach a view of the river and some of the boats docked at the marina. Turn left, following the trail. (Alternatively, turn right, walk out to the trail bridge and back.) The landscaping along this trail includes daffodils, ornamental grasses, woody plants, and a variety of trees; it is done very nicely, allowing views of the river along much of its distance. There are also benches conveniently placed at intervals.

There are a couple of trail-access points that meet the path from the left. While walking, you'll notice that the well-planned flora and distance of the buildings from the path render them to the unseen background for most of the walk. The atmosphere here also makes this island a desirable place to work. The landscaping appears to have been done with great care on both sides of the trail and is maintained throughout much of the walk. It appears that even an eastern white pine, the largest conifer in Pennsylvania, has been included. This type of conifer was formerly the dominant tree in Pennsylvania and the backbone of the timber industry; it was known as the Monarch of the Trees. Efforts are underway to restore its place in Pennsylvania's habitat. By the way, the eastern white pine is a favorite nesting tree for bald eagles.

Also to be found are ferns, daylilies, sweet gum trees, and honey locust trees, so-called because of the sweet, yellowish substance found in its seedpods. Flowering trees have been included in the landscaping as well.

At about 0.25 miles, you'll walk underneath an old railroad bridge. Not long after, the path passes briefly along the sidewall of an office building.

At 0.36 miles, make a right down the stairs to the overlook. You may catch a sighting of one of the many sculling teams rowing down the river. Pittsburgh's rivers have made it a natural favorite for competitive rowing. Before 1860, there were 11 rowing clubs in the area; as one of the first sports to attract women, it was also one of the first to reward them with cash and other prizes, as well as celebrity. Between the 1850s and 1880s, rowing competitions drew large crowds, and thousands came to witness the races via railroads, trolley cars, and boats. Pittsburgh's heavy industrial past caused the sport's decline in this area, but as the city changed, the sport experienced a dramatic resurgence. The Three Rivers Rowing Association is located on the island and has played an important role in establishing Pittsburgh as one of the nation's top rowing-competition hosts.

When you return to the trail, you'll see trellises alongside the entire back of the last office building. Each building on the island has been built to work in synergy with the new environment. As a result, their presence is not at all obtrusive. The island space on the left opens after the office buildings end, and a wide grassy field leads to five tennis courts on the left. After passing the tennis courts and an open field, there are several curved walls designed as an outdoor amphitheater. This also appears to be a nice spot for relaxation and contemplation. Coming up is a rock sculpture donated by The Pittsburgh Foundation and the Three Rivers Rowing Association.

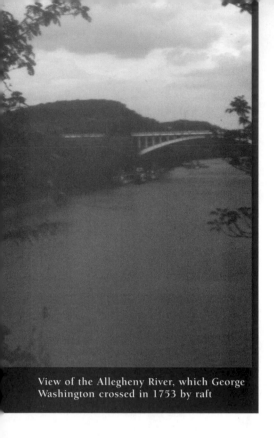

View of the Allegheny River, which George Washington crossed in 1753 by raft

The path then reaches a small garden area that indicates you are close to the end of the island; walk through it and out to an information plaque.

Here, you have a wonderful view of the river and can walk down the stairs, which lead to a more expansive view. From there, you can see the 40th Street Bridge, marked "Washington's Crossing" in memory of George Washington's 1753 crossing of the river as a young soldier who was then on his first diplomatic mission. Washington crossed the Allegheny on a raft with Christopher Gist and was thrown into the icy water as the pole he was using to guide the raft was knocked from him by floating ice. Unable to reach either shore, the two found refuge for the night on what was once variously known as Wainwright's, McCollough's, or Good Liquor Island near midstream. That island has disappeared because of changes in the river.

When finished, continue on the trail using the walking path along the other side of the island. The landscaping on this side is more intermittent. On the right, the drop-off of the hillside and proximity to the water offer views to this back channel of the Allegheny. Once the trail curves left to pass in front of buildings, you are walking on a sidewalk for a bit. Walk past the Three Rivers Rowing Club, which is likely busy with activity, and then past the building of the Department of Environmental Protection and the Department of Conservation and Natural Resources; this restored island seems a fitting place for their location. Even this short portion along the sidewalk is pleasant. Both sides of the street are lined with young maples.

Turn right past the building to return to the crushed-stone path. At the Y, veer left (going right leads to the back of the Three Rivers Rowing Club). This area of the path is also nicely landscaped and there are many birds enjoying it as well. Once beyond the last of the buildings, the parking lot comes into view.

▶ NEARBY ATTRACTIONS

Troll's restaurant is located on the island and is shown on the map. The island is close to the North Side and the Strip District; both areas offer numerous restaurants.

For more walks close by, see North Shore: River, Memorial, and Sports Walk (hike 15); Point State Park: History and Three Rivers Walk (hike 16); and Downtown Historic Walk (hike 3).

TOWNSEND PARK LOOP

▶ IN BRIEF

Townsend Park offers short but pleasant hiking trails, a pond with a picnic shelter, and accessibility for the handicapped for both fishing and picnicking. It also has two gardens, one with benches, the other with a gazebo.

▶ DESCRIPTION

This small park is very well maintained and pleasant to enter. The landscaped gardens and seating complement the hiking trails and pond, creating a mix of amenities that should accommodate most needs for a few hours or so of outdoor enjoyment. The hike begins along a path that passes through the first garden and ends next to the pond.

Walk through the Rotary Garden and around the gazebo. The sign for the Ron Stoll Trail is on the left side of the trail and will become obvious after you pass the gazebo. Walk up the gravel path, following it into the woods. The gravel gives way to nature, allowing you to hike on the woodsy dirt trail that starts with a slight ascent but quickly levels. Follow the wide trail through a mix of lower brush and deciduous trees.

In less than a quarter mile, make a right onto Pine Grove Trail; there is a sign. The green-blazed trail narrows as the surrounding atmosphere immediately changes. The trail is now padded with fallen needles, muffling any noises from the community that might have been heard

▶ KEY AT-A-GLANCE INFORMATION

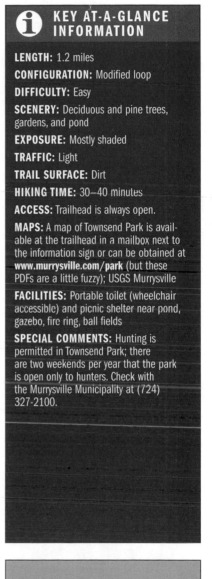

LENGTH: 1.2 miles

CONFIGURATION: Modified loop

DIFFICULTY: Easy

SCENERY: Deciduous and pine trees, gardens, and pond

EXPOSURE: Mostly shaded

TRAFFIC: Light

TRAIL SURFACE: Dirt

HIKING TIME: 30–40 minutes

ACCESS: Trailhead is always open.

MAPS: A map of Townsend Park is available at the trailhead in a mailbox next to the information sign or can be obtained at www.murrysville.com/park (but these PDFs are a little fuzzy); USGS Murrysville

FACILITIES: Portable toilet (wheelchair accessible) and picnic shelter near pond, gazebo, fire ring, ball fields

SPECIAL COMMENTS: Hunting is permitted in Townsend Park; there are two weekends per year that the park is open only to hunters. Check with the Murrysville Municipality at (724) 327-2100.

▶ DIRECTIONS

From Pittsburgh, take Interstate 376 East to the second Monroeville exit. Turn left onto PA 22 East and travel approximately 3.5 miles. Make a left onto Vincent Hall Street (turns into Sardis Road) and travel approximately 3.2 miles. Turn left onto Twin Oaks Drive and travel less than a half mile. Make a left onto Townsend Park Court. Pull in and park in the upper lot.

Townsend Park Loop

UTM Zone (WGS84)   17T

Easting   612461

Northing   4479863

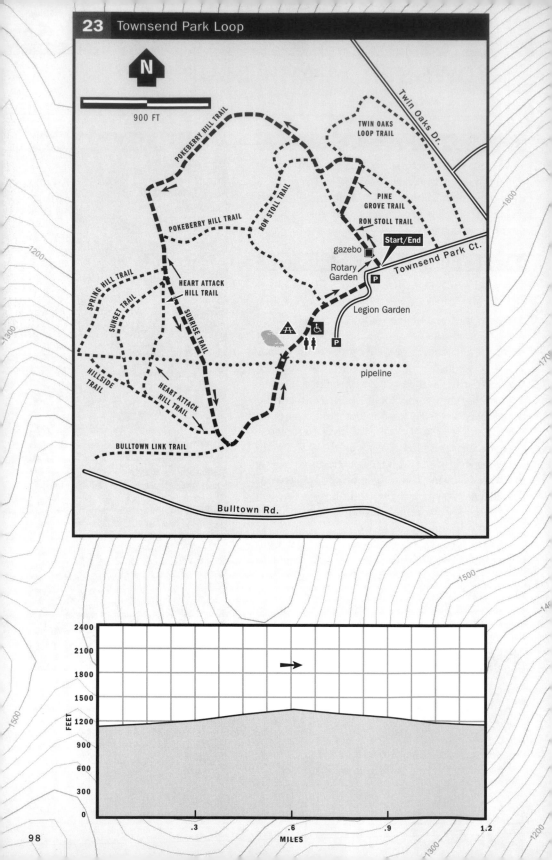

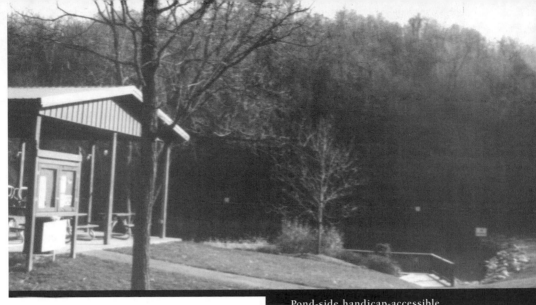

and filling the olfactory senses with the smell of pine. If you made this turn with your eyes closed, there would still be no mistaking that you're in a pine grove. It is a pleasant surprise in this community park.

Continue past the intersecting Twin Oaks Loop Trail (no sign), remaining in the pine grove and walking deeper into the woods. Walk up a slight incline and enjoy the grove while it lasts. It seems over too soon when arriving again at the Ron Stoll Trail; turn right. In just a few hundred feet, there is a choice to turn right again. The park map labels this connector trail Spicebush Loop, but the sign at this intersection in the park is Pokeberry Hill. Make a right at this sign. Shortly after, there is another right but no sign. Make the right. This is actually the Pokeberry Hill Trail.

You'll find that Pokeberry Hill lives up to its name as you ascend for about 150 feet. The trail is enjoyable, the little bit of exercise keeps the hike interesting, and the elevation out of the lower woods provides access to viewing more of the sky and feeling more of the sun. Once the knob of the hill is reached, the trail curves left around it, meanders, and eventually begins to descend through a mixture of hardwoods and long-needled pines.

Arrive at a choice of trails and turn right onto Heart Attack Hill (left continues on Pokeberry and returns to the Ron Stoll Trail), which sharply descends. It would be great exercise in the other direction; still, downhill is good for the hamstrings. Pass the right for the Spring Hill Trail and continue to the Sunrise Trail, which is marked with a sign.

Make a left onto Sunrise Trail (straight continues with an ascent of Heart Attack Hill and right is the Sunset Trail). The Sunrise Trail is somewhat of a stroll with a slight descent until the trail meets again with the Heart Attack Hill Trail (no sign). Make a left to continue downhill and in just another 100 feet come to the sign. Continue left, remaining on the Heart Attack Hill Trail (right is Bulltown Link Trail, which leads to Bulltown Road). The descent on this section is steep. The bottom of the trail leads across a short bridge and to a sign marking the end of Heart Attack Hill Trail. Walking up and to the left, find a pond furnished with a picnic shelter and a picnic table on the platform by the pond. The entire area here is handicap accessible, including the portable toilet to the right. An information board and memorial are also found up the path. Walk to the left of the lower parking lot and follow the road up to the upper parking lot. Stop and admire the Legion Garden on your way.

▶ NEARBY ATTRACTIONS

The Murrysville Municipality Building can't be missed along Sardis Road (on the right as you head back toward US 22). Stop in for information on other parks and hiking in the area. There are many eating establishments on Old William Penn Highway (crossed just before you get to US 22) and on US 22. For other hikes in the area from this book, try Boyce Park Log Cabin Expanded Loop (hike 2) or Bushy Run History Loop (hike 24).

WESTMORELAND COUNTY

BUSHY RUN HISTORY LOOP

KEY AT-A-GLANCE INFORMATION

LENGTH: 1 mile

CONFIGURATION: Loop

DIFFICULTY: Easy

SCENERY: Ligonier Blue Rock marker, Bushy Run battlefield; eastern hemlock, oak, birch, and dogwood trees

EXPOSURE: Mostly shaded

TRAFFIC: Moderate

TRAIL SURFACE: Dirt

HIKING TIME: 1 hour

ACCESS: The park is open year-round, Wednesday–Sunday, 9 a.m.–5 p.m.; see Nearby Attractions (following the Description) for visitor's center and museum hours

MAPS: Overview maps with information about stops on the various trails are available at the visitor's center at no charge; USGS Irwin and Greensburg

FACILITIES: Restroom facilities are available near the parking lot and inside the visitor's center; picnic pavilion is located by the parking lot.

SPECIAL COMMENTS: There is an admission charge for the museum: adults, $3; seniors and groups, $2.50; children ages 6–17, $2 (visitor's center is free).

Bushy Run History Loop

UTM Zone (WGS84)   **17T**

Easting   **616721**

Northing   **4468483**

IN BRIEF

Bushy Run is perfect for history buffs, families, and anyone who enjoys a pleasant hike. Combining a tour of the museum inside the visitor's center with a hike through history makes a great way to spend a few hours in the morning or afternoon.

DESCRIPTION

Before hitting the trail, learn about the role of the Bushy Run Battlefield during Pontiac's War in 1763. The Bushy Run Museum is a very good way to begin, and, although not large, it houses enough interesting artifacts to be worth paying the small fee. There are even some interactive displays where children (or adults if they have a mind to) can dress in some of the uniform garb of the soldiers and are encouraged to touch some of the other items on display.

If you would like to visit the museum during docent hours, when a guide is available, call ahead. The docent that caught up with me provided additional insight into the history of both the battle and the area, and her guidance provided enjoyable conversation. I learned, for example, that a man had to have one bottom and one top front tooth that lined up in his mouth to qualify for service in the American provincial army. Why? So he could bite the end of the paper gunpowder pouch off, hence the common saying "Bite the bullet." With the help of the docent, I also learned that the beautifully chiseled stone relief found in the great room of the museum came from one of Pittsburgh's bridge renovations

DIRECTIONS

From Pittsburgh, take Interstate 376 East to the Murrysville exit. Follow PA 22 East through Murrysville and make a right onto Harrison City Export Road. Make a left at the T onto PA 993 and follow to the left into Bushy Run.

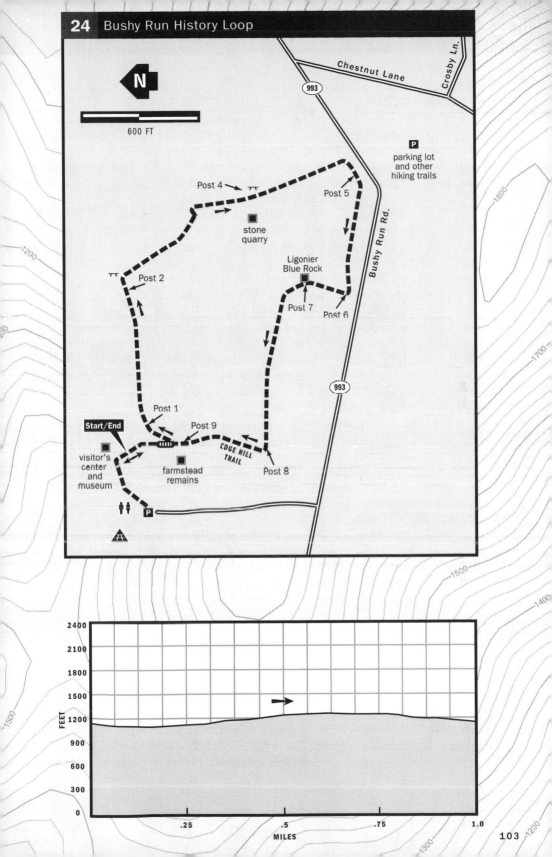

N

600 FT

Chestnut Lane

993

Crosby Ln.

P
parking lot
and other
hiking trails

Post 4

Post 5

stone
quarry

Bushy Run Rd.

Post 2

Ligonier
Blue Rock

Post 7   Post 6

Post 1

Start/End

Post 9

visitor's
center
and
museum

farmstead
remains

EDGE HILL
TRAIL

Post 8

993

P

2400

2100

1800

1500

1200

900

600

300

0

FEET

.25   .5   .75   1.0
MILES

and that there is a mistake in it: Native Americans are depicted riding on horses, which were not found in this area at the time of Pontiac's War.

Once you have completed your indoor history tour, choose a trail. This description is the hike on the Edge Hill Trail, which circles the main battlefield area. Step out of the visitor's center and to the right a short way. Look to your left for a pair of steps and descend them all the way to the bottom for the Edge Hill Trail. Before starting, though, try to place yourself in the predicament of that time. Posts on the trail will guide you on this journey through time.

The roots of Pontiac's War lie in the broken Treaty of Easton. The British had agreed to guarantee the Native Americans a homeland west of the Allegheny Mountains, free from the encroaching settlements that brought with them the loss of land and two of the greatest threats to the Native Americans at that time—smallpox and measles. The treaty also aimed to guarantee the halt of alcohol trade with Native Americans. It was thought that their bodies were unable to adapt to the drug, and many lives were lost to its effect. Even though the Native Americans had kept their part of the treaty, which was to stop hostilities against the British and to offer their assistance as scouts to the French, the British failed the Native Americans. Consequently, Chief Pontiac, the great warrior and orator, united many tribes, including those of the Great Lakes, and began the well-organized war with an attack on the British-held Fort Detroit on May 8, 1763. Within two months Native Americans controlled an immense land area from Michigan to Pennsylvania.

On June 2, 1763, a party from a local tribe warned the owners of a Bushy Run way station (the Byerly family) to abandon it or be killed in four days. The station was abandoned and burned to the ground, but it remained the destination of Colonel Henry Bouquet and 450 soldiers on their way to defend Fort Pitt. Thus it happened that on August 5, 1763, Bouquet and his soldiers were attacked and forced to retreat to a hilltop from which the battle resumed early in the morning on August 6. Turn left and walk to Post 1.

Native Americans controlled the valley surrounding this area after forcing the British troops to retreat using a horseshoe-shaped formation and hit-and-run tactics. Walking along the wide path toward Post 2, you'll notice the many pine needles mixed with the debris of the deciduous forest. From written accounts of the 1700s, this area was covered with a mature virgin forest consisting of oaks and chestnut trees, often six to seven feet in diameter. Their size provided a canopy that prevented much sunlight from reaching the forest floor. Although those trees have been cut down, the surrounding eastern hemlocks, oaks, and birch trees simulate the shaded environment of long ago. However, the fields and dense brush seen here today would not have been a factor in the forest battlefield in 1763.

Continue on, passing Post 3, and note that the tradition of carving names in trees, although seeming to offer timelessness to the carver, is deadly to the trees themselves. The stone quarry at Post 4 is a remnant of the changing times. The British won the battle of Bushy Run, and Pontiac's War eventually failed the Native Americans. Thus, quarries such as this sandstone excavation into the hillside became more common as settlers used the natural surroundings to provide shelter in the form of homes and other buildings. Take a rest on the bench at this pretty spot if you like as your hike continues with a slight upgrade before leveling out at the battlefield area.

When you're ready, continue along, watching carefully for a right as you near Bouquet's Road (Post 5), a southern fork of Forbes Road, which Colonel Bouquet used instead of the main Forbes Road in hopes that it would speed his troops' journey. Turn right before reaching PA 993 (Bushy Run Road). There are no clear indicators to show the location of Post 6, but to get to it stay left near Bushy Run Road and walk to the large oak tree; the post is at the oak tree. It is at Post 6 that, according to a survey map created in 1765, Colonel Bouquet's convoy was maintained. Turn right and head to the large blue rock surrounded by a wrought iron fence; this is Post 7.

This is a slice of Ligonier "Blue Rock" and it marks the site where Colonel Bouquet and his soldiers erected a defense using flour sacks to protect the wounded; some stuffed flour sacks lay near the marker. Look at the plaques within the wrought iron fence to review a relief map of the battlefield and letters written by Colonel Bouquet about what was occurring at the time, as well as a historical summary. It was at this spot that the British troops both had a visual advantage and a water disadvantage. It's also the location from which British companies maneuvered to flank the Native Americans by feigning a retreat and then swinging back to chase the exposed Native Americans into the woods.

When finished, look to the left of the woods for a faint sign of a path in the grass. This is the direction to walk, not into the woods (that avenue is part of the Flour Sack Trail). Post 8 is the last spot on this hike to take in a good view of the battlefield.

To reach Post 9 and the end of the loop, turn right. You will come upon the remains of a springhouse that was once a part of the Lewis Wanamaker Farm. He was the principle owner of Bushy Run and sold it to the Commonwealth of Pennsylvania in 1941. This ends a brief but pleasant tour though a significant turning point in the history of this country. Continuing straight you'll come upon the end of the loop. Turn left and head up the steps.

▶ NEARBY ATTRACTIONS

The visitor's center and museum are open April 1 through October 31, Wednesdays through Saturdays from 9 a.m. to 5 p.m. and Sundays, noon to 5 p.m.; the facility is closed Mondays and Tuesdays. From November 1 through March 31 the center and museum are open Saturdays from 9 a.m. to 5 p.m., Sundays from 1 to 5 p.m., and closed all other days of the week. Call the visitor's center at (724) 527-5584 for information concerning guided tours, special events, reenactments, and use of the facilities.

CEDAR CREEK PARK: GORGE TRAIL LOOP

KEY AT-A-GLANCE INFORMATION

LENGTH: 1.5 miles

CONFIGURATION: Loop

DIFFICULTY: Easy

SCENERY: Youghiogheny River, Cedar Creek, deciduous woodlands

EXPOSURE: Mostly shaded

TRAFFIC: Light

TRAIL SURFACE: Dirt

HIKING TIME: 45 minutes

ACCESS: Park hours are 9 a.m. to sunset

MAPS: Available at Cedar Creek Station for overall park (the trail is shown but not in correct detail); USGS Donora

FACILITIES: Restrooms, food, and beverages are available at Cedar Creek Station by the parking area; there is a water fountain in the far parking lot.

SPECIAL COMMENTS: This trail is a short, easy escape into the woodlands and to Cedar Creek, where children can explore its banks and shallow waters.
  You can hike or bike the nearby Youghiogheny River Trail. Bicycle rentals are available at Cedar Creek Station, as are snacks, drinks, maps, fishing bait, ice, and souvenirs; call (724) 930-7004 for more information. River access, a boat launch, 19 pavilions, group-camping areas, and picnic areas are also available. For information on the park's Summer Concert Series and August Fun Fest, or use of facilities, call the Westmoreland County Bureau of Parks and Recreation at (724) 830-3950 or (800) 442-6926, x3950.

Cedar Creek Park: Gorge Trail Loop

UTM Zone (WGS84)   17T

Easting   603986

Northing   4448301

IN BRIEF

The trailhead is within spitting distance of the Youghiogheny River Trail and a stone's throw to the Youghiogheny River. This hike can be easily combined with other outdoor activities or relaxation (see Special Comments in the Key At-a-Glance Information).

DESCRIPTION

The trailhead is located at the end of the far parking lot, near the Youghiogheny River, on the river side (eastern) of the Youghiogheny River Trail. There is a sign at the trailhead for the Cedar Creek Gorge Trail and a picnic bench and grill next to the trailhead by the river. Look beyond these, to the right of the trail, and you'll see a large silver maple. The Cedar Creek Gorge Trail passes underneath the Youghiogheny River Trail and winds southwest to a plaque claiming there's a 109-year-old apple tree nearby. We had no luck finding it; perhaps you will have better fortune.

Along this beginning section, we did find mountain maple and jewelweed. The trail quickly meets up with Cedar Creek. Bypass two mountain bike trails and cross the first of two suspension bridges over Cedar Creek at 0.13 miles. There is a large sign directing hikers of the Cedar Creek Trail to turn left at its end. Turn left, bypassing the trail straight ahead and another on your right after

DIRECTIONS

From Pittsburgh, take PA 51 South and drive 21.5 miles. Turn left at the small sign for Cedar Creek Park. (Note that the turn is 0.25 miles before PA 51 intersects with Interstate 70.) Drive 0.2 miles, turn left on Port Royal Road, and follow 0.1 mile. Turn right at the stop sign and drive 0.5 miles to reach the beginning of the park. Travel an additional 0.1 mile, turn left onto Timm's Lane (no sign), and follow 0.9 miles to the parking area.

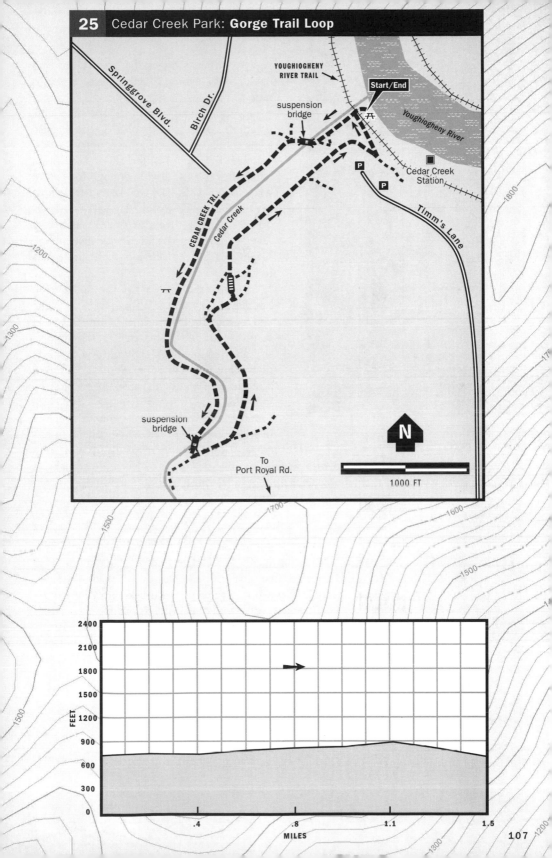

YOUGHIOGHENY
RIVER TRAIL

Start/End

Youghiogheny River

Springgrove Blvd.

Birch Dr.

suspension
bridge

CEDAR CREEK TRL.

Cedar Creek

Cedar Creek
Station

P

P

Timm's Lane

suspension
bridge

To
Port Royal Rd.

N

1000 FT

2400
2100
1800
1500
1200
900
600
300
0

FEET

.4   .8   1.1   1.5
MILES

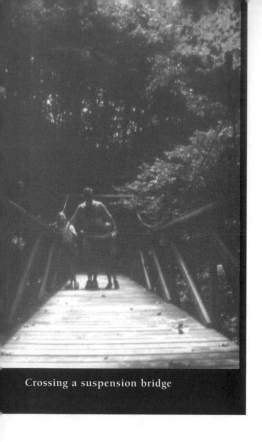
Crossing a suspension bridge

you've turned. The main trail is flat and obvious, following Cedar Creek, which is now to your left.

Among the trees in the area are sycamore, oaks, and maples. There are also a few wildflowers, even in late summer. Find a bench at 0.43 miles, where the trail becomes narrower but is still wide enough for two to walk side by side. The trail veers left, following the natural flow of the creek. Water flows down large flat sheets of shale, which step down the creek bed, and provide just enough height for small (one-foot-high) waterfalls to form.

Cross the second of the suspension bridges at 0.71 miles. Walk up the hill at the end of the bridge. At the T, turn left and continue uphill. In this area find Solomon's seal and red maple. At 0.8 miles there is a Y: the trail to the right appears to lead uphill to a model-airplane field; continue straight by following the leftmost branch. The trail becomes level as it travels the side of the hill. Two trails lead down at 1 mile; you can go left and down here to avoid a bit of a steeper descent and meet up with where this hike descends or continue straight. If continuing straight, just after a slight uphill grade, you'll find another choice to continue straight and uphill or go left on a lower trail. Take the lower trail to begin traveling down the hillside back toward the creek. This leads down a set of trail steps that are not well maintained. At the bottom of these stairs, turn right.

Along this section of the trail, find pin oak, witch hazel, and beech trees. Bypass another trail coming down the hill from the right and shortly after, at 1.33 miles (almost directly in line with the first suspension bridge now in view below)—you can't miss the huge American basswood tree with six trunks growing from a single point on your left. The lightweight, soft wood of this tree is commonly used for carving. Native Americans once used its fibrous inner bark to make rope, baskets, and mats. Bees produce a high-quality honey from the nectar of this tree's fragrant flowers. If you missed it, there is another, also with six trunks, at 1.37 miles, just before the trail veers right. Beyond this, you can go left downhill to make a steep descent or straight. Go straight for an easier way to meet up with a lower trail that parallels the Youghiogheny River Trail. Turn left when you reach it.

Depart the woods and walk uphill to the Youghiogheny River Trail. If you parked in the far parking lot near the trailhead, turn left and complete the loop. If you parked in the parking lot closer to the bike concession, you can turn right. The parking lot is within view.

(See Special Comments for nearby attractions.)

FORBES STATE FOREST: LAUREL SUMMIT— SPRUCE FLATS BOG AND WILDLIFE AREA LOOP

▶ IN BRIEF

You can walk the short distance to the bog and out, or combine a visit to the bog with the loop in this hike. Bring a picnic basket and relax, or hike to Wolf Rocks (see the Wolf Rocks Overlook Loop [hike 27] in this book).

▶ DESCRIPTION

To begin this hike, walk past the restrooms to the trailhead sign, which points the way straight on the wide grass path to Spruce Flats Bog. Milkweed, daisies, and many ferns are growing along the first exposed portion of the trail. The path quickly narrows to a dirt trail where witch hazel, various maple and oak trees, and conifers are growing.

At just 0.12 miles, you'll see the Picnic Area Trail branching on the right. You'll come back to this to hike the loop but continue straight to see the bog, which is just a short walk away. Veering left with the trail, follow the walkway out to the bog overlook platform. Bogs usually result from glacial activity that creates a recess suitable for the formation of a pond. After a glacier recedes and the remaining basin fills with water, it takes centuries before conditions turn it into a bog. The pond must first be stocked with a bountiful supply of living organisms. Once this happens, the organisms slowly use all of the minerals of the surrounding rock and soil. An acidic environment is created, and pond water turns murky brown as organic matter collects; only plants that are able to tolerate the acidic conditions survive.

▶ DIRECTIONS

From Pittsburgh, take Interstate 376 East and enter the Pennsylvania Turnpike I-76 East (a toll road). Take the Irwin exit to PA 30 East and travel 2 miles past Ligonier. At the intersection of PA 381, turn south for 2.9 miles and then left on Linn Run Road at the small town of Rector. Travel on Linn Run Road for 7.5 miles and turn left into the parking area for the Laurel Summit Picnic Area.

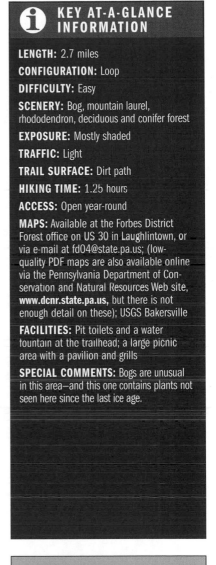

ⓘ KEY AT-A-GLANCE INFORMATION

LENGTH: 2.7 miles

CONFIGURATION: Loop

DIFFICULTY: Easy

SCENERY: Bog, mountain laurel, rhododendron, deciduous and conifer forest

EXPOSURE: Mostly shaded

TRAFFIC: Light

TRAIL SURFACE: Dirt path

HIKING TIME: 1.25 hours

ACCESS: Open year-round

MAPS: Available at the Forbes District Forest office on US 30 in Laughlintown, or via e-mail at fd04@state.pa.us; (low-quality PDF maps are also available online via the Pennsylvania Department of Conservation and Natural Resources Web site, **www.dcnr.state.pa.us,** but there is not enough detail on these); USGS Bakersville

FACILITIES: Pit toilets and a water fountain at the trailhead; a large picnic area with a pavilion and grills

SPECIAL COMMENTS: Bogs are unusual in this area—and this one contains plants not seen here since the last ice age.

Forbes State Forest:
Laurel Summit—Spruce Flats Bog and Wildlife Area Loop

UTM Zone (WGS84)   17T

Easting   655436

Northing   4442443

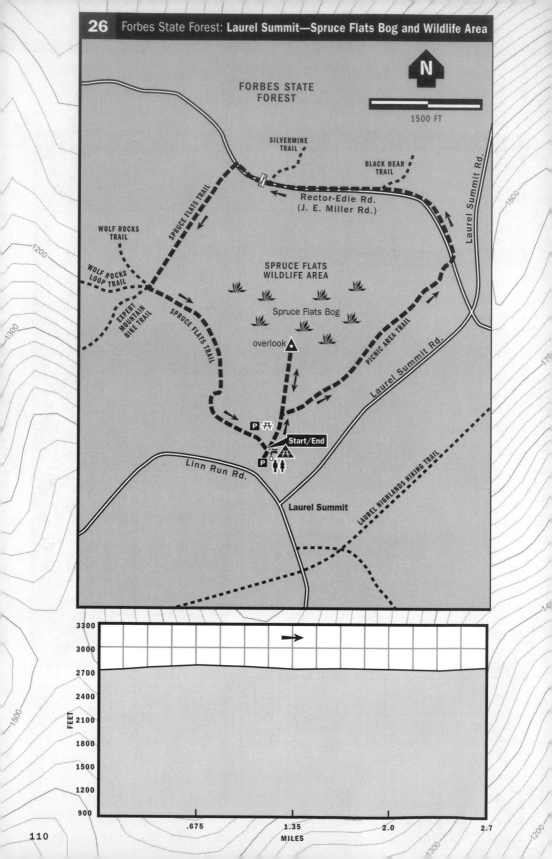

N

1500 FT

FORBES STATE FOREST

SILVERMINE TRAIL

BLACK BEAR TRAIL

Laurel Summit Rd.

Rector-Edie Rd. (J. E. Miller Rd.)

SPRUCE FLATS TRAIL

WOLF ROCKS TRAIL

SPRUCE FLATS WILDLIFE AREA

Spruce Flats Bog

WOLF ROCKS LOOP TRAIL

EXPERT MOUNTAIN BIKE TRAIL

SPRUCE FLATS TRAIL

overlook

PICNIC AREA TRAIL

Laurel Summit Rd.

P

Start/End

P

Linn Run Rd.

LAUREL HIGHLANDS HIKING TRAIL

Laurel Summit

3300
3000
2700
2400
2100
1800
1500
1200
900

FEET

.675   1.35   2.0   2.7
MILES

Gradually, the pond is filled with dead, undecomposed plant matter; then plants grow across the water's surface, creating a thick mat. Over time, the bog becomes a meadow and then a forest. When this area was cut by lumbermen in 1908, what they first found was a virgin hemlock forest (the name Spruce Flats was a misnomer). There was no evidence of a bog, although the land was described as swampy. It is thought that fires may have followed the timber harvest, causing the forest to revert back to a bog.

If you look out over the bog in June or later in the summer you may see pitcher plants, with their insect-devouring red and yellow flowers. You also may see sundews, tiny plants with delicate flowers that grow no more than an inch high; this innocent-looking plant devours insects, too, in order to retrieve the nitrogen from the insects' bodies. As all plants need nitrogen and it is not available in bogs, these plants developed the survival skill of luring (with smell), trapping (with sticky or recurved hairs), and devouring (with digestive enzymes) insects. Cranberries are plentiful (I've picked them here) and grow throughout this bog as well; they are mature in November.

When you've finished at the bog, retrace your steps to the Picnic Trail, where you make a left; the trail is marked with red blazes. It is very level, but the surface is somewhat uneven with small pieces of broken shale and other rock. At 1.05 miles, you'll reach Rector-Edie Road (also shown as J. E. Miller Road on some maps), a dirt road for which there is no sign. Turn left, and walk northward. The sides of the road are adorned with ferns, boulders, and mixed deciduous and conifer forest. At 1.15 miles, you'll notice a clearing where the ground on the left is boggy, indicating the outer reaches of an arm of the bog. Pass Black Bear Trail on the right at 1.28 miles and continue to pass some large flat boulders and then the Silvermine Trail at 1.60 miles. Walk around the gate immediately following to the trailhead sign for the Spruce Flats and Wolf Rocks trails at 1.71 miles; turn left.

There are a lot of striped maples and ferns along this trail, which turns into a single track for a while and is lined closely with grasses. At about 1.9 miles, walk through a small boulder area and over a large flat rock; there are several spots like this. Reach an intersection and a decision at 2.10 miles. Spruce Flats Trail continues to the left, leading back to the parking and picnic area. But if you wish to hike to Wolf Rocks, which offers a panoramic overlook to be viewed from a large rock outcropping, you can turn right; read the Wolf Rocks Overlook Loop (hike 27) write-up in this book. Beginning the Wolf Rocks hike from here shaves off 1.2 miles from that hike. It is a scenic trail and the overlook and front-row rock seating are worth the walk.

If you're returning to the parking and picnic areas, turn left. The trail along this section is dotted with conifers and mountain laurel; at 2.34 miles, rhododendrons hug its sides and many of the rocks are covered with moss. As you walk in and out of sections such as this, long-needled pine branches sometimes hang out over the trail. This ends when you enter a clearing. The trail then reenters the woods and finishes in a clearing for picnicking and parking. Walk through here to the parking area at the trailhead below.

▶ NEARBY ATTRACTIONS

In addition to Wolf Rocks (hike 27), there are many other hikes in this area. You can continue driving on Linn Run Road to Laurel Summit Road (turn left, heading north, and drive to the warming hut) and hike any of the numerous trails in that area (see hike 28 in this book, or pick up a map at the warming hut). Other areas close by include Linn Run State Park and Powdermill Nature Reserve, hikes 31 and 32, respectively, in this book.

FORBES STATE FOREST: LAUREL SUMMIT—WOLF ROCKS OVERLOOK LOOP

 ## KEY AT-A-GLANCE INFORMATION

LENGTH: 4.4 miles

CONFIGURATION: Balloon

DIFFICULTY: Easy

SCENERY: Overlook, mountain laurel, rhododendron, mixed deciduous-and-conifer forest

EXPOSURE: Mostly shaded

TRAFFIC: Light

TRAIL SURFACE: Dirt path

HIKING TIME: 2.5 hours

ACCESS: Open year-round

MAPS: Available at the Forbes District Forest office on US 30 in Laughlintown, (724) 238-1200, or via e-mail at fd04@state.pa.us; (low-quality PDF maps are also available online via the Pennsylvania Department of Conservation and Natural Resources Web site, **www.dcnr.state.pa.us,** but there is not enough detail on these); USGS Bakersville

FACILITIES: Pit toilets, water fountain, large picnic pavilion and grills are located by the first parking area.

SPECIAL COMMENTS: Combine this hike with the Spruce Flats Bog and Wildlife Area Loop (hike 26) for a look at the unique bog found in this area.

Forbes State Forest: Laurel Summit—Wolf Rocks Overlook Loop

UTM Zone (WGS84)   17T

Easting   655382

Northing   4442508

▶ IN BRIEF

Wolf Rocks Overlook offers a spectacular 180-degree view, and the hike to it is just as spectacular as the overlook itself.

▶ DESCRIPTION

If you've parked in the first parking area near the restrooms, turn left and walk through the second parking area, looking left for the trailhead sign for Wolf Rocks Trail. The first 0.6 miles of this trail, although signed here as the Wolf Rocks Trail, is actually the Spruce Flats Trail, according to a sign later found at an intersection at 0.6 miles. In this write-up and on the map, it is referred to as the Spruce Flats Trail. The confusion of the signs and the fact that one-half of the Wolf Rocks Loop is called just that while the other half is named just Wolf Rocks Trail likely stems from the fact that the eastern portion was added later to create a cross-country skiing loop.

If you are combining this hike with the Spruce Flats Bog and Wildlife Area Loop (hike 26), begin at the trailhead there. Upon reaching the intersection for the Wolf Rocks Loop, use this hike description beginning at the 0.6-mile intersection below.

From the trailhead, walk into the woods along this red-blazed trail and enjoy the shade created by the mixed forest. A variety of maple trees including striped and red maples, along with oaks

▶ DIRECTIONS

From Pittsburgh, take Interstate 376 East and enter the Pennsylvania Turnpike I-76 East (a toll road). Take the Irwin exit to PA 30 East and travel 2 miles past Ligonier. At the intersection of PA 381, turn south for 2.9 miles and then left on Linn Run Road at the small town of Rector. Travel on Linn Run Road for 7.5 miles and turn left into the parking area for the Laurel Summit Picnic Area.

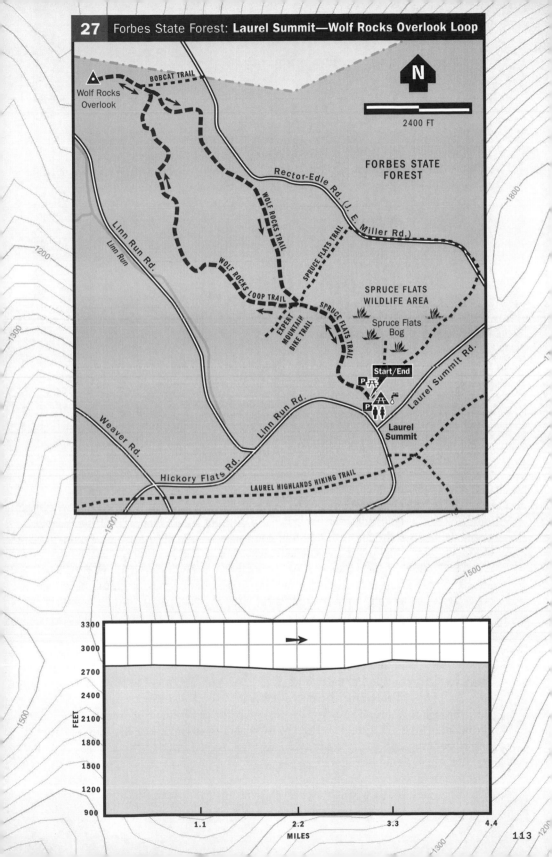

N

2400 FT

Wolf Rocks
Overlook

BOBCAT TRAIL

FORBES STATE
FOREST

Rector-Edie Rd. (J. E. Miller Rd.)

WOLF ROCKS TRAIL

SPRUCE FLATS TRAIL

SPRUCE FLATS
WILDLIFE AREA

Spruce Flats
Bog

Linn Run Rd.

Linn Run

WOLF ROCKS LOOP TRAIL

EXPERT MOUNTAIN BIKE TRAIL

SPRUCE FLATS TRAIL

Start/End

P

P

Laurel Summit Rd.

Laurel
Summit

Weaver Rd.

Linn Run Rd.

Hickory Flats Rd.

LAUREL HIGHLANDS HIKING TRAIL

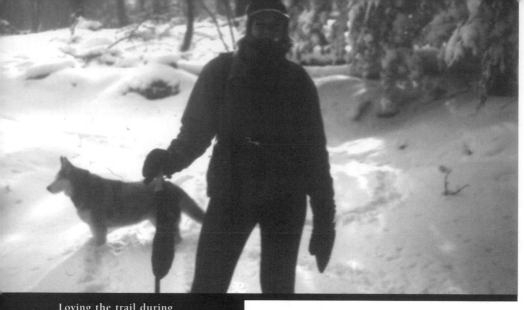

Loving the trail during
Siberian-husky weather

and witch hazel are among the specimens you'll find here. Pass through a clearing and back into the woods. Here, the overhanging branches of long-needled pines sometimes arch partway over the rocky trail, which is lined with rhododendron and mountain laurel. The root systems of conifers, rhododendrons, and mountain laurel are shallow, and your boots visit them frequently; watch your step if it's wet. This trail is the most popular access to Wolf Rocks and it is more heavily used, but not enough so it appears the least bit disturbed. Relish in the tranquility as you walk through sections where rhododendrons hug the trail on either side and pine needles soften your steps.

At 0.6 miles, come to an intersection where the trail branches in a Y in front of you. There is a sign indicating Wolf Rocks Loop is a soft left and Wolf Rocks Trail a soft right. Also, the Spruce Flats Trail continues with a sharp right and an expert mountain-biking trail is a sharp left. Take the left branch of the Y onto the Wolf Rocks Loop Trail to hike a clockwise loop. Walk over the large boulder and follow the single-track trail that is lined with grasses and ferns. Deciduous trees including beech are mixed with conifers and soon the trail is carpeted in small pieces of their wood. The myriad plant growth along the forest floor includes fan and other mosses, wildflowers, and berry plants.

At 0.9 miles, notice the large swaths of moss that are growing across the wide, flat boulders lining this popular trail. It's somewhat amazing that it endures in such a healthy state, considering the many soles it must pad throughout the hiking season.

Soon the forest around you opens out, and if you are fortunate a soft breeze will blow through it. Catbrier, also known as greenbrier, grows along the trail and has all but taken over at 1.15 miles. For the most part, its growth across the trail has been controlled but watch out for your legs if a stray thorny branch or two wanders across the trail.

You may have noticed that the trail has been less rocky for a bit but this soon ends. The careful footing you must make as you pick your way along the many rocks cropping up from the trail's surface is rewarded with the site of their gray roughness against the variety of green and brown hues of color that surround them. Four-foot high boulders can be seen to the right of the trail at 1.54 miles; at least you don't have to scale any of these to get around.

Shortly after, cross a small waterway at a low point in the trail. After a very low-grade down-and-uphill jaunt, you'll reach a trail sign (at 2.02 miles) that marks the trail you have just been hiking and Wolf Rocks Trail behind and to the right. There is no indication of Wolf Rocks Overlook, however, until you walk straight ahead another 160 feet. There you'll find a sign indicating that Wolf Rocks are straight ahead and Bobcat Trail is to the right. Go straight, veering left to follow the trail back over and through boulders to Wolf Rocks. When you reach them, relax and take in the view, which allows you to see up Fish Run Valley to the top of Laurel Hill. Looking west, gaze down Linn Run Valley across to Chestnut Ridge. This is a nice place to break for lunch, unless you plan to picnic back at the tables later. In any case, enjoy one of the rather rare rock outcroppings that afford such views in this area before turning around to hike back.

Once back on the trail, retrace your steps to the sign for Wolf Rocks Trail, and veer left at the Y onto it. The scenery along this trail is much like that of the first half of the loop, although the trail itself is much less rocky and therefore, easier on the feet. The deciduous forest contains tulip, pin oak, and mountain ash trees. Just after 3 miles, walk through an area where the forest is thinner and views into it include large boulders upon which some rhododendrons have found foothold. At 3.6 miles the trail is completely surrounded by ferns, and you'll approach the intersection with the Spruce Flats Trail, connecting this loop with the parking area, which you will follow to the picnic area clearing.

▶ NEARBY ATTRACTIONS

There are many hikes in this area in addition to the Spruce Flats Bog and Wildlife Area Loop (hike 26) mentioned above. You can continue driving on Linn Run Road to Laurel Summit Road (turn left, heading north, and drive to the warming hut) and hike any of the numerous trails in that area; see the Laurel Summit Loop (hike 28) write-up in this book or pick up a map at the warming hut. Other areas close by include Linn Run State Park and Powdermill Nature Reserve; see hikes 31 and 32, respectively, in this book.

FORBES STATE FOREST: LAUREL SUMMIT LOOP

KEY AT-A-GLANCE INFORMATION

LENGTH: 6.8 miles

CONFIGURATION: Loop

DIFFICULTY: Easy to moderate

SCENERY: Mountain laurel, pines, and boulders

EXPOSURE: Mostly shaded

TRAFFIC: Light to moderate

TRAIL SURFACE: Dirt path, sometimes rocky

HIKING TIME: 3.5 hours

ACCESS: Open year-round

MAPS: Available at the Forbes District Forest office on US 30 in Laughlintown (724) 238-1200, at the warming hut near the trailhead, via e-mail at fd04@state.pa.us, or online (in PDF format) via the Pennsylvania Department of Conservation and Natural Resources Web site, **www.dcnr.state.pa.us;** USGS Ligonier

FACILITIES: Warming hut is open all week; a concession inside the hut is open on weekends; there are portable toilets near the warming hut

SPECIAL COMMENTS: This is a beautiful trail. It can be hiked any time of the year; snowshoeing is how I did it. The trails at the summit are also perfect for cross-country skiing. If hiking in warmer weather, wear sturdy boots.

Forbes State Forest:
Laurel Summit Loop

UTM Zone (WGS84)   17T

Easting   657548

Northing   4446824

IN BRIEF

Laurel Summit State Park is part of the Forbes State Forest system. It is a spectacular place and has something for every level hiker. Mountain laurel, Pennsylvania's state flower, is abundant, as are large boulders. Hiking in western Pennsylvania doesn't get much prettier than this.

DESCRIPTION

To begin this hike, walk approximately 1,000 feet past the warming hut and turn right on Ben Albert's Trail. The hike begins on flat terrain that soon turns into a gradual incline, passing through hardwoods and mountain laurel. The incline continues as you reach the Towhee Trail at 0.3 miles; turn left at the sign that marks this trail. Meander along the now more level route, as the mountain laurel recedes and hardwoods encompass the view. At 0.75 miles you'll see a sign for Lippo's Loop to the right; continue straight on Towhee. After the sign, a small stream trickles along the right-hand side of the trail for a while. Begin to descend slightly with the trail as it curves to the left. When the trail veers sharply right, find yourself enjoying about 100 feet of mountain laurel. The short stature of some of the laurel is likely due to wind on the summit; the tallest thus far has been about six or seven feet high along this somewhat rocky trail.

Soon you'll come to an intersection with the Spruce Run Trail, marked also with the Summit Trail to which it connects. Continue straight on

DIRECTIONS

From Pittsburgh, take Interstate 376 East to enter the Pennsylvania Turnpike I-76 East. Take Exit 89, Irwin, to PA 30 East and follow it past Laughlintown. Turn right (before Jennerstown) on Laurel Summit Road (there is a sign). Follow it to the parking area. The warming hut is on the left, and there is an information board on the right.

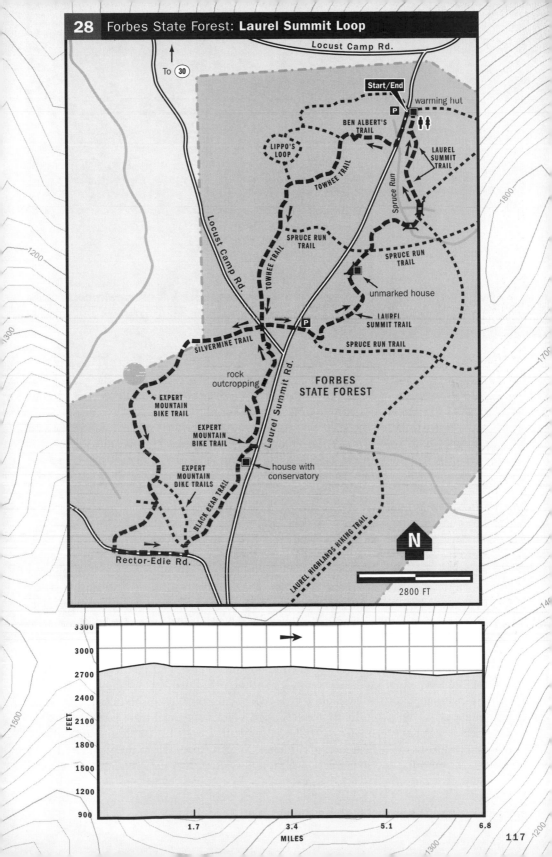

Locust Camp Rd.

To 30

Start/End

warming hut

P

BEN ALBERT'S TRAIL

LIPPO'S LOOP

LAUREL SUMMIT TRAIL

TOWHEE TRAIL

Spruce Run

TOWHEE TRAIL

SPRUCE RUN TRAIL

SPRUCE RUN TRAIL

unmarked house

LAUREL SUMMIT TRAIL

P

Locust Camp Rd.

SILVERMINE TRAIL

SPRUCE RUN TRAIL

rock outcropping

FORBES STATE FOREST

EXPERT MOUNTAIN BIKE TRAIL

Laurel Summit Rd.

EXPERT MOUNTAIN BIKE TRAIL

EXPERT MOUNTAIN BIKE TRAILS

house with conservatory

BLACK BEAR TRAIL

N

Rector-Edie Rd.

LAUREL HIGHLANDS HIKING TRAIL

2800 FT

FEET

3300
3000
2700
2400
2100
1800
1500
1200
900

1.7   3.4   5.1   6.8
MILES

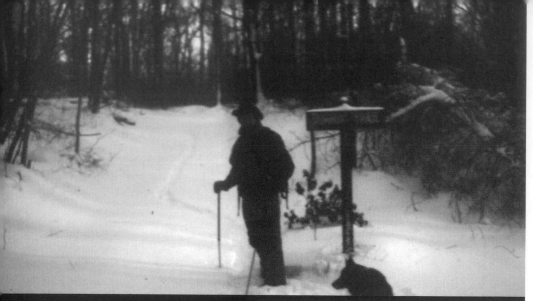

the Towhee Trail. The scenery changes slightly as the trail widens, the older hardwoods disappear, and small pine trees and thorny underbrush line it. At 1.2 miles begin a steep descent that would prove great fun on skis.

Following this, the trail view expands as grasses line it and lead outward to expanses of hardwoods and closes up once more with young growth. At this point, the trail veers right and you are nearing Locust Camp Road at 1.5 miles. Walking straight across the marked road, take the Silvermine Trail; the sign is posted about 30 feet back from the trailhead. This trail looks more like an old road in the beginning and is picturesque with pines interspersed often among the hardwoods. In the winter snow I hiked in, they are drooping with gobs of the compacted wet flakes and it is beautiful. Boulders become apparent more and more frequently—a prettier setting for a Pennsylvania hike couldn't be expected. At about 2 miles, you'll arrive at an open area; there is a pond to the right and an expert mountain-biking trail marked to the left. Walk straight to continue on the Silvermine Trail. Here the trail narrows and you begin to ascend once more. For about one-quarter mile during my trip, the trail is surrounded by a forest of pines so heavy with snow I must duck beneath their branches in places. The pines thin again as the hardwoods and mountain laurel take precedence.

Continue straight past another intersection with an expert mountain-biking trail, underneath the pines, through the mountain laurel, and over a small stream as the trail veers right. At 3 miles, turn left on the pine-lined Rector-Edie Road and follow it for approximately one-third mile, where you turn left on the Black Bear Trail. In about 0.1 mile, the trail intersects once again with two expert mountain-biking trails. Veer right to remain on the Black Bear Trail. The trail is scenic and not difficult and begins to more closely parallel Laurel Summit Road. Off to the right along it, a house with what appears to be a small round conservatory for a top floor comes into view. At 4 miles you'll reach the next branch for an expert mountain-biking trail, turn left to follow this trail; this is still the Black Bear Trail and it is the alternative to reaching and walking on Laurel Summit Road.

The trail narrows and becomes much rockier. During my winter trek, I am sliding on a couple of the larger rocks even though there is at least a foot of snow and I am wearing snowshoes. On this portion of the trail, look left periodically and you'll notice the large rock outcropping that serves as sentry from the wind for quite a portion of this branch.

At 4.7 miles, you'll reach the intersection with Locust Camp Road. Cross the road and arrive at an intersection with signage for the Towhee and Spruce Run trails. Take Spruce Run Trail to the right, which leads shortly to Laurel Summit Road; cross over it. There is a parking area and signs for both the Spruce Run Trail and Summit Trail. Walk around the gate and take the Summit Trail.

This trail is by far the most varied and scenic of this loop. It boasts bountiful mountain laurel and plenty of twists and turns through rocky outcroppings. At 5.2 miles begin a slow descent of approximately 150 feet over the course of a mile. At 5.6 miles, there is a home to the right of the trail in a gorgeous setting of pine draping over the bridge you'll cross. At 5.7 miles, you'll arrive at an unmarked intersection and make a right to remain on the trail. (Going straight will take you to Laurel Summit Road.) In about 100 feet you'll get to a sign that marks the trail. Take the left branch to follow Summit Trail; going straight is the Spruce Run Trail, which will not return you to the warming hut but loops to the right and south, and would put you back farther on the Summit Trail.

This portion of the trail is just a pleasant and spectacularly beautiful ending to a most enjoyable hike. I think it should be visited in both winter and summer, when the mountain laurel is in bloom. In another quarter mile cross a bridge. Just before the next bridge is an intersection with the Laurel Highlands Trail; this joins the Laurel Summit Trail to share the bridge and cross over Spruce Run before turning right once again (this portion is marked with yellow blazes). Continue straight on Laurel Summit Trail. Finish the hike with a slight ascent, passing the sign for the warming hut and reaching the hut at 6.76 miles.

▶ NEARBY ATTRACTIONS

There are two overlooks of note nearby. To see them both, drive south on Laurel Summit Road. The closest is Beam Rocks, which can be enjoyed via a short jaunt from a parking area on Laurel Summit Road. To see the other, Wolf Rocks, either turn right onto J. E. Miller Road (the same as Rector-Edie Road but changes names on the western side of Laurel Summit Road) and hike 2 miles from a parking area, or park at the Laurel Summit State Park picnic area just a little farther south on Laurel Summit Road and hike the Laurel Summit Wolf Rocks Overlook Loop (hike 27) in this book.

You can also enjoy hot chocolate or some lunch in winter at The Springs at Laurel Mountain, a downhill-skiing resort once known as the ski capital of Pennsylvania and owned and operated by General Richard K. Mellon. It is located in bordering Laurel Mountain State Park. General Mellon gave the property to the commonwealth in 1964. Linn Run State Park (hike 31) is also nearby.

FORBES STATE FOREST: ROARING RUN NATURAL AREA LOOP

KEY AT-A-GLANCE INFORMATION

LENGTH: 7.8 miles

CONFIGURATION: Balloon

DIFFICULTY: Moderate

SCENERY: Roaring Run, deciduous forest, wildflowers, berries, rock outcroppings, mountain laurel, rhododendron

EXPOSURE: Mostly shaded

TRAFFIC: Light

TRAIL SURFACE: Dirt path, often rocky

HIKING TIME: 4.5 hours

ACCESS: Open year-round

MAPS: Available at the Forbes District Forest office on US 30 in Laughlintown, (724) 238-1200, or via e-mail at fd04@state.pa.us (low-quality PDF maps are also available online via the Pennsylvania Department of Conservation and Natural Resources Web site, **www.dcnr.state.pa.us,** but there is not enough detail on these); USGS Seven Springs

FACILITIES: None

SPECIAL COMMENTS: Wear boots and take walking poles for the many stream crossings and rocky descent, and wear long pants for the greenbrier. Camping is not permitted.

Forbes State Forest:
Roaring Run Natural Area Loop

UTM Zone (WGS84)   17T

Easting   641228

Northing   4434693

IN BRIEF

The first portion of this hike crosses Roaring Run 32 times (including tributaries) at my count; I've read 28 in other places. Either way, it's quite a few. Some of these crossings may prove challenging. I recommend this hike in early autumn when the water is lower and the steep, scenic descent of the second portion features spectacularly colorful views of the valley.

DESCRIPTION

The Roaring Run Natural Area is named for its complete mountain stream and watershed, which are protected within this 3,593-acre natural area, the largest in Pennsylvania. Located along the western slope of Laurel Ridge, it has a history of repeated logging. Today, it is slowly returning to its natural state, and only the varied age of the trees, former logging roads, and old railroad grades provide clues that humans once removed its valuable timber.

The trailhead is at the right-hand end of the parking area, closer to County Line Road. Take this access trail to 0.3 miles, where you'll reach a Y. The right branch is the South Loop Trail (there is a sign up on a tree to the right), which travels uphill; the left branch is Roaring Run Trail (there is not sign for it here). Take the left branch and follow this former logging railroad grade as it makes its way with a slow, steady descent toward Roaring Run, which is soon within earshot. There

DIRECTIONS

From Pittsburgh, take Interstate 376 East and enter the Pennsylvania Turnpike I-76 East (toll road). Take Exit 91, Ligonier–Uniontown. Turn left onto PA 31 East. Go straight for 2.1 miles and then right onto PA 711–PA 381 South and follow for 1.2 miles; turn left on County Line Road. At 1.8 miles, turn left into the parking area.

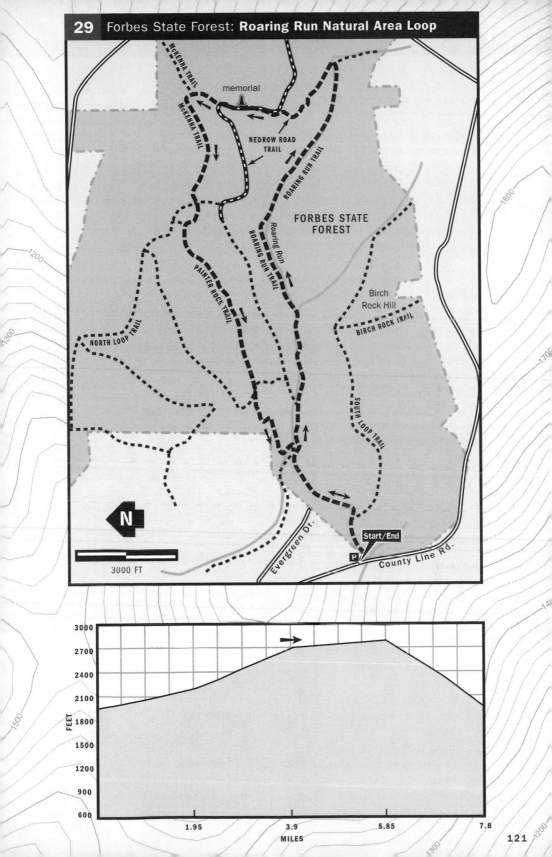

McKENNA TRAIL

memorial

McKENNA TRAIL

NEDROW ROAD TRAIL

ROARING RUN TRAIL

Roaring Run

ROARING RUN TRAIL

PAINTER ROCK TRAIL

NORTH LOOP TRAIL

FORBES STATE FOREST

Birch Rock Hill

BIRCH ROCK TRAIL

SOUTH LOOP TRAIL

N

3000 FT

Evergreen Dr.

Start/End
P
County Line Rd.

is a patch of blackberries on the way, before you reach an unmarked trail leading off to the left (at 0.9 miles) and an intersection with Painter Rock Trail almost immediately after. Turn right, staying on Roaring Run Trail. You'll notice a campsite here (and more later), but camping is not allowed. The trail leads over a rock bed that may be wet or dry and to the first crossing over Roaring Run. After crossing the run, which is now on the right, you'll arrive at a trail that seems to lead straight ahead; veer right and follow the blue blazes to stay on the main trail. Cross the water again, putting it to your left. (Note that if the water is high and you have trouble with these first crossings, you may want to turn back and follow South Loop Trail, which will also lead to the second half of the hike via the Tower Road Trail.)

Another crossing at 1.37 miles puts the run on your right, taking you through some rhododendron and American beech trees and marking where the frequency of the water crossings begins to pick up. You'll see more patches of blackberries and jewelweed as the trail leads slightly away from the main run and through a short, narrow section before crossing tributaries from the south, after which the trail widens again. Cross the run again, putting it on your right. It can be a little difficult through here to know whether you are crossing the main run or tributaries as the trail meanders back and forth across the water and sometimes between runoffs on both sides. Just follow the blue blazes as you zigzag your way along, making a slow ascent up the valley via the streambed's path. You are treated to hemlocks, moss-covered rocks, oaks, and sassafras. After the trail veers south, you'll continue to cross and recross the main run—its course adorned at times with ferns, more patches of blackberries, hawthorns, and basswood. The crossings of Roaring Run are almost at an end at 3.3 miles, where you'll have a choice to continue straight ahead and up a steeper ascent, or turn left. Turn left onto the Nedrow Road Trail (marked just Nedrow Trail on the Bureau of Forestry map) and cross the run twice more.

Now your boots have a chance to dry out as you turn north, leaving Roaring Run behind. For a bit, your climb is steeper and the trail surface is embedded with rocks and roots over which you must make your way. It is a lovely section and worth the climb. It levels out shortly to become a rolling stroll through a pleasant forested section that leads to a clearing and an information board at 3.82 miles. Turn left along the gravel road, which is marked on maps as both Nedrow Road and Painter Rock Road. (For clarity with the trail signs, which have all been marked Nedrow Road Trail, that is what the trail is called in this book's description and map.) Shortly, you'll arrive at a sign for Nedrow Road Trail. Continue straight on it to find a stone memorial (off to the right at 4.02 miles) that's dedicated to three children who died in January 1896; rumor has it that they died while riding in a sleigh.

Just ahead at 4.15 miles, the Nedrow Road Trail makes a sharp left. Continue straight, now on the McKenna Trail. Where the trail splits (4.28 miles); veer left. The trail narrows as you traverse the hillside with its ridge to your right, and through a long stretch of ferns. McKenna Trail ends when you reach Painter Rock Trail; continue straight, now on Painter Rock Trail.

Be sure to look for the oak tree that appears old enough to have escaped the logger's cut; it is located only about a third of a mile beyond the sign and before reaching another connector trail on the left that goes to Nedrow Road Trail.

Continue ahead on Painter Rock Trail for a real treat, passing the junction (at

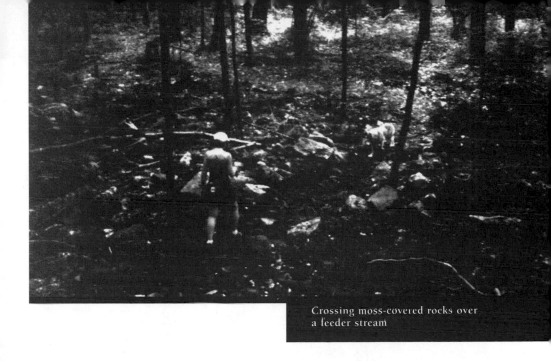

Crossing moss-covered rocks over
a feeder stream

5.18 miles), with the North Loop Trail on the right. You'll begin walking along the top of the ridge through a grassy section and then descending through boulders. There is an unmarked trail on the left that leads to a couple of large boulder outcroppings at 5.81 miles. You might wish to take a look. The boulders are interesting, and the side trail appears to continue down. Step back up to the main trail, though, or you'll miss some lovely views across the valley that can be enjoyed when there are no leaves on the trees. Just a short distance away, you'll see another connector trail from the right (this one signed) that leads to North Loop Trail.

The sign for Painter Rock Trail directs you straight ahead. The trail is very pretty here with its combination of greenery, strewn leaves, and gray boulders. Greenbrier thrives in places, but fortunately volunteers sometimes come through and cut back the clawing thorny vine. At about 6 miles, the descent becomes noticeably steeper; it veers sharply south at 6.42 miles. Pass through patches of mountain laurel and large boulders. The trail veers west but continues to be somewhat steep until you reach another bend to the south, which leads to a lovely view of a water seepage over which moss-covered rocks have been placed.

You are approaching Roaring Run once more; cross a couple of feeders and look for a sharp right (there is not a double blaze). Make the right to cross Roaring Run and look for another unmarked sharp right, which leads you past a campsite you'd have seen on the way in and to the junction with Roaring Run Trail. Turn right and retrace your steps on the access trail to the parking lot.

▶ NEARBY ATTRACTIONS

There are many hiking opportunities in this area, including Kooser State Park (hike 53), Laurel Hill State Park (hikes 54, 55, and 56), and Powdermill Nature Reserve (hike 32), which appear in this book. Numerous eating establishments are found along PA 31, and Sarinelli's (on the corner of PA 711–PA 381 and PA 31) sells some hot and cold ready-to-eat foods in addition to groceries.

KEYSTONE STATE PARK: STONE LODGE TRAIL

 KEY AT-A-GLANCE INFORMATION

LENGTH: 1.5 miles

CONFIGURATION: Loop

DIFFICULTY: Easy

SCENERY: Mainly deciduous forest, view of Keystone Lake

EXPOSURE: Mostly shaded

TRAFFIC: Light use

TRAIL SURFACE: Dirt

HIKING TIME: 1 hour

ACCESS: Park is open year-round.

MAPS: Available at the visitor's center or the park office (see Nearby Attractions following the Description for phone numbers); maps in PDF format are also available online via the Pennsylvania Department of Conservation and Natural Resources Web site, **www.dcnr.state.pa.us;** USGS Latrobe

FACILITIES: Restroom facilities available inside visitor's center, picnic areas, fishing, boating, beach

SPECIAL COMMENTS: If visiting in warm weather, leave some additional time for a swim at the beach. Also, the picnic areas allow visitors to make a day of it.

IN BRIEF

Don't let the ascent at the beginning of this hike scare you. The trail is relatively flat along most of the route and offers a very peaceful stroll in the sometimes busy park. The visitor's center is worth spending a little time in before or after hiking.

DESCRIPTION

Keystone State Park's existence may well be credited in part to the park's lake's beginnings as part of the endeavors of the Keystone Coal and Coke Company. Owners of the company purchased the land from several farmers in 1909 and created the lake to serve as a reservoir and guard against drought. Originally, water from the reservoir was used to wash the coal mined from the land that today makes up much of Keystone State Park. Water from the reservoir flowed by gravity through wooden pipes to Salemville, where it was used to wash sulfur from the coal and to cool it after it was baked to make coke.

In 1945, with a strong belief in the preservation of land for public use, James A. Kell, then secretary of Pennsylvania's Department of Forests and Waters, fought hard for the purchase of the land and the lake for a state park. He won that fight and Keystone State Park was born. Today, swimmers, boaters, and those who love to fish enjoy the reservoir, which was dug out with horse-drawn scoops and allowed to fill freely with the water of nearby springs and streams.

The Keystone Coal and Coke Company also

Keystone State Park: Stone Lodge Trail

UTM Zone (WGS84) **17T**

Easting **636968**

Northing **4470324**

DIRECTIONS

From Pittsburgh, take Interstate 376 East to the Murrysville exit. Follow PA 22 East to New Alexandria. Turn right onto PA 981. Make the second left for Keystone State Park on Slag Road and a right on Stone Lodge Road. Follow it to the visitor's center parking lot.

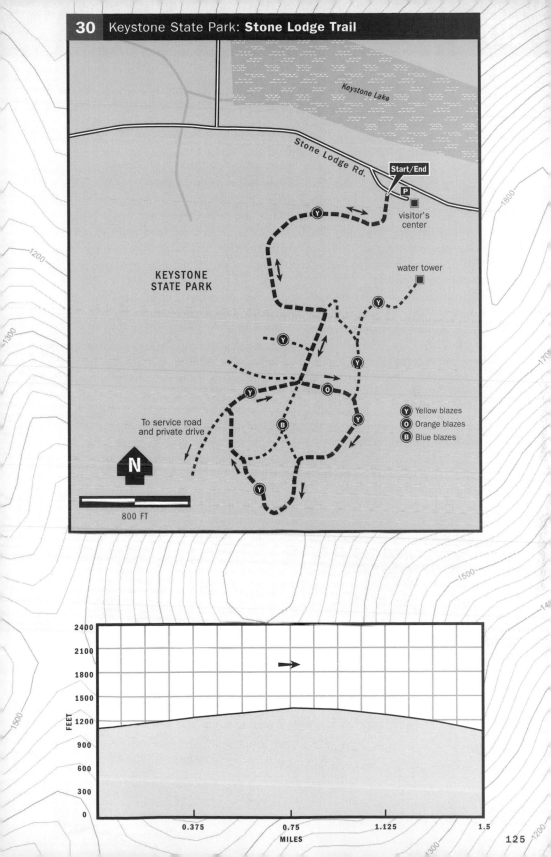

Keystone Lake

Stone Lodge Rd.

Start/End

P

visitor's center

water tower

KEYSTONE STATE PARK

To service road and private drive

Y Yellow blazes
O Orange blazes
B Blue blazes

N

800 FT

built the present-day visitor's center: a stone building from which the park staff provides interesting interpretations of both the natural surroundings and the historic artifacts housed inside, allowing a connection to the park's mining roots.

From the visitor's center, access the trail by walking across the parking lot. As soon as you step onto the trail, turn left and begin an ascent that slowly climbs the hillside. This portion of the trail is marked with yellow blazes. In just a few hundred feet, the trail turns right and briefly levels. If you are hiking when the leaves are down or sparse, enjoy a good view of Keystone Lake.

As the trail turns away from the lake, you'll begin another low-angle ascent that continues for approximately 500 feet, until you reach the loop that follows the outskirts of the hilltop. At the T, turn right. The trail opens out wide and relatively flat, resulting in a stroll along the hilltop. Bypass a spur trail on the right and pass a long row of evergreens.

At the four-way intersection, make a left onto the orange-blazed trail to begin a clockwise loop. If hiking in the fall, there will be fiery orange maple leaves to match the blazes on this pleasant trail. Soon you'll reach a T with the yellow trail. Turn right to continue the loop. (The left leads to either a water tower or the visitor's center, depending on later turns). As you continue hiking, ignore faded blue blazes that are visible on some of the trees; the yellow blazes are obviously more recently painted so hikers shouldn't doubt the course.

You'll arrive at another juncture with the blue trail; continue straight on yellow. You're about halfway through the hike when the trail circles right in a U-turn where club moss, young and full-grown oaks, maples, hickory, and evergreens are evident.

Immediately after the turn, a very slight descent begins and you'll encounter another blue-blazed trail on the right that is not marked on the park map; continue straight on yellow. At almost 1 mile is another T; turn right to close the loop (the left leads to a service road and a private drive). At just beyond 1 mile, look left to view a very large and beautiful hemlock. Soon you'll reach the point where the orange trail was originally met; make a left to exit the loop the way you entered it. Continue past the unmarked trail (now on the left) passed on the way in. Pay attention to avoid missing the left-hand turn onto the narrow path that leads downhill to the parking lot (where you turned right on the way up; continuing straight on the wide path loops back up the hill).

▶ NEARBY ATTRACTIONS

Call (724) 668-2566 to contact the visitor's center about hours of operation and special programs. Call the park office at (724) 668-2939 or e-mail keystone@dcnr.state.pa.us for information concerning other park uses. The park offers rustic cabins, and camping. For reservations for overnight stays and pavilions, call (888) 727-2757 Monday through Saturday, 7 a.m. to 5 p.m.

LINN RUN STATE PARK: GROVE RUN LOOP

▶ IN BRIEF

If you enjoy bird-watching, bring your binoculars; you may spot a sharp-shinned hawk, vultures, warblers, or thrushes. If trout fishing is more your idea of a challenge, bring your pole if you want to try your luck; the park allows angling in Linn Run.

▶ DESCRIPTION

Linn Run State Park is 612 acres of lush second-growth forest. When it was first purchased by the Commonwealth of Pennsylvania in 1909, it was known as a wasteland, cluttered with cast-off tree tops and devastated by the many severe wildfires caused by the railroad that once hauled timber and other products through the landscape. There is little evidence of that history left today. Traces of the old railroad can be seen along Fish Run Trail (which connects to Grove Run Trail and does not loop; it is not a part of this hike.)

You'll begin with a walk through the Grove Run picnic area to the trailhead; there is a sign. A few steps in on this level start, look up and to the right to see the remnants of a fireplace. Ahead, light-blue blazes mark the way. Although there is no marker on the trail to indicate a boundary, most of this hike actually takes place in Forbes State Forest. The trail exits Linn Run State Park in less than a quarter mile.

At 0.25 miles begin a slight incline that continues to take you up, with dips and flat portions,

▶ DIRECTIONS

From Pittsburgh, take Interstate 376 East and enter the Pennsylvania Turnpike I-76 East (toll road). Take Exit 89, Irwin, to PA 30 East; follow 2 miles past Ligonier. At the intersection of PA 381, turn south for 2.9 miles and then left on Linn Run Road at the small town of Rector. Travel on Linn Run Road 3 miles to reach the parking area.

❶ KEY AT-A-GLANCE INFORMATION

LENGTH: 4 miles

CONFIGURATION: Loop

DIFFICULTY: Moderate

SCENERY: Grove Run, Linn Run, and a variety of hardwoods

EXPOSURE: Sunny when the leaves are down

TRAFFIC: Light

TRAIL SURFACE: Dirt and rock

HIKING TIME: 2.5 hours

ACCESS: Open year-round

MAPS: Available at the Forbes District Forest office on US 30 in Laughlintown, (724) 238-1200, or at the park office on Linn Run Road, located approximately 0.5 miles west of the trailhead; maps in PDF format are also available online via the Pennsylvania Department of Conservation and Natural Resources Web site, **www.dcnr.state.pa.us;** USGS Ligonier

FACILITIES: Restrooms, picnic tables, drinking water, and a playground within the picnic area surrounding the trailhead. Cabins and picnic pavilions may be reserved by calling (888) 727-2757 7 a.m.–5 p.m., Monday–Saturday, or by visiting **www.visitpa.com.**

SPECIAL COMMENTS: The trail becomes very narrow in spots while traversing a hillside. Hiking poles might be helpful, and long pants are recommended due to patches of greenbrier.

Linn Run State Park: Grove Run Loop

UTM Zone (WGS84)   17T

Easting   651051

Northing   4446128

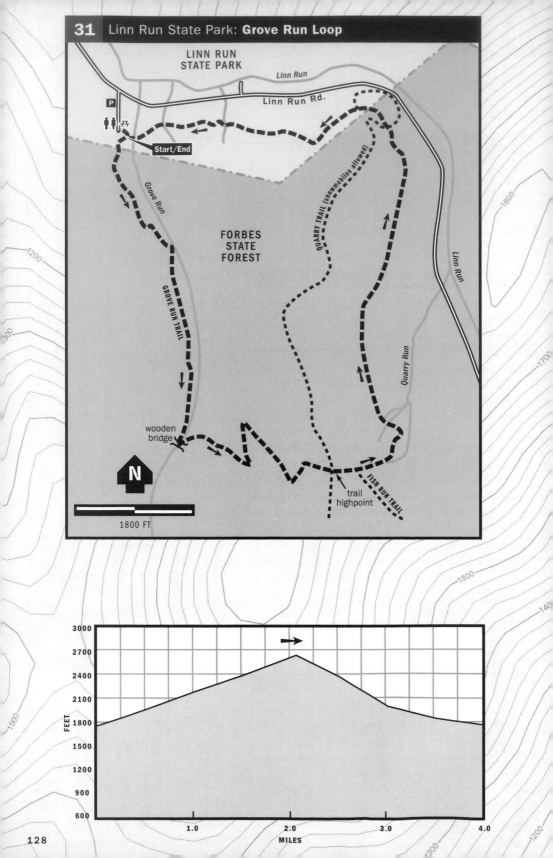

LINN RUN
STATE PARK

Linn Run

Linn Run Rd.

P

Start/End

Grove Run

FORBES
STATE
FOREST

GROVE RUN TRAIL

QUARRY TRAIL (snowmobiles allowed)

Linn Run

Quarry Run

wooden
bridge

N

1800 FT

trail
highpoint

FISH RUN TRAIL

3000
2700
2400
2100
1800
1500
1200
900
600

FEET

1.0   2.0   3.0   4.0

MILES

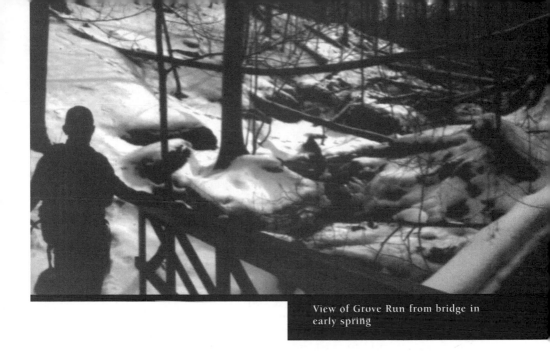

View of Grove Run from bridge in early spring

to an elevation of 2,665 feet. The trail climbs very gradually until the first mile is completed as it is tucked between two ridges following Grove Run, a tributary to Linn Run that sometimes flows underground through this lower section. At 1 mile, there is a wooden bridge crossing over Grove Run, allowing a view of the water rushing over and between the rocks.

The sharp left turn at the end of the bridge marks the trail's departure from the run. Now it's time to pump your quadriceps and gluteus muscles. At the point where the trail dips and is about to wrap toward the right, you can look down and see a branch of water feeding into Grove Run. There are many small runoffs throughout this hike, at least during the time of year I visited (April).

Although it is still a bit early for most spring blossoms, hiking on the still-cold days of early spring treated me to small dripping icicles hanging over some of the rocks near runoffs. Every time of year has something to offer anyone willing to venture a little into the woods. At 1.25 miles, cross over one of the larger runoffs. Just after this point, multitudes of greenbrier line the trail. The trail becomes pretty rocky here and stands of hardwoods including beech; striped, red, and sugar maples; and basswood command the view. Although the greenbrier may not be pleasant for a hiker who diverges from the trail, it is a good food source for bear, deer, turkey, and other animals.

At 1.6 miles you'll see a weatherworn, illegible sign. Here, the trail veers left, and you are now walking along the ridge you were looking at to the left of the trail when hiking in along Grove Run. At 1.8 miles, you'll arrive at an intersection with the Quarry Trail—a designated snowmobile trail that is part of the Laurel Highlands snowmobile-trail system. This is the highest point of the hike and where you will notice a break in the greenbrier. Most of the remainder of the hike is downhill. In less than a tenth of a mile come to and bypass the turnoff for Fish Run Trail. At just about 2 miles, cross over Quarry Run.

As you descend and veer left, look to your right for the half-cut log alongside the trail with the water of Quarry Run flowing over its length. After this, the grade of the descent becomes a bit higher and Quarry Run heads down the hill on the right. The descent is not very steep, but be careful; the trail becomes fairly narrow and runs along the outside of the hill. With snow still on the trail during my trip, it occurred to me that hiking poles would have been wise as there are several spots to negotiate down tree roots or over rocks and the trail is a little slanted.

At 2.7 miles, carefully work your way over rocks and roots as you veer right with the trail. Now you are nearing Linn Run, which becomes obvious with the sound of rushing water. At 3 miles, there is break enough in the trees for a view of the run just beyond Linn Run Road. Soon you'll cross over Quarry Trail again; there is a large sign indicating where to pick up Grove Run Trail directly across it. Shortly after this trail crossing, you'll reenter Linn Run State Park and the Quarry Trail meets the Grove Run Trail again on the right. Continue on Grove Run to traverse left across the hillside and complete the loop.

At 3.6 miles and again at 3.8 miles, cross over two larger water runoffs and at 3.9 miles use the rocks to cross Grove Run once more. If the water is high, you can go downstream and use the road bridge instead. The trail ends back in the Grove Run picnic area.

▶ NEARBY ATTRACTIONS

Many other natural areas surround this state park. The closest hikes included in this book are those on Laurel Summit (hikes 26, 27, and 28). For something short, try Powdermill Nature Reserve (hike 32).

POWDERMILL NATURE RESERVE TOUR

▶ IN BRIEF

This is an especially enjoyable place for children who are fascinated with the animals (not live) on display within the Nimick Nature Center as well as the many butterflies at the butterfly bush on the side of the building.

▶ DESCRIPTION

The Powdermill Nature Reserve is a research station of Carnegie Museum that was established in 1956, when General and Mrs. Richard K. Mellon and Mr. and Mrs. Alan M. Scaife presented 1,160 acres of land to the Carnegie Institute for the use of its Natural History Museum. Over the next several years, additional acreage was added through other gifts, providing the reserve with more than 2,200 acres of woodlands, streams, open fields, ponds, and thickets.

The Natural History Museum uses the reserve to study changes in bird and mammal life, as well as annual changes in weather conditions. Powdermill Run is one of the few unpolluted streams available for ongoing studies of aquatic life. To study avian migration, survival, and other factors in avian population, a bird-banding program was started in 1961 at the Powdermill Avian Research Center (located elsewhere on the reserve). The center is not open for random public tours but can be contacted concerning visits or volunteerism (see Special Comments at right). The bird-banding program is the longest-running continuous study of its kind in the country.

ℹ KEY AT-A-GLANCE INFORMATION

LENGTH: 0.5 miles

CONFIGURATION: Loop

DIFFICULTY: Easy

SCENERY: Nature center, butterflies, deciduous woodlands, stream

EXPOSURE: Mostly shaded

TRAFFIC: Light

TRAIL SURFACE: Dirt

HIKING TIME: 20 minutes

ACCESS: Trail open year-round; see Special Comments below for nature center hours

MAPS: A map with an interpretive guide is available at the Nimick Nature Center; USGS Stahlstown

FACILITIES: Restrooms are available at the nature center

SPECIAL COMMENTS: If you'd like, pick up an interpretive guide and map for the trail and a guide for the herbal garden at the Nimick Nature Center.
  The Nimick Nature Center is open April–October, Wednesday–Saturday, 8 a.m.–4 p.m., Sundays 12–5 p.m.; and November–March, Monday–Friday, 8 a.m.–4 p.m., and Sundays during program times. For information about the center's various programs, call (724) 593-6405 or visit **www.powdermill.org.** To learn more about the Powdermill Avian Research Center, visit the Web site above, or call (724) 593-4070 to learn about volunteer opportunities.

▶ DIRECTIONS

From Pittsburgh, take Interstate 376 East and enter the Pennsylvania Turnpike I-76 East (toll road). Take Exit 91, Ligonier–Uniontown. Turn left onto PA 31 East. Drive 2.8 miles and turn left onto PA 381 North. Drive 6.4 miles and turn left into the parking area for Powdermill Nature Reserve.

Powdermill Nature Reserve Tour

UTM Zone (WGS84)   17T

Easting   647175

Northing   4446972

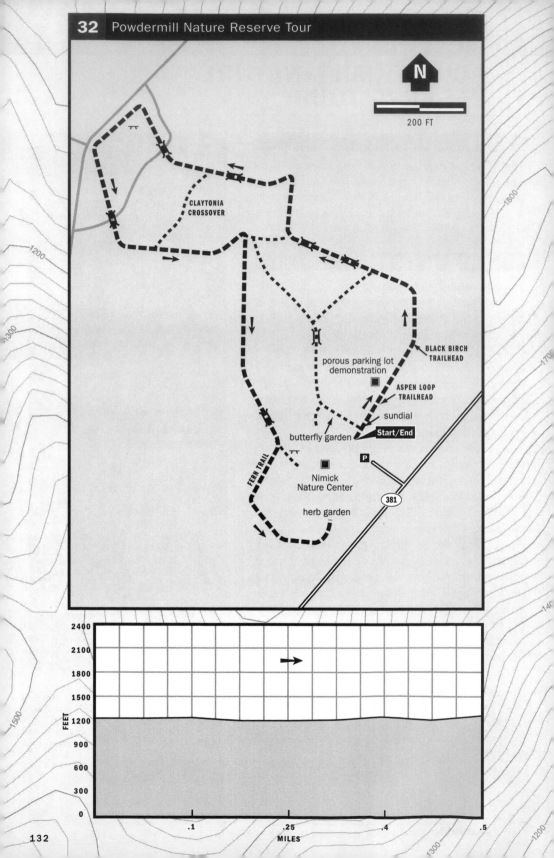

N

200 FT

CLAYTONIA
CROSSOVER

porous parking lot
demonstration

BLACK BIRCH
TRAILHEAD

ASPEN LOOP
TRAILHEAD

sundial

butterfly garden

Start/End

FERN TRAIL

P

Nimick
Nature Center

381

herb garden

FEET

2400
2100
1800
1500
1200
900
600
300
0

.1 .25 .4 .5
MILES

While the reserve provides a place for long-term research of the life histories, behaviors, and ecological relationships of nonhuman natural populations, it also serves as a haven for these plants and animals, and for human visitors as well.

After enjoying a tour of the Nimick Nature Center (be sure to watch the video), begin this hike by walking to the edge of the parking lot, away from the nature center and toward the porous parking lot demonstration (on the left past the butterfly garden); stop and read the information plaque. The parking lot demonstration shows how the surface can be reinforced to support the weight of vehicles while also using porous materials to avoid polluted water from running off unfiltered and into our waterways. This certainly appears to be a more intelligent design, as well as being more aesthetically pleasing than conventional parking lots.

When you've finished reading, continue past the lot to the Black Birch Trail sign, and turn left onto the trail. During this hike you'll see big-toothed aspen, ironwood, black birch, black cherry, tulip, and white and red oak trees; you'll also notice that some of the trees along the trail are labeled. Very quickly arrive at a junction; pass the connector trail on the left and continue straight to walk down the trail steps and cross the short bridge.

Pass the left-hand turn for the Claytonia Crossover, and continue straight, to cross a second short bridge. In this area find skunk cabbage and an enormous American beech tree. At 0.22 miles, a stream that appears to be a runoff from Powdermill Run begins to parallel the trail on the right. If you'd like, take a seat on the bench around the bend and enjoy the sound of the water as it is near to the trail for about 300 feet or so. While doing so you may spot the red maple and white ash trees found in this area.

Cross another small bridge and head up the short set of trail steps. Notice the Claytonia Crossover feeding in from the left at 0.31 miles. Shortly after, the trail veers left and meets with the Aspen Loop Trail. Turn right to continue on the Black Birch Trail. Along this section of the trail find tulip and musclewood trees; also find jewelweed and ferns. A final short set of trail steps take you to the last bridge.

Just after, make a right onto the Fern Trail, which is very short but does feature several kinds of ferns (some are labeled). This trail ends at the herb garden. When you reach the garden, walk around to the trellis, which is found at the entrance nearest to the nature center. Here, a map is posted that depicts the layout of the garden, which contains beds for ornamental, medicinal, and culinary herbs, among others. If you haven't picked up a pamphlet about the herb garden in the nature center, you may wish to do so and learn about the many attractive herbs, both flowering and nonflowering. It can be enjoyed while resting on the bench found in the back of the garden. The pamphlet also has a couple of recipes on the last page.

This concludes the hike. It is worthwhile to relax in the area of the nature center before driving off, though; this is a peaceful and beautiful environment. There is another bench behind the nature center, near the butterfly bush, which is located on the side of the building facing the parking lot. Just look for the butterflies. Children love to see them flit about and take in flower nectar. There is also a short walk around the butterfly garden on that side of the center, near the Aspen Loop trailhead.

▶ NEARBY ATTRACTIONS

There are many other hikes in this area. Those on Laurel Summit (hikes 26, 27, and 28) and in Linn Run State Park (hike 31) and Kooser State Park (hike 53) are the closest. There are also many eating establishments and shops along PA 31.

TWIN LAKES PARK: LOOP THE LAKES

KEY AT-A-GLANCE INFORMATION

LENGTH: 2.3 miles

CONFIGURATION: Loop

DIFFICULTY: Easy

SCENERY: Lakes, ducks and geese, variety of deciduous and conifer trees, garden and wildflowers, sculpture and two memorials

EXPOSURE: Half shaded, half exposed

TRAFFIC: Moderate

TRAIL SURFACE: Fitted brick

HIKING TIME: 1.25 hours

ACCESS: Park hours are 9 a.m.–sunset

MAPS: Available at the boat and ski concession or by calling the Westmoreland County Bureau of Parks and Recreation at (724) 830-3950 or (800) 442-6926 ext. 3950; USGS Latrobe

FACILITIES: Restrooms and drinking water throughout the park, picnic pavilions, boat and ski concession, food and vending machines at concession, fishing, World Trail fitness route (Upper Lake), and playgrounds

SPECIAL COMMENTS: This path is suitable for walking, pushing a stroller or wheelchair, jogging, biking, or skiing. Loop one lake or both.

Twin Lakes Park: Loop the Lakes

UTM Zone (WGS84)   17T

Easting   629553

Northing   4464247

IN BRIEF

This is an extremely well-maintained park with pleasant views of the lake during most of the walk. A stroll around the lakes' perimeters can be a wonderful way to end a stressful day, or begin a peaceful one.

DESCRIPTION

From the upper parking lot, walk down the park road. If you wish to add a fitness workout, the World Trail begins at the first workout area on the right along this road and continues on the Upper Lake portion of the hike.

At the end of the road turn right on the fitted brick pathway to loop the lakes counterclockwise. The rustic and well-kept pavilion and playground facilities, combined with a grand view of the upper lake and the deciduous and conifer trees that greet your entrance, are a preview of this nicely planned and maintained park. Follow this mixed deciduous and conifer woodland along the right-hand edge of the trail, and you'll notice the stand of pines ahead that line your path to the dam. You quickly arrive at the dam dividing the two lakes. This hike is described by continuing on this side of the lakes and veering right to continue along the path leading to the lower lake. If you wish to reduce the mileage, you can cross the dam and loop just the upper lake by turning left at the end of the dam.

DIRECTIONS

From Pittsburgh, take Interstate 376 East, enter Pennsylvania Turnpike I-76 East (toll road), and take Exit 89, Irwin. Follow US 30 East toward Greensburg 10.8 miles; turn left onto Donohoe Road. At 0.1 mile, curve right to follow Donohoe Road for 2.2 miles (through a light and two stop signs). Turn left into parking lot for Twin Lakes Park. Handicap-accessible parking is available in lower lot (drive down park road and turn left.)

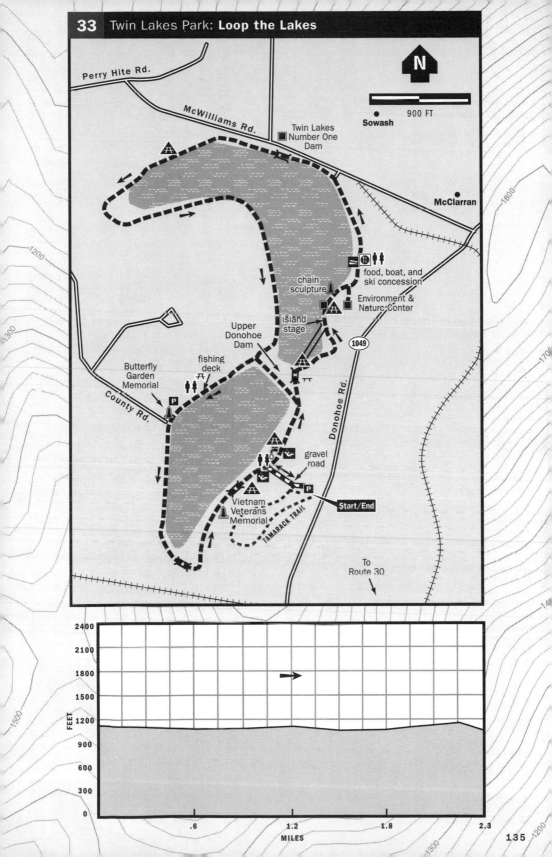

Perry Hite Rd.

McWilliams Rd.

N

900 FT

Sowash

Twin Lakes
Number One
Dam

McClarran

1800

1200

chain
sculpture

food, boat, and
ski concession

1700

island
stage

Environment &
Nature Center

1049

Upper
Donohoe
Dam

fishing
deck

Butterfly
Garden
Memorial

County Rd.

Donohoe Rd.

P

gravel
road

Vietnam
Veterans
Memorial

P

Start/End

TAMARACK TRAIL

To
Route 30

1500

1400

1300

1200

FEET				
2400				
2100				
1800		→		
1500				
1200				
900				
600				
300				
0	.6	1.2	1.8	2.3

MILES

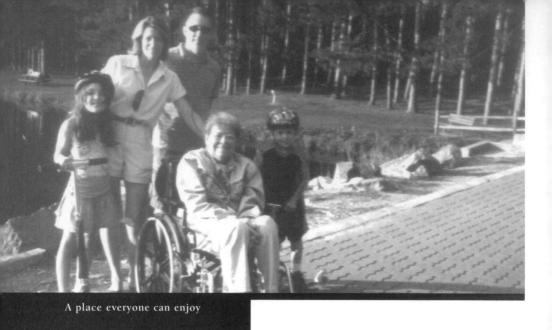

A place everyone can enjoy

To follow this description, veer right, walking downhill on the path and over a small bridge to reach the lower lake's edge. Just after, at 0.2 miles, you can diverge left to go out and visit the pavilion over the lake and then, if you wish, use the bridge from the pavilion to meet up with the main path again at 0.32 miles or stay right. I stayed right, walking through a section with planted rhododendrons and then over a raised wooden walkway through marshlands with a pretty view of pussy willows, milkweed, and a weeping willow hanging its branches close to the rails. There are pines, mature maples, young oaks, and daylilies, among other trees and flowers, following the marshland.

At 0.37 miles you can't miss the Lower Lake Island Stage where the park hosts a free Sunday concert series every summer. When not protecting musicians from rain or sun, its cover is used by others for comfortable fishing. Following this is a sculpture made of chain shaped into human form; called *La Familia,* it honors the Westmoreland Arts and Heritage Festival, which is also hosted at Twin Lakes Park. The festival has been named one of the top 100 events in North America. Along this section of the lake, flowerbeds have been planted, adding to the pleasant scenery. After curving right with the lake, find the Environment and Nature Center up a pathway on the right. The rough-hewn plank building fits in beautifully with the park's environment.

Continuing along the edge of the lower lake, where ducks enjoy hanging out, the path leads directly to the park's concession area, where you can rent canoes, paddle boats, and row boats in the warm months and cross-country skis in the cold ones. A snack bar is inside and vending machines are outside on the right of the building.

After passing the concession, continue along the lake's edge and pass the walkway at 0.54 miles to stay close to the lake. At 0.66 miles, pass another walkway; this one, although laid in brick the same as the main walkway, just leads to the road, runs along its side a short way, and then stops. The lower lake is in full view around this northern perimeter, and there are many benches to sit on and enjoy if you like. As you round the end of the lake, find what looks like the northern version of the catalpa tree on the right.

By this time you'll have noticed how many people enjoy fishing in these lakes. A friendly fisherman told me that bass, perch, bluegill, trout, sunfish, and many other species swim the waters of these lakes—and he'd already caught one for dinner. The Pennsylvania Fish and Boat Commission stocks the lakes, even in winter to the delight of ice-fishing enthusiasts.

After about 1 mile, the trail leaves the immediate side of the lake and the typical growth of marshland is found again along the left-hand side of the path, followed by an array of wildflowers. Among these are purple aster, common sunflower (tall plant but miniature flower compared with the domesticated form), and jewelweed. Also find Solomon's seal, ferns, and some mosses. The trees include black locust, striped maple, black maple, shagbark hickory, and oaks. After the split-rail fencing stops and you reach 1.3 miles, the lake becomes more visible through the trees as the trail travels close to its side again.

There is a very slight uphill grade as you approach the southern end of the lower lake and reach the dam and the upper lake at 1.64 miles. Again, you can reduce the mileage by crossing the dam, turning right, and following the path back to the parking lot. To complete the Upper Lake Loop, continue straight. This lake is smaller than the lower lake but also very pleasant to circle and it has other things to offer. At 1.74 miles, notice the picnic and fishing deck that is built over the water; these platforms and pavilions that place one over the water seem a wonderful idea, and many people use them.

In this area, you'll see Norway spruce and other conifers mixed in with the deciduous trees. After passing a parking lot on the right, find the Butterfly Garden Memorial at 1.81 miles. Leave the path to take a look at this touching memorial dedicated by Compassionate Friends to parents who have lost children. The use of butterflies to symbolize rebirth is an ancient custom that is continued in this pleasant garden. Back on the trail are maple and tulip trees.

As you round the southern end of the upper lake, the trail leads a bit away from the lake's edge at about 2 miles. Just after you walk over a wooden bridge the trail makes a sharp turn north and shortly, at 2.2 miles, you'll arrive at a chiseled-granite Vietnam Veterans Memorial dedicated to those from Westmoreland County who served. When you are ready to leave the memorial and have returned to the path, you'll pass a playground for small children and cross a shorter wooden bridge. Pass another playground consisting mainly of slides and round it with the walkway to complete the trail. Walk back up the road and to your car.

▶ NEARBY ATTRACTIONS

You can hike the Tamarack Trail, a half-mile learning loop through the woods, which begins at the edge of the parking lot on the left-hand side of the park's road entrance. For information on the Sunday concert series and the use of park facilities, call the Westmoreland County Bureau of Parks and Recreation at (724) 830-3950 or (800) 442-6926, x3950. To learn about the Westmoreland County Arts and Heritage Festival, call (724) 834-7474 or visit **www.artsandheritage.com.** Call the concession for seasonal hours and rates for boat or ski rental at (724) 832-7735. For children's camp and family programs held by the Environment and Nature Center visit **www.co.westmore land.pa.us** or call (724) 830-3962.

LAWRENCE, BEAVER, AND WASHINGTON COUNTIES

McCONNELLS MILL: ALPHA PASS TO KILDOO LOOP

KEY AT-A-GLANCE INFORMATION

LENGTH: 3.4 miles

CONFIGURATION: Balloon

DIFFICULTY: Moderate

SCENERY: Slippery Rock creek and gorge, McConnells Mill, covered bridge, numerous waterfalls, boulders, moss, ferns, and evergreens

EXPOSURE: Mostly shaded

TRAFFIC: Busy near the mill, light farther away

TRAIL SURFACE: Dirt, sometimes very rocky

HIKING TIME: 2 hours

ACCESS: Open year-round, except if too icy or washed out in winter

MAPS: Available at the park office (see Nearby Attractions following the Description for phone numbers); PDF maps are also available online via the Pennsylvania Department of Conservation and Natural Resources Web site, **www.dcnr.state.pa.us;** USGS Portersville

FACILITIES: Restrooms, picnic areas, playground, first aid

SPECIAL COMMENTS: This hike is abundant in beauty and combines the Alpha Pass and Kildoo trails to form a 3.4-mile loop. Wear sturdy boots or trail shoes due to the rocky terrain.

McConnells Mill:
Alpha Pass to Kildoo Loop

UTM Zone (WGS84)   17T

Easting   569939

Northing   4534646

IN BRIEF

If you want to shorten the hike, park near McConnells Mill either at the mill, which is very limited, or in the parking area above it on McConnells Mill Road. From the mill, visitors of all ages and abilities can enjoy both the Kildoo and Alpha Pass trails. The first 200 yards of the Kildoo Trail is paved and suitable for wheelchairs and strollers. Tours of the mill are conducted (see Nearby Attractions following the Description) and worth spending the time. The covered bridge is charming, and there is an overlook of the dam.

DESCRIPTION

McConnells Mill State Park encompasses 2,546 acres of the Slippery Rock Creek Gorge. The geology of this area formed the gorge, providing the path for the 49-mile-long Slippery Rock Creek and the environment for the formation of the many waterfalls and rock outcroppings.

For the 3.4-mile loop, park at the trailhead on McConnells Mill Road. From the trailhead, follow the dirt path down the steps and become immediately immersed in the sound of water cascading over Alpha Pass. Stop at the end of the railing and turn to the right to look behind you for a view of the falls. The path veers left at the bottom of the stairs. The Alpha Pass portion of the trail is marked with blue blazes, indicating its role as part of the North Country National Scenic Trail. The rushing water of Slippery Rock Creek is heard before it is seen but soon becomes visible. In this

DIRECTIONS

From Pittsburgh, take Interstate 279 North to I-79 North. Take Exit 96, Prospect–Portersville; turn left on US 488. Turn right on US 19; follow for approximately 2.7 miles. Turn left on Johnson Road and right on McConnells Mill Road. The trailhead parking area for Alpha Pass is on the left.

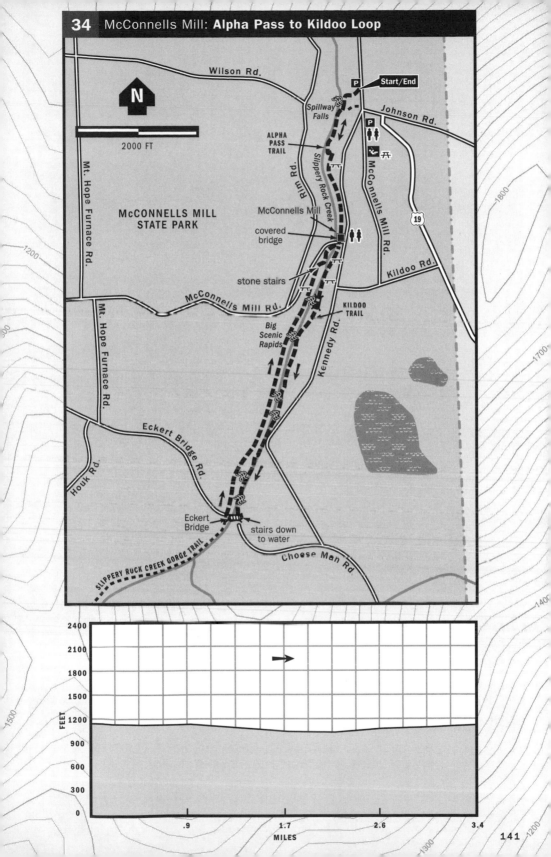

Wilson Rd.

P Start/End

Johnson Rd.

N

2000 FT

Spillway Falls

ALPHA PASS TRAIL

Rim Rd.

Slippery Rock Creek

McConnells Mill Rd.

19

McCONNELLS MILL STATE PARK

Mt. Hope Furnace Rd.

McConnells Mill

covered bridge

stone stairs

McConnells Mill Rd.

Kildoo Rd.

KILDOO TRAIL

Mt. Hope Furnace Rd.

Big Scenic Rapids

Kennedy Rd.

Eckert Bridge Rd.

Houk Rd.

Eckert Bridge

stairs down to water

Choose Man Rd.

SLIPPERY ROCK CREEK GORGE TRAIL

1800

1700

1200

1400

1300

2400
2100
1800
1500
1200
900
600
300
0

FEET

.9   1.7   2.6   3.4
MILES

1500

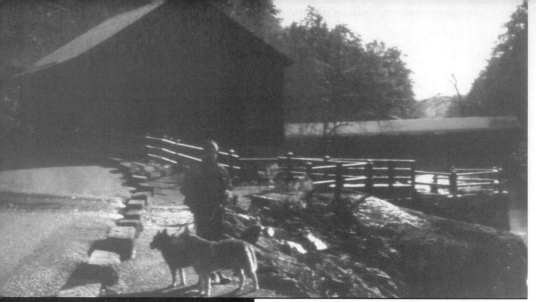

View of mill and covered bridge
at end of Alpha Pass Trail

section, the creek is about 40 to 50 feet wide and the gorge through which this creek flows is 400 feet deep.

At approximately 0.15 miles are a parking area, restrooms, picnic area, and playground up and to the left of the trail. Even this short distance in, it is already obvious that this is a very scenic hike. Evergreens are abundant, and it seems when there isn't an evergreen there's a boulder covered in moss and sprouts of ferns instead. The weaving of the trail, to and fro from the water, allows wonderful views of the creek's flow over and around the rocks.

Directly across from what should be the second bench along the trail is a huge rapid, one that would prove challenging to most boaters (note the lifesaver hanging nearby on a post). Don't forget to look inland as well and notice the gorge's landscape, such as the enormous boulder about 100 feet beyond the bench.

As you continue, the trail and the road above it come together in a V and join in the vicinity of McConnells Mill. When the trail joins the sidewalk, there are restrooms up the hill and an information board on the left. The mill, located straight ahead, is worth a visit and tour if you have the time or have timed it well. There is an informative sign just beyond the mill depicting what the typical whitewater rapid kayaker wears. If the water is up, you may see some kayakers preparing to run the rapids.

Cross the road; the trail can be hiked beginning on either side of the bridge but this description follows the mill side. The McConnells Mill covered bridge dates to 1874 and is one of two in Lawrence County; it is a registered National Historic Landmark. Don't be concerned about missing a walk through the bridge, as you will cross it at the end of the Kildoo Trail.

To start the Kildoo Trail portion of the hike, pass the bridge and pick up the trail at the trailhead, which is marked with a sign. This trail is paved for the first 200 feet, providing access for those who may have a more difficult time on rockier sections. The Kildoo Trail runs very close to the water with open views and is quite pleasant. If you are hiking after a heavy rain or snowfall with some runoff (as I was), the water will be high and moving very fast. This portion of the trail is easy enough for small children, but handholding is recommended. You'll arrive at another bench at about 0.8 miles, across from more wildly churning rapids. Soon, stop in the center of the 15-foot wooden bridge that crosses the pretty waterfall cascading from Kildoo Run. Looking up for its source will allow you to spot the blue Kildoo Bridge above.

Beyond this point the trail winds up and down for a bit and then meanders back close to the water. It is extremely easy to follow, and as its width and height vary, so does the scenery. At about 1.2 miles, you'll come to a large flat rock overlooking the water. This makes a great spot to take a break in the sun. For lunch, though, you may wish to wait to reach the larger rock outcropping in just another 0.3 miles.

At 1.3 miles is an area that is sometimes washed out by heavy rains. Almost immediately after, look for another large waterfall. The trail's surface here is rock, so if you've worn your sturdy trail shoes or boots you'll be happy; if not, watch your ankles. At 1.5 miles is a huge flat-rock outcropping that makes for an ideal lunch spot. The view is open across the water, and the return trail for this loop can be seen on the other side. (When I was there it was several feet underwater.) Not far beyond this, you'll come to a waterfall over a huge flat rock jutting out into the water; it is about 50 feet from where you stand on the trail.

Once past the waterfall, Eckert Bridge comes into view; on the near side of the bridge are steps that lead down to the water. Cross the bridge and turn right to pick up the trail on the other side of Slippery Rock Creek (turning left at the end of the bridge leads to Slippery Rock Gorge Trail, hike 35 in this book). At 1.8 miles is another waterfall; stepping back a little allows a better view of its tall height. Shortly thereafter, cross a small beach and look for the double blue blazes at its far end, indicating that the trail veers left, slightly away from and above the water.

In the high water during my hike, the washed out section of the trail on this side was encountered at 2 miles. After a little climbing the hillside to go around it, where there is another waterfall to enjoy. Soon the trail becomes wider and there is yet another waterfall.

For almost a half mile, the hiking is a slow, steady incline. But this ends briefly across from "Island Rock," which can be seen in the middle of the creek. From this area and side of the trail, the effect of the large rocks jutting out from the other side of the creek and those in the creek becomes more apparent. Only an experienced whitewater boater would want to be out in these rapids when the water is moving fast. If you're lucky, you will be able to watch some of the kayakers make their way through them.

On the trail, you'll come to another waterfall before reaching a set of stone stairs at 2.5 miles. Notice the picturesque boulders covered with moss and fern off to the left just a tenth of a mile beyond the bottom of the steps. When the bench at 2.6 miles is reached, the red covered bridge is back in sight. Cross the bridge and turn left, passing the front of the mill to return via the Alpha Pass Trail.

▶ NEARBY ATTRACTIONS

Guided tours of the restored gristmill are conducted daily, 10:30 a.m. to 5:30 p.m., from Memorial Day through Labor Day, and off-season by appointment. Call (724) 368-8811 (McConnells Mill State Park care of Moraine State Park) for more information, or e-mail morainesp@state.pa.us. For other nearby attractions visit Moraine State Park. Other tourism opportunities can be found at **www.lawrencecounty.com/tourism** or by calling (724) 654-8408.

McCONNELLS MILL: SLIPPERY ROCK GORGE TRAIL

KEY AT-A-GLANCE INFORMATION

LENGTH: 12.4 miles (6.2 miles if using car shuttle)

CONFIGURATION: Out-and-back or car shuttle

DIFFICULTY: Moderate to difficult

SCENERY: Slippery Rock creek and gorge, old-growth oak, hemlock, maple, and beech trees

EXPOSURE: Mostly shaded

TRAFFIC: Light

TRAIL SURFACE: Dirt, sometimes very rocky

HIKING TIME: 4 hours one way

ACCESS: Open year-round

MAPS: Available at park office (see Nearby Attractions following Description for phone numbers); PDF maps are also available online via the Pennsylvania Department of Conservation and Natural Resources Web site, **www.dcnr.state.pa.us;** USGS Portersville

FACILITIES: Nearest restrooms are located at McConnells Mill.

SPECIAL COMMENTS: Wear sturdy boots or trail shoes due to the rocky terrain. Stop in and tour McConnells Mill (see Nearby Attractions).

**McConnells Mill:
Slippery Rock Gorge Trail**

UTM Zone (WGS84)   17T

Easting   563991

Northing   4531410

IN BRIEF

Bring your camera. The gorge itself, cut in just a few thousand years by the force of the meltwater of three glacial lakes, is surrounded by large trees (some virgin), waterfalls, and at least 69 species of wildflowers. Its rugged beauty made it one of the selections of trails that make up the North Country National Scenic Trail.

DESCRIPTION

McConnells Mill State Park encompasses 2,546 acres around the Slippery Rock Creek Gorge. The 930-acre Slippery Rock Creek Gorge was designated a Natural National Landmark in 1974 and became a State Park Natural Area in 1988. Through the gorge flows the 49-mile-long Slippery Rock Creek, which begets its name from a time when a Native American trail crossed the creek across a sandstone shelf over which a natural oil seep flowed. The shelf is located below the Armstrong Bridge on the southern end of the

DIRECTIONS

From Pittsburgh, take Interstate 279 North to I-79 North. Take Exit 96, Prospect–Portersville; turn left onto US 488 and right onto US 19. If hiking from Hell's Hollow, at 2.7 miles turn left on Johnson Road, drive to mill, then follow directions below. To hike from Eckert Bridge, about 0.5 miles from US 19 turn left onto Cheese Man Road; follow about 2 miles to turn right into Eckert Bridge–Breakneck Bridge parking area. If setting up a shuttle, drive back up Cheese Man Road, turn left on Kennedy Road, and follow past mill and over covered bridge. At about 1 mile from bridge, turn left on Mount Hope Furnace Road; at about 0.4 miles, turn right on Eckert Bridge Road; at about 0.2 miles, turn left on Houk Road; and at about 3.2 miles, turn left on Shaffer Road. At about 0.5 miles, turn left into parking area for Hell's Hollow.

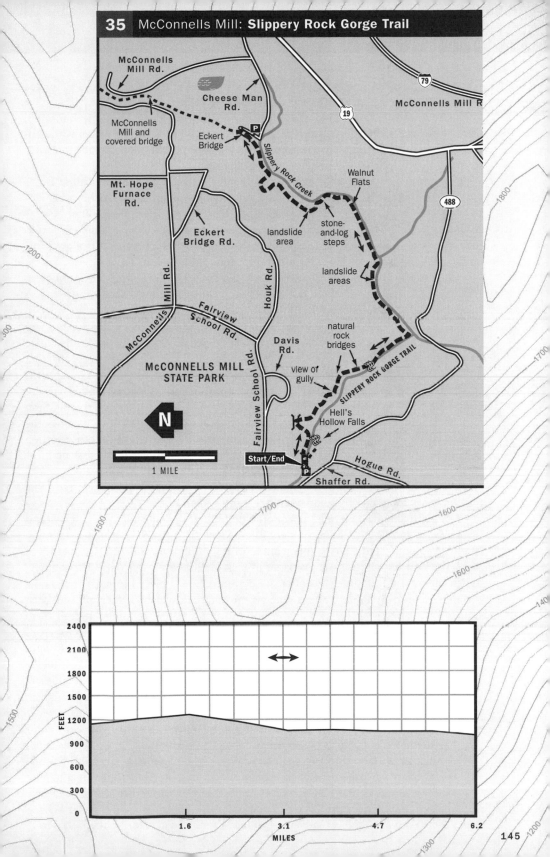

McConnells Mill Rd.

Cheese Man Rd.

79

19

McConnells Mill R

McConnells Mill and covered bridge

P

Eckert Bridge

Slippery Rock Creek

Walnut Flats

488

Mt. Hope Furnace Rd.

Eckert Bridge Rd.

landslide area

stone-and-log steps

Houk Rd.

landslide areas

McConnells Mill Rd.

Fairview School Rd.

Davis Rd.

natural rock bridges

SLIPPERY ROCK GORGE TRAIL

McCONNELLS MILL STATE PARK

Fairview School Rd.

view of gully

Hell's Hollow Falls

N

1 MILE

Start/End

P

Hogue Rd.

Shaffer Rd.

2400
2100
1800
1500
1200
900
600
300
0

FEET

1.6   3.1   4.7   6.2

MILES

gorge; and the oil seep was drained by oil wells drilled in the late 1800s, which were shortly abandoned as groundwater swiftly invaded them.

Credit for the existence of this spectacular trail goes to the Keystone Trails Trail Care Team, the Shenango Outing Club, and various Pittsburgh volunteers who conceived the trail and completed it from 1990 to 1994. Having done some trail work myself, I appreciate the difficulty of cutting this one.

The trail can be hiked from either end, but I started it at the trailhead at Hell's Hollow. The trail begins jointly with the Hell's Hollow Trail on a wide, flat path and over a small footbridge that crosses Hell Run. The Slippery Rock Gorge Trail departs to the left just before the second footbridge. If you don't mind an extra mile added to the hike, take the 0.5-mile level walk back to admire cascading Hell's Hollow Falls, enjoy a wide array of wildflowers, and look for an old lime kiln.

Upon returning to the Slippery Rock Gorge Trail, you'll find it continues to remain relatively flat until about 0.6 miles where, after crossing a small bridge over a water runoff that flows to Hell Run, a short but steep climb takes you to the ridge of the hillside. Mountain laurels and chestnut oaks can be found along this section. For almost a half mile, descend approximately 150 feet to an opening that affords a nice view of the ravine. The trail then leads through hemlocks growing so closely together and to the trail that they appear to form a tunnel. Hiking with a significant other turns this into a great spot to steal a kiss. A break in the hemlocks allows another view of the ravine before a turn in the trail at 1.4 miles leads to yet another visual treat. Stop here to take a look at the natural-rock bridge before crossing it. As you cross the bridge, take in the view of the water rushing underneath. Following is another section of hemlocks and another natural bridge where a side stream has dissolved the limestone underneath the trail. Rock outcroppings and shale are found along this section, and a waterfall on the right of the trail cascades down a steep drop in the terrain. The trail becomes more cumbersome with rocks and roots.

At approximately 2.4 miles is a short side trail on the right that you can descend for a view of Hell Run entering Slippery Rock Creek. Return to the trail and follow it carefully. You may find yourself following reroutes around blowdowns.

The trail has a lot of sun exposure in this section, even this deep in the gorge. At 2.6 miles, you'll find a series of cross-sections of trees placed to keep your boots out of the mud. At about 3 miles emerge into an area in which the trail has been somewhat washed away by mudslide. Round a narrow curve heading left, and tread carefully over water running down a shelf of rocks. Look for the blue blazes to regain the trail. Make a sharp right, dropping down to cross over more water runoff. Slippery Rock Creek comes into better view. Initially it is wide and calm, but quickly shifts into high gear as the depth changes and the water crashes around the boulders in the creek. Once again make your way over water runoff, and then you'll head back into the woods to be surrounded by mixed forest with a floor where moss-covered rocks and logs are frequent. The trail is flatter here and easier to navigate.

At 3.6 miles the land is separated in sections on the hillside, caused by more landsliding; the packed earth is literally cracked in sections horizontal to the hillside. Hikers are well rewarded for the navigation around cracks and fallen trees by the pure beauty to be found here. Be sure to avoid the thorny underbrush and look closely near the water's edge for evidence of busy beavers. At 4 miles, you'll reach Walnut Flats; there's no sign here to indicate it, but it should be evident by the rather level walk along the creek. Across the creek and up the side of the gorge is Cleland Rock. About 140,000 years ago, small Lake Prouty was formed by a glacial dam and eventually spilled over the ridge to begin the carving of the gorge. This caused Lake Watts (a smaller version is what we now know as Lake Arthur in Moraine State Park) to eventually spill into the channel. The third contributor, Lake Edmund, finally scoured the gorge to its 400-foot depth.

After another mile, the ascent away from the water is marked by a climb up stone steps supported by some logs. At the top, look for the double blue blazes marking the sharp left turn in the trail. Continue the steep ascent from Walnut Flats. The climb lets off a little where large flat boulders come into view. I also noticed a number of pretty wildflowers blooming in early spring. At about 5 miles there is a waterfall caused by water running from the top of the ridge. This kind of water flow is partially what is responsible for the number of landslides that occur along this trail, including the one you should be arriving at now, which occurred in 1990 and has devastated the hillside. Beyond it, reaching unaffected forest provides a reference for the magnitude of the damage.

Eventually you'll round a bend toward the west, and the sound of the creek greets your approach. Looking down to try and see it gives an appreciation of how far you have now climbed above it. Enjoy the brief level section, crossing a few more runoffs and switching back left and then right to reach 5.6 miles. A steep descent leads back to the creek along which most of the remainder of the hike takes place. The trail along the descent is well supported to avoid its collapse. Notice the trail construction as you descend, and also the waterfalls along the way.

A set of double blue blazes at the bottom marks an obvious but sharp left turn. Pass another waterfall and pay attention to the trail, as the many rocks and tree roots require careful footing. At almost 6 miles, flatter rocks cover the trail and it is worthwhile to look around and take in the waterfalls, conifers, and deciduous trees that complement the sound and sight of the beautiful Slippery Rock Creek. Just after, the trail veers once more away from the creek affording another viewpoint and then rejoins it again following a stone trail. Not long after being on this section, at 6.05 miles, look across the creek for an inlet to see a low but wide waterfall flowing over boulders into the creek. The trail ends as scenically as it had begun. An old millstone mounted on a pedestal marks the trailhead on the Eckert Bridge side. If you shuttled a vehicle, make the 0.4-mile walk up to the parking area. If not, take a nice break and retrace the trail back.

▶ NEARBY ATTRACTIONS

Guided tours of the restored gristmill are daily, 10:30 a.m. to 5:30 p.m., from Memorial Day through Labor Day, and off-season by appointment. Call (724) 368-8811 (McConnells Mill State Park care of Moraine State Park) for more information, or e-mail morainesp@state.pa.us. The covered bridge next to the mill is a registered National Historic Landmark. For other attractions, visit Moraine State Park. Additional tourism opportunities can found at **www.lawrencecounty.com/tourism** or by calling (724) 654-8408.

MINGO CREEK COUNTY PARK LOOP

KEY AT-A-GLANCE INFORMATION

LENGTH: 5 miles

CONFIGURATION: Loop

DIFFICULTY: Moderate to difficult

SCENERY: Covered bridge, pond, wildflowers, deciduous woods, fields, and meadows

EXPOSURE: Half shaded, half exposed

TRAFFIC: Light

TRAIL SURFACE: Dirt

HIKING TIME: 3 hours

ACCESS: Park hours are 7 a.m.–8 p.m.

MAPS: An overview map of the park's trails (not as detailed for this hike) is available by calling the Washington County Department of Parks and Recreation at (724) 228-6867; also available in PDF format at www.co.washington.pa.us; USGS Hackett

FACILITIES: Restrooms, fountains, picnic shelters, and grills are found during the first part of the hike, along the paved walkway; picnic tables are also at the pond.

SPECIAL COMMENTS: The paved portion of the walk is wheelchair and stroller accessible and leads to picnic facilities and the Ebenezer Covered Bridge.

Mingo Creek County Park Loop

UTM Zone (WGS84) 17T

Easting 580782

Northing 4449654

IN BRIEF

For a short 1.4-mile walk, follow the paved path to the Ebenezer Covered Bridge and turn around for an out-and-back. The remainder of the hike is hilly and can be muddy, but it's a good workout with pretty views.

DESCRIPTION

From the parking area, walk across the road to the beginning of the paved path, passing a picnic bench. The path veers left, paralleling Mingo Creek. You may be as fortunate as we were and see a great blue heron flying above it. There are many picnic tables, grills, fountains, pumps, and restrooms along the paved pathway. Cross Park Road at 0.26 miles, walk through a large picnic area, and pass the trail turning right toward a bridge over the creek at 0.42 miles. Through this area see conifer trees, berry bushes, wildflowers, and deciduous trees such as red maple, black cherry, crab apple, and oaks.

The paved path leads over a bridge and through a parking lot, from which you can see two small footbridges and the Ebenezer Covered Bridge at 0.7 miles. You can check out the bridge and turn around here for a 1.4-mile out-and-back hike. To continue, turn right and begin walking up the

DIRECTIONS

From Pittsburgh, take Interstate 279 South to Interstate 79 South; from the end of Fort Pitt Tunnels drive 20.8 miles and take Exit 43, Houston–Eighty-Four. Turn right on US 519 South and follow 7 miles. Turn left on US 136 East and follow 4.4 miles; turn left onto Sichi Hill (sign for Mingo Creek County Park). In 0.4 miles turn right at the park's entrance sign and turn right onto Mingo Creek Road (almost immediately). Follow it 0.2 miles and turn left into a parking area, just beyond the information board on the right.

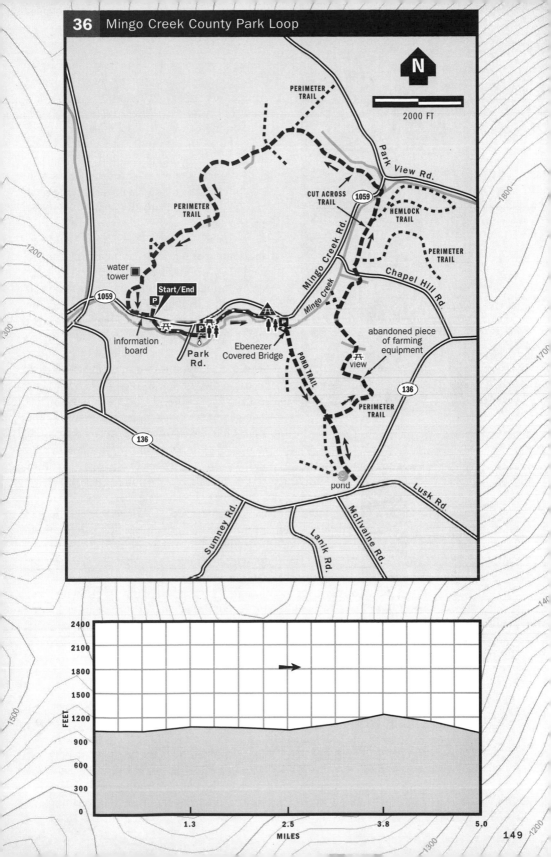

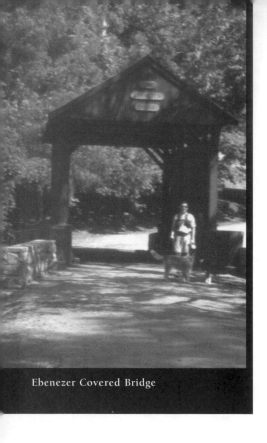
Ebenezer Covered Bridge

grown-over asphalt road on the right, directly across from the Ebenezer Covered Bridge. On the Washington County Park map this is called the Pond Trail, but it is not marked with a sign. Follow it straight uphill and come to a split in the road at 0.82 miles. Continue straight uphill and an open field comes into view shortly afterward; it was filled with goldenrod in early September and is likely sprouting all kinds of wildflowers in spring.

Black walnut, crab apple, and an abundance of black cherry trees line the old road. Pass the trail on the left at 1.1 miles and continue straight at the intersection at 1.14 miles if you want to go and see the pond; if not, turn left here. Walking straight ahead, pass the wide mowed swath on the left at 1.35 miles and turn right at the intersection at 1.39 miles for the short walk back to the pond. Be forewarned that at the time of my visit the pond was a stagnant, mostly algae-filled muck hole; nonetheless, the great blue heron was there, and it was grand to watch the bird gracefully glide and flap its large sleek body over and around the pond. When you return to the old road, turn left and retrace your steps to the intersection passed at 1.14 miles and turn right. This is part of the park's Perimeter Trail (no sign). The dirt path is narrow but the right side opens to a field; goldenrod, daisies, thistle, Queen Anne's lace, and berries grow in the ample sunlight. Shortly after, at 1.8 miles, cross open fields that appear to be former farmer's fields and follow the trail back into the woods.

Once back under the trees, faded orange blazes mark this trail. An old piece of farming equipment abandoned in the woods on the right verifies the former use of this land. Again, the woods give way to open fields where there is a picnic bench and a view. The trail continues leading into and out of the woods, at times granting wonderful views of the distant hillside, where you'll see a water tower. Trees, sky, and goldenrod fill your field of vision. Back in the woods and traveling downhill, cross a water runoff at 2.19 miles. You'll reach a Y at 2.37 miles. The left branch crosses a water runoff and then splits, likely leading back down to Mingo Creek. Take the right branch toward the field.

The trail leads into the woods again, where you cross a water runoff and then Chapel Hill Road. Walk left on the other side to pick up the trail and reenter the woods. Not long after, the trail splits. Go straight, using what is called the Cut Across Trail on the park map (the Perimeter Trail continues with the right-hand branch). There are no signs but the Cut Across Trail is eventually blazed in blue. Look for some very large old oak, shagbark and shellbark hickory, and American beech trees in this area. At 2.83 miles a hikers-only trail, called the Hemlock Trail on the park map, branches off to the right. The trail name is not displayed but signs on a post indicate that bikes and horses are not permitted. It is a loop that returns to this spot (according to the park map) if you want extra mileage. Otherwise, continue straight. Shortly after, at 2.9 miles, is another path leading straight into an open field; follow the main trail as it veers right. There are faded blue blazes after this. Cross a water runoff just after turning.

This leads out into an open field where you can see a road (SR 1059/Mingo Creek Road), and blue blazes leading diagonally right to cross Mingo Creek and SR 1059. Three blue circles on a tree across the road mark where the trail continues on the other side. There is a Y almost immediately; take the left branch uphill (the right just loops around to meet the left branch). There are a couple of places where short diversions branch off and meet up with the main trail as you make your way up the hill. Soon you'll see a rope swing down the hill over the gully on the right at 3.25 miles. You don't have to go down there to use it though—there are some great sturdy vines hanging from an enormous old maple; they are able to hold adults for a swing right next to the trail on a level section at 3.32 miles. We had great fun testing it.

You'll pass a narrow trail on the right when you reach a brief break in the woods and the top of the hill at 3.46 miles. Here the trail splits again. Straight is less obvious, if you see it and do walk straight, though, turn left at the next junction to go downhill and south. (If you miss the path straight ahead and turn right, you'll come to a T where a large blue arrow is painted on a tree pointing right; turn left to wind back around to where you can see the way you came up and veer right, heading downhill and south.)

Continue downhill and at 3.62 miles reach a T. Turn left, following the orange arrow. You are now back on the Perimeter Trail. Walk along the dirt road briefly until you see the break in the woods with an orange arrow pointing right at 3.73 miles. Turn right and continue downhill, following the wide path to cross a water runoff. After the crossing, head back uphill to reach the top at 4.03 miles. Along the way you'll find American bladdernut, pin oak, striped maple, and sassafras trees. The trail travels up and down for the next half mile, but the grades are gentler. Cross another water runoff and go straight through the intersection at 4.43 miles. At 4.53 and 4.6 miles, go straight again, passing the left branches (the first may be a shortcut to the second). Come out of the woods at 4.72 miles and walk with the woods to your right and a pleasant open meadow to the left.

On the way downhill, pass a water tower and long-needled pines, and walk once more through the woods. When you come out of the woods again, your vehicle will be within sight. Walk down to the road and turn left to reach it.

▶ NEARBY ATTRACTIONS

Learn about the Annual Covered Bridge Festival, held in September that includes eight bridges in Washington and Greene counties, including the two in Mingo Creek County Park at **www.washpatourism.org** or call (800) 531-4114. Other activities within Washington County can be found at **www.washwow.com** or by calling (866) 927-4969.

RACCOON CREEK STATE PARK: LAKE-FOREST LOOP

KEY AT-A-GLANCE INFORMATION

LENGTH: 4 miles

CONFIGURATION: Loop

DIFFICULTY: Easy to moderate

SCENERY: Mixed deciduous-and-conifer forest, wildflowers, valley fields, Raccoon Lake

EXPOSURE: Mostly shaded

TRAFFIC: Light

TRAIL SURFACE: Short gravel and pavement section, mostly dirt

HIKING TIME: 2 hours

ACCESS: Open year-round

MAPS: Available at park office (call [724] 899-2200 or see Directions); PDF maps are also available online via the Pennsylvania Department of Conservation and Natural Resources Web site, **www.dcnr .state.pa.us;** USGS Hookstown

FACILITIES: Portable toilet and water fountain in the trailhead parking area; restrooms, water fountain, and vending machines are located at the park office (see Nearby Attractions following the Description for other park facilities).

SPECIAL COMMENTS: Swimming, fishing, and boating are permitted in Raccoon Lake. Concession and changing facilities are available at the public beach. Boat rentals are available, too. (See Nearby Attractions for more information.)

IN BRIEF

This loop explores both lakeside and upland-forest habitats. On a hot day, the trail near the lake can be muggy and a little buggy; the second portion has some hill climbing. Bring your swimsuit for a refreshing dip in the lake after the hike.

DESCRIPTION

At 7,572 acres, Raccoon Creek State Park is one of the largest state parks in Pennsylvania. It began in the 1930s as the Raccoon Creek National Recreation Demonstration Area, created by the National Park Service and developed with sweat equity from the Civilian Conservation Corps (CCC) and the Works Progress Administration (WPA). These groups built some of the still-existing recreation facilities and provided conservation planning and labor.

Raccoon Creek State Park became an official state park in 1945 and has continued to develop from its roots to include the 101-acre Raccoon Lake; an 800-foot-long beach with changing, restroom, shower, first aid, and concession facilities; cabins; Lakeside Lodge; a recreation hall; campsites; and numerous picnic areas and pavilions.

This hike provides a short tour of both the lakeside and forested areas of the park. To begin, turn right from the parking area and walk up the road a short distance to the trailhead entrance on the left; it is distinguished by a small footbridge crossing Traverse Creek and a sign on the other

---

Raccoon Creek State Park: Lake-Forest Loop

UTM Zone (WGS84)   17T

Easting   548943

Northing   4483607

DIRECTIONS

From Pittsburgh, take Interstate 279 South to US 22–30 West (roads split; continue on US 22 West); follow 14.1 miles. Take the exit for PA 18 North; follow 5.9 miles. To go directly to trailhead, make a right, follow 0.1 mile, and turn right into the roadside parking area. For the park office, pass the right-hand turn and turn left in 0.1 mile.

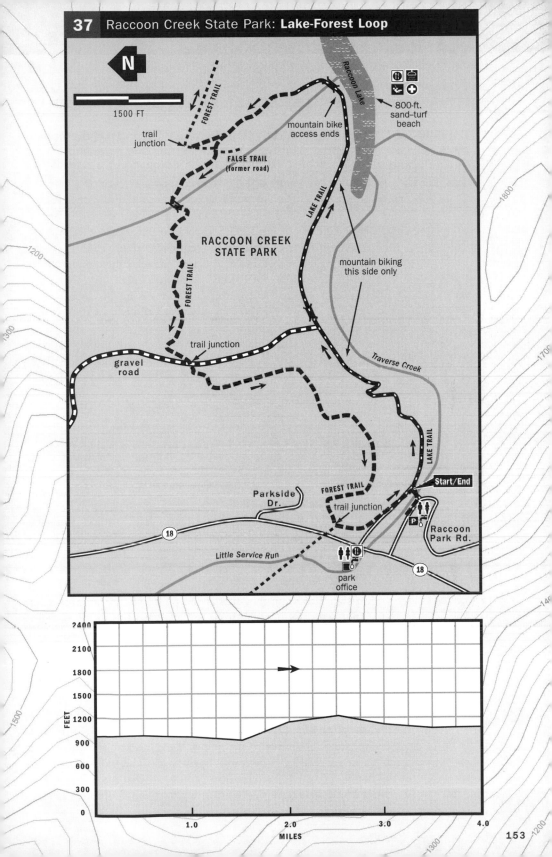

N

1500 FT

FOREST TRAIL

trail
junction

FALSE TRAIL
(former road)

mountain bike
access ends

Raccoon Lake

800-ft.
sand–turf
beach

**RACCOON CREEK
STATE PARK**

LAKE TRAIL

FOREST TRAIL

mountain biking
this side only

gravel
road

trail junction

Traverse Creek

FOREST TRAIL

trail junction

Parkside
Dr.

LAKE TRAIL

Start/End

P

Raccoon
Park Rd.

18

Little Service Run

park
office

18

2400
2100
1800
1500
1200
900
600
300
0

FEET

1.0   2.0   3.0   4.0
MILES

side for the Lake Trail. After crossing the footbridge, turn right on the blue-blazed Lake Trail, which begins on a former road. (Biking is allowed on this wide path, but only up to the lake.)

During the 1800s, this area was known as Traverse Valley and was the location of several pioneer homesteads and gristmills. Both the trail and surrounding flora allude to the area's history. The trail is wide, flat, and roadlike, and its rather level surface had been paved at some point. Brief paved sections are revealed where the plant life has not yet overtaken it. The surrounding forest is thin and mainly young. In the beginning portion of the hike, there are many flowering trees and shrubs, including pie cherry, growing close to trailside. Shortly into the hike, a rock wall on the left, still in good repair, provides evidence of someone's hard labor.

As you continue, brief glimpses of Traverse Creek can be caught periodically and at about 0.65 miles the terrain on both sides of the trail opens out, allowing a better chance of spotting various birds and butterflies. Flowers in this area include phlox and dame's rocket. You can tell the difference between the two by the number of petals—dame's rocket has only four; phlox five.

Norway pines and sycamores also grow here. Sycamores are known for pioneering on exposed sites. Its wood is used for many functions such as furniture parts, flooring, butcher blocks, and even particleboard. The huge hollow trunks of former giant Norways are often homes for many animals and birds.

At 0.83 miles, you'll cross a short bridge over a feeder stream and perhaps spot cream violets. Don't miss the pretty sight of water trickling down the hillside on the left, either. Afterward, find mayapples and ferns on the right. The birdsong is noticeable and interrupted with the sounds of ducks and geese floating up from the water. Trees to be seen in the area include maples, hickories, and oaks, including the large swamp white oak. With slight inclines, the trail rises above Traverse Creek. Enjoy pleasant hiking above its edge before it gradually drops back down to reach Raccoon Lake. During the warm months, a view of the lake is preceded by voices from the beach. By 1.25 miles the trail runs directly along the lake's edge and the beach across the water comes into view.

Along the lake's edge, you'll see black locust and American bladdernut trees and bluets, tiny, beautiful, delicate bluish violet–colored flowers. At 1.47 miles, cross a wooden bridge with a sign indicating that this is the point where trail access for bicycles ends and the trail veers north, away from the lake. For the next half mile, hike a steady incline into a forestland ecosystem. Along the way, find purple and cream violets, whirled milkwort, moss, mountain laurel, and a large variety of trees including blue beech, horse chestnut, and ironwood.

The junction that marks the end of the Lake Trail and a T with the Forest Trail is reached at 1.92 miles. There is a sign indicating that the Forest Trail travels both right and left. Turn left on the white-blazed Forest Trail (turning right takes you to the dam for Raccoon Lake and the eastern end of the Forest Trail). This is a sharp U-turn that leads down the hillside you just climbed. The yellow hairy hawkweed (with many spiked flower petals on a long stalk) can be found in this area. The trail switchbacks down; watch for the double blazes. At 2 miles, don't go left at what looks like a false trail and may be part of an old road that is still struggling to retain its former identity.

Cross a short wooden bridge at 2.2 miles and veer left with the trail, beginning another climb. Skunk cabbage is near this feeder stream and soon knee- and hip-high ferns begin to appear in abundance, growing close to the trail and sometimes stretching into the forest as far as the eye can see; white asterlike flowers dot the floor in spots.

At 2.7 miles, don't miss the group of three large red oaks to the left of the trail as you begin another descent. Veer left with the trail at 2.75 miles and reach a junction at 2.76 miles where two posts indicate that the Forest Trail continues straight. The intersecting trail appears to be a former access road. You'll also notice the young swamp white oaks at the turn.

Shortly after, cross two small feeder streams and begin using switchbacks to climb the other side. When the trail becomes more level again, fields of fern appear once more, intermixed with tall grasses and other undergrowth. I was surprised to find myself suddenly immersed in a pine forest at about 3.17 miles. It only lasted for approximately 200 feet, but afterward I was treated to blue-eyed grasses—these small, six-petal violet or bluish flowers grow atop stalks surrounded by grasslike leaves; underneath the flower a small pod can be found.

Another short section of conifers includes black spruce and red pines and is followed by mixed deciduous and conifer forest. Various mosses decorate the trailside, and yellow common cinquefoil is among the wildflowers in this area. I found this to be the most peaceful section of the trail.

The trail begins to distinctly drop down the hillside at about 3.62 miles and some low-level road noise interrupts the tranquility. There is another junction with the Lake Trail at 3.74 miles, allowing the loop to be completed. Turn left on the blue-blazed Lake Trail (Forest Trail is a 6.2-mile trail that continues to the right).

There is some boot-sucking mud on the trail, but that ends when you rejoin the road portion of Lake Trail at 3.91 miles. Turn left on the road to reach the footbridge you crossed to reach the trailhead. Cross the footbridge and turn right to reach the parking area.

▶ NEARBY ATTRACTIONS

For information concerning fishing, swimming, boat rentals, cabin or campsite rentals, or other information about Raccoon Creek State Park and its facilities, call the park office at (724) 899-2200, or e-mail raccooncreeksp@state.pa.us. For other hikes, see the park map or the Raccoon Creek State Park Wildflower Reserve Loop hike (hike 38) in this book.

RACCOON CREEK STATE PARK: WILDFLOWER RESERVE LOOP

KEY AT-A-GLANCE INFORMATION

LENGTH: 2.6 miles

CONFIGURATION: Loop

DIFFICULTY: Easy to moderate

SCENERY: Numerous wildflowers, Raccoon Creek, boulders, deciduous forest

EXPOSURE: Mostly shaded

TRAFFIC: Light

TRAIL SURFACE: Dirt

HIKING TIME: 2 hours

ACCESS: Open year-round, 8 a.m.–sunset

MAPS: A map specifically for the Wildflower Reserve is available at the Wildflower Reserve Interpretive Center (some are posted outside) and at the park office (see Nearby Attractions following the Description for contact information); USGS Aliquippa

FACILITIES: Restrooms and a water fountain are located in the Wildlife Reserve Interpretive Center.

SPECIAL COMMENTS: Neither dogs nor smoking is permitted on the reserve grounds. Peak wildflowers are in April and August.

Raccoon Creek State Park:
Wildflower Reserve Loop

UTM Zone (WGS84)   17T

Easting   553925

Northing   4484174

IN BRIEF

This hike loops through the higher grounds and meadows of the wildflower reserve and the lowlands near Raccoon Creek. The abundance and diversity of wildflowers is truly a treat.

DESCRIPTION

The Wildflower Reserve of Raccoon Creek State Park contains more than 500 species of identified plants. The Western Pennsylvania Conservancy originally purchased this 314-acre tract in 1962; the property was transferred to the state and became a part of the park in 1971.

To begin the hike, locate the path on the far end of the parking lot; it's to the right of the sidewalk that leads to the interpretive center. You'll see a sign for Jennings Trail and Hungerford Cabin; the hike begins on the grassy path of the Jennings Trail. A little into the woods, you'll see bluets and an interesting intertwining of a conifer and a deciduous tree to the right that make the pair appear as one new hybrid. There are many bird boxes, and the sounds and sights of many birds in the area indicates that a number of them may be happily inhabited. There are also ferns, cream violets, and daisy fleabane, the latter noted for the numerous white rays encircling its yellow center.

Once you've climbed this short hill, reach Hungerford Cabin. The trail veers left around the cabin, which was unlocked during my visit. Take a

DIRECTIONS

From Pittsburgh, take Interstate 279 South to the Clinton exit. Turn left onto Clinton Road and follow 1 mile. Take US 30 West and follow 4.8 miles to the Raccoon Creek State Park Wildflower Reserve. Turn right onto the road and into the parking area. Note that the reserve sign is easy to miss; there's a much larger state-park sign shortly after where you can turn left and turn around if you missed the reserve sign.

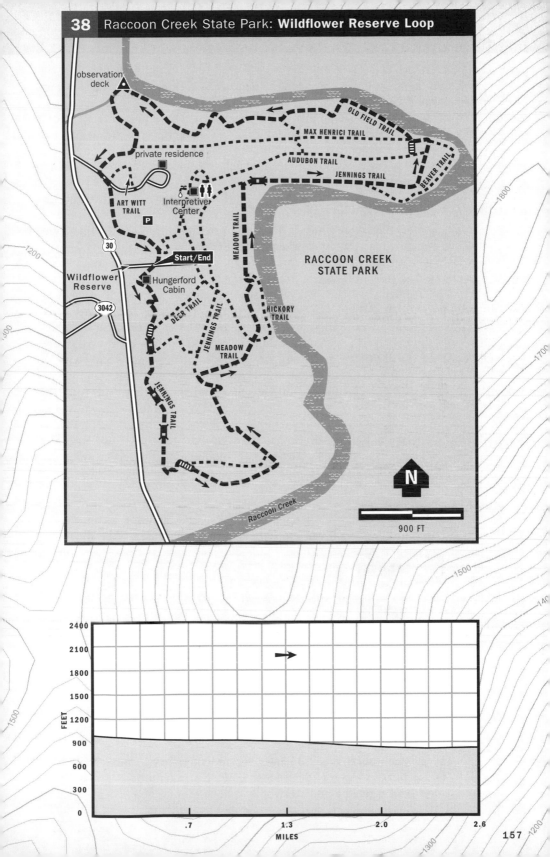

look inside at this modest former second home of Cyrus Hungerford, an award-winning cartoonist for the *Pittsburgh Post-Gazette* from 1927 to 1977. The home appears to be used for some park storage, so there is not much to see. But a peek reveals a nice fireplace and the fact that a second home did not mean luxury on the inside. For nature lovers, the luxury is found in the surroundings. This was one of many private second homes located in the area. (More private homes, inhabited, are located off the northeast parking area.)

Leaving the cabin and continuing, you'll pass between a slightly dilapidated bench and a sign indicating that you are on Jennings Trail. You'll see mayapples once you've gone beyond the clearing. At 0.2 miles, you'll pass the Deer Trail juncture on the left. Walk over the boardwalk where you'll find many varieties of fern. This is followed by a bridge and then another trail leading off to the left, this one unmarked. Per the reserve map, this is a shortcut to the other side of the Jennings Trail.

Walking along, you are likely to be accompanied by the sounds of many birds and some sightings—warblers, crows, and catbirds are among those I heard. Look for gray-headed coneflowers (yellow petals extend down, lower than the center), Virginia waterleaf (purple bells), and unique fungus growing in this area. Cross another bridge over a feeder stream and head slightly uphill where you are greeted with beautiful wild geranium, club moss, and a variety of ferns only an expert could identify.

At about 0.5 miles the trail briefly splits (and then rejoins). I went right to descend a set of steps to a wider loop on the trail. Watch your step if the stairs are muddy. Water may be pooled at the bottom; if it is, look for frogs (I saw a number of them). Along the left-hand side of the trail is shelved rock decorated with lots of moss; you may see appendaged waterleaf, very similar to its Virginia counterpart but with a wider leaf base and flowers that are more upright and not so tightly grouped. Dwarf or spring larkspur also grows in this area; the purple flower is a member of the buttercup family.

Through this section the trees are widely spaced, allowing for much undergrowth. At about 0.7 miles is what appears to be an established trail heading right; it leads to a network of unmarked trails and floodplains near the creek side. Don't turn here but use the established trail of this hike to avoid additional damage. Just beyond, the upper and lower portions of the Jennings Trail meet again. The fact that this is a floodplain is made evident with the bogs of water and washed-out sections to the right. Skunk cabbage as high as your hip is abundant, as are huge maple sycamores.

At 0.94 miles turn right onto the signed Meadow Trail, with its fields of gray-headed coneflowers and small groups of cream violets. There is a juncture with the Hickory Trail at 1.06 miles. You can take this 0.16-mile trail closer to the creek if you wish; it rejoins Meadow Trail at 1.19 miles. I headed straight to get a look at the other flowers of the meadow. The trail surroundings do indeed offer a meadow, and the trail itself is narrow and grassy through it. Many bird boxes dot the way; birdsong fills the air; goldenrod and white and purple violets are visible, while honeysuckle and flowering trees provide fragrance.

This pleasant trail ends at 1.33 miles, where it meets the Jennings Trail again. At this T, turn right and cross over the wooden plank bridge for a walk close to Raccoon Creek. More wild geranium and signs of beavers are found here. Nice views of the creek are on the right, and a high sandstone cliff lines the trail to the left. Boulders change the terrain scenery, and among the deciduous trees you'll find are poplar and old oaks. In this very wide section of Raccoon Creek, you may have luck and see the mink, muskrat, or beavers that reside in stream valleys in this more remote area of the park. Along here find the beautiful wild stonecrop; these star-shaped white flowers with red tips on their sepals appear to sprout straight up from the rock's mossy outcroppings. You also see white asters. Notice their many-rayed flower heads and grasslike leaves. Also in the area is cut-leaved toothwort, many with white or pale lavender flowers.

Continue straight where the Beaver Trail veers off to the right, unless you wish to take this 0.2-mile trail. It looked washed out when I was hiking, so I bypassed it and continued alongside the sandstone cliff wall. At about 1.7 miles the Beaver Trail meets with Jennings Trail again and the Jennings Trail turns left, rounding the sandstone cliff. Along this find Virginia bluebells, toadshade, and jack-in-the-pulpit. Shortly after, ignore the unmarked spur to the right and reach the end of the Jennings Trail. Here, the Max Henrici Trail goes up the hill to the left and Old Field Trail is a turn to the right. Turn right onto Old Field Trail.

At this point Raccoon Creek is not nearly as wide as it was, and the trail is narrower as well. Smooth phlox grows here, and the undergrowth grows very close to the trail. At 2 miles is a spur trail with a sign to go to Max Henrici Trial. Continue right on Old Field Trail. You may see deer in this more wooded area, as I did. The deer must be somewhat accustomed to visitors and their protected status, as this one never felt threatened enough to run far.

You'll see a fallen observation deck at the top of a short pair of stairs at 2.35 miles. Its supports may have been washed away in flooding waters and perhaps will be restored. Walk down another set of short wooden stairs and continue, finding yellow cinquefoil along the way. You may spot some mallard ducks in the water before you turn away from it, heading left and inland.

Old Field Trail ends at a juncture with the Max Henrici Trail. Turn right on Max Henrici Trail (there is a sign) to head toward the parking lot. This trail provides a deviation from the level hiking as it leads back to the uplands. The trail is wide and lined with thigh-high ferns and moss along the hillside. At almost the top of this incline, the slight elevation change offers some change in flora; pines are in sight once again. When you reach the paved road, turn left. The Art Witt Trail intersects with the road. Stay on the road until you reach the parking lot.

▶ NEARBY ATTRACTIONS

The Wildflower Reserve Interpretive Center has year-round programs and exhibits and brochures on natural history and historical areas of the park. Call (724) 899-2200. For more information on the remainder of Raccoon Creek State Park, call (724) 899-2200, e-mail raccooncreeksp@state.pa.us, or see the Raccoon Creek State Park: Lake-Forest Loop hike(hike 37) in this book.

BUTLER, ARMSTRONG, AND INDIANA COUNTIES

BAKER TRAIL:
CROOKED CREEK LAKE AREA

 KEY AT-A-GLANCE INFORMATION

LENGTH: 7 miles

CONFIGURATION: Out-and-back

DIFFICULTY: Moderate

SCENERY: Crooked Creek Lake, covered bridge

EXPOSURE: Mostly shaded

TRAFFIC: Light

TRAIL SURFACE: Dirt, pavement, gravel

HIKING TIME: 3.5 hours

ACCESS: Open year-round

MAPS: A guide for the entire 141-mile Baker Trail is available by sending a check for $12.70 to The Rachel Carson Trails Conservancy, P.O. Box 35, Warrendale, PA 15086; go to **www.rachelcarsontrails.org** to ensure current pricing and information; USGS Leechburg and Whitesburg

FACILITIES: Restrooms, drinking water, picnic shelters, grills, playgrounds, concession area, campgrounds, and boat launches are available in Crooked Creek Lake Park.

SPECIAL COMMENTS: Horse paths (marked with white circles) periodically crisscross the Baker Trail throughout this section; be careful not to follow them.

Baker Trail:
Crooked Creek Lake Area

UTM Zone (WGS84)   17T

Easting   626542

Northing   4508405

IN BRIEF

This hike is part of the 141-mile Baker Trail, which begins in Freeport and ends in Allegheny National Forest, and is continually threatened by encroaching development. Very short portions of this segment have been rerouted to road, which turned out to be pleasant, as locals were welcoming.

DESCRIPTION

The Baker Trail began as an idea conceived in 1948 by Tony Pronses, the first chairman of the Pittsburgh chapter of the American Youth Hostels. The Board of the Pittsburgh Council authorized construction of the extended trail to connect Pittsburgh and Cook Forest via forest paths, old jeep roads, and some dirt roads through woods and farmlands. The trail was named the Horace Forbes Baker Trail to honor the prominent Pittsburgh attorney who had been instrumental in establishing the Pittsburgh Council in 1948.

Volunteers and scout troops performed all of the trail's development, and this continues to be the method by which the trail is maintained. The Baker Trail is included on the Pennsylvania Recreational Guide and Highway Map. Despite this status, it has no overseeing government protection. Its maintenance had always been led by the American Youth Hostels but the current status of the Pittsburgh chapter does not allow its management.

DIRECTIONS

From Pittsburgh, take PA 28 to US 422 toward Kittanning to PA 66 South toward Ford City, making the immediate right at the end of the bridge. Pass the first entrance to Crooked Creek at 5 miles; at 6.4 miles from the bridge, turn left at the Crooked Creek Market onto SR 2019. Pass the environmental center and park office, drive over the dam, and make a left into the parking area where there is a restroom.

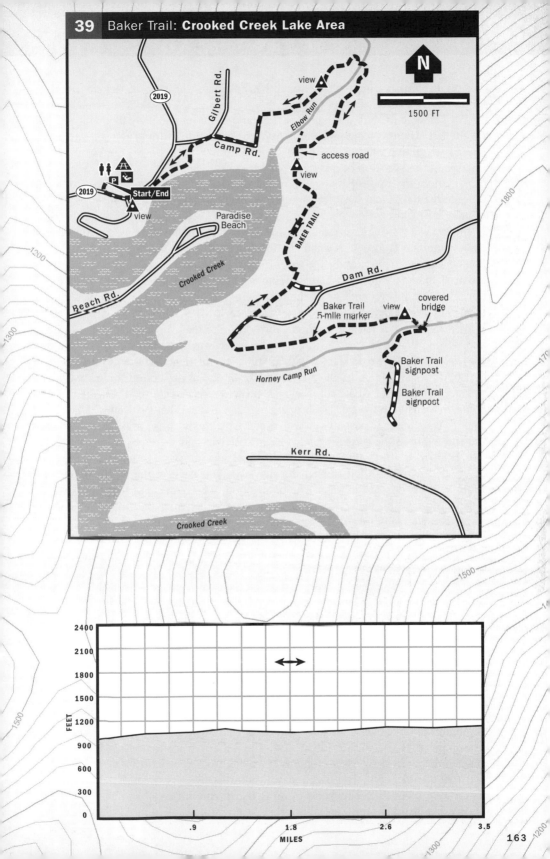

N

1500 FT

2019

Gilbert Rd.

view

Elbow Run

access road

view

Camp Rd.

2019

Start/End

view

Paradise Beach

BAKER TRAIL

Crooked Creek

Dam Rd.

covered bridge

Baker Trail 5-mile marker

view

Beach Rd.

Horney Camp Run

Baker Trail signpost

Baker Trail signpost

Kerr Rd.

Crooked Creek

1800

1300

1200

1500

1700

1300

1500

1500

FEET				
2400				
2100				
1800				
1500				
1200				
900				
600				
300				
0	.9	1.8	2.6	3.5

MILES

The Rachel Carson Trails Conservancy has taken stewardship of the trail, and the entire trail is blazed with yellow rectangles.

I parked and started the hike at the parking lot immediately following the dam on the left. There is a sign for the Baker Trail before this turn. The trail can also be started by pulling off in a lot just 0.25 miles down the road on the right, but the mileage in this write-up begins at the upper parking lot.

Exiting the upper parking lot, make a left on SR 2019, and follow it for 0.25 miles to the Baker Trail sign. Turn south toward the lake at a small drainage ditch; look up and left for the yellow blaze that indicates your rocky ascent to acquire the ridge. At the top is a view of Crooked Creek Lake, and the trail becomes a dirt path through some mountain laurel. After walking a few hundred feet along the ridge, look for the double blaze at 0.35 miles for the left turn in the trail. In about 200 feet another double blaze marks a right turn. Ridge hiking is often pleasant and this one is no exception; however, it soon ends when the trail meets a road in less than 0.5 miles to avoid traversing private property.

A sign to your left marks a right turn onto the road. I thought I really wouldn't like walking this road, but the way is well marked with yellow blazes on intermittent telephone poles. The road is lined with tall pines on the right and woods on the left and the sounds of songbirds fill the air. A resident of one of the homes smiled and waved and assured me that I would soon be back in the woods just around the bend. The final home on the left has a large "No Trespassing" sign and another that states "Hikers Welcome." Walk straight past this house and up its grassy drive; another yellow blaze shows you are in the correct place. Look to the right and see a post style that should look familiar by now—at the top is a Baker Trail sign and arrow pointing left.

At 0.75 miles, a left turn at the sign puts you back in the woods, where you attain another view of the water. The orange boundary markers of the Army Corps of Engineers are visible below you on the hillside. Wait for the Baker Trail double yellow blaze soon after, and turn right. In spring, mayapples are found in this section. Don't forget to take a peek underneath to see if their so-called apples are there or their pretty white flowers have bloomed; each produces only one flower, but it's a beauty. A double blaze marks another right to begin switchbacks down the steep hillside. After the last left switchback here, step over a log (which my 12.5-year-old dog leaped like a show horse), cross a water runoff, and walk along the neighboring hillside.

Keep your eyes open for the many wildflowers to be found if you are fortunate enough to be here in the spring. Come to a stack of two trees fallen one atop the other; I found it easiest to squeeze between them. At just about 1 mile, a lovely view of Elbow Run comes within sight below and to the right. In another 500 feet I saw double blazes indicating a turn but also single blazes ahead. The path clearly was straight, so if the false double blazes remain when you are hiking watch this spot and stay straight on the trail. The hiking since descending the hillside has been rather easygoing and relatively flat and continues that way during a slow descent over rolling hills that lead toward Elbow Run. Along the way are some large rock outcroppings and then a sharp right along an open field. Look around to see a Baker Trail sign that is currently falling over but still pointing in the correct direction. A quick observation reveals a yellow blaze to verify the direction.

Watch your footing, as it is rather steep initially. A double blaze leads the switchbacks right and then another left, where you follow the trail closely around a tree. At the bottom, head left and cross a muddy area and then Elbow Run. Look up to see the blazes marking the trail over a third feeder stream and go right. Pass through the abundant skunk cabbage and begin a steep incline. Horseshoe around the large fallen tree. Although trail maintenance is difficult and trees may lie in the way in places, the trail itself has remained easy to follow. In this area though, dirt bikers chew up the trail so it will likely be a bit muddy. Mixed deciduous and conifer woods, mayapples, and trillium are some of the surrounding flora.

At 1.5 miles be sure to notice the double blaze and make the right rather than following the trail straight. Curve right with the trail into the conifers. At the T, turn left and walk under tall hemlocks, through some very young growth, and back under hemlocks. At 1.6 miles follow the trail downhill, passing the access road to the left and enjoying the view of the lake on the right. Just beyond this are a 6-mile marker and a rotted bench displaying Baker Trail on its front. As the trail dips down a bit farther I'm greeted by the rising sound of geese and another great view of the lake before it becomes shrouded with the branches of more hemlocks. For the next 0.5 miles, the trail traverses the hillside on the opposite side of the lake from which the hike began. During this portion views of the lake come and go and come again. Rolling hills take you through alternating rusty-colored and clear water, over a small log bridge surrounded by black shale, through mud patches and dry ground, and through deciduous and conifer sections.

At 2.06 miles are a gravel road to the left and a Baker Trail sign pointing right. Follow the direction of the sign and turn right again when you reach a residential road. The hiking remains quite peaceful here. At 2.23 miles is another Baker Trail sign for a left turn back into the woods. Here you'll find a gorgeous section of level walking through more mountain laurel and then evergreens and mixed woodlands along a wide path that follows Horney Camp Run. After passing the 5-mile Baker Trail marker, you should be able to see a covered bridge over Horney Camp Run down the hill on the right. Shortly after, a double blaze indicates your right turn to go to it.

After reaching the covered bridge, a structure built as part of the Baker Trail, and perhaps taking a break at this lovely run, you may choose this as a good turnaround point, as the remainder of this hike leads to another residential area. The covered bridge is located about 3 miles from the starting point.

If you choose to go on, continue straight, passing the horse trail to the right and climb the hill. Pass another horse trail connection on the left at a Y and continue straight. The trail becomes grass and leads to a gravel road. Turn right on the road. Along the top of the hill it appears that the surrounding land is all privately owned. There are several covered pavilions up here and a restroom, but these are not likely for public use. I turned around at 3.5 miles and retraced my steps.

Be careful on the return to pay attention to the double blazes and turns to follow the Baker Trail; otherwise, you may find yourself backtracking to it from a horse path.

▶ NEARBY ATTRACTIONS

Crooked Creek Lake has a beach with a concession stand, in addition to the facilities mentioned in the At-a-Glance Information for this hike. To reserve a pavilion or campsite or acquire more information, call (724) 763-2764 or visit **www.lrp.usace .army.mil.** The Crooked Creek Market and restaurants are found on PA 66.

BLACKLICK VALLEY NATURAL AREA: PARKER TRACT HIKE

KEY AT-A-GLANCE INFORMATION

LENGTH: 3.5 miles

CONFIGURATION: Balloon

DIFFICULTY: Moderate

SCENERY: Views via power-line clearings, Blacklick Creek, meadows, wetland

EXPOSURE: Half shaded, half exposed

TRAFFIC: Light

TRAIL SURFACE: Dirt and grass

HIKING TIME: 2–2.5 hours

ACCESS: Open year-round

MAPS: Available online at **www.indiana countyparks.org** or by calling Indiana Parks and Trails at (724) 463-8636; USGS Vintondale. You can also obtain an explanatory guide with a map for Points of Interest marked with numbered posts by calling the above number.

FACILITIES: None

SPECIAL COMMENTS: The flat portions of the hike are well marked. The orange blazes on the wooded section of the hike are faded but legible.

Blacklick Valley Natural Area:
Parker Tract Hike

UTM Zone (WGS84)   17T

Easting   670037

Northing   4480944

IN BRIEF

This hike provides two views via power-line clearings obtained by climbing through pretty wooded sections, as well as a walk through meadows and along Blacklick Creek and a wetland. The uphill hike can be reduced or even avoided by following other trails and giving up the view.

DESCRIPTION

The Blacklick Valley Natural Area is divided into three tracts, encompassing a total of 713 acres, 300 of which make up the Parker Tract. (The other two tracts do not have developed trails.) According to Indiana County Park literature, the first recorded owner of what is now the Parker Tract was William Bracken, who purchased 309 acres from the Commonwealth of Pennsylvania in 1786. The property has since changed hands many times and was donated to Indiana County parks in 1995 by Penny and David Russell.

You'll see a map on an information board at the head of the parking area. This hike begins on the trail called Parker Lane, which begins on the right end of the parking lot (there is not a sign). Go around the gate and begin on the wide, open, grass-covered lane. True to Indiana County's fame as the Christmas tree capital of the world, spruce trees are found growing along the sides of the lane. There are also crab apple trees, elderberry, and a plethora of small fruiting and blooming trees along this meadow opening.

At 0.29 miles, you'll reach a five-way intersection. The soft right is the branch to take; the two lefts are connector trails that lead to the Wetland and Blacklick trails, and the hard right is not

DIRECTIONS

From Pittsburgh, take US 22 East 1.09 miles past the PA 403 Dilltown–Johnstown exit and turn left onto McFeaters Road, which is a dead-end road that leads directly to the parking lot in 0.7 miles.

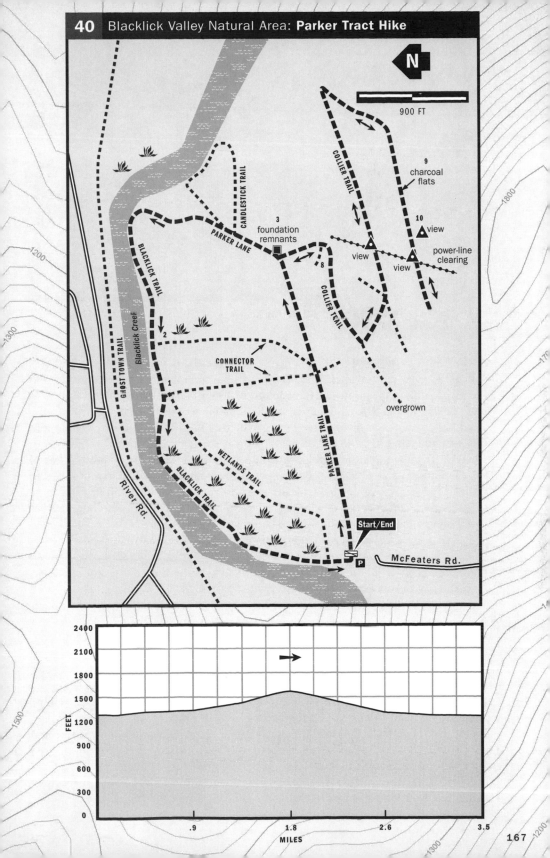

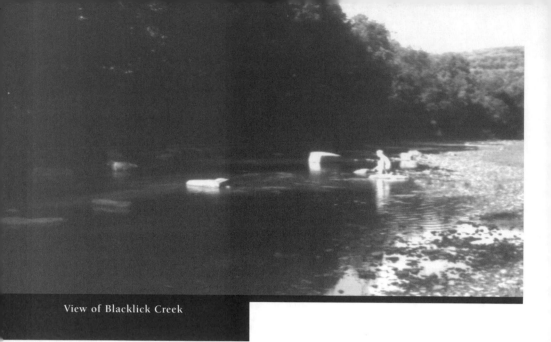

View of Blacklick Creek

identified on the county map. There are many blue spruce trees as you continue, and the meadow flowers and plants to be found will depend on the season. In late summer, joe-pye weed (blooms August through September) can be found. There's milkweed, too, which is in bloom June through August. Both plants are very common in this area and are 2 to 5 feet tall, depending on the species, and their flowers grow in clusters. If you are interested in knowing the difference, joe-pye weed and milkweed can be a bit difficult to discern. Both have species that are white. When it comes to colors, though, joe-pye weed is typically pale to deep purple, while milkweed can be pink, magenta, and varying shades of purples, usually duller. Both also have species with hollow stems. If you really want to be sure of which one is which, only milkweed produces a thick, milky juice when its stem is broken. Watch out though, it's sticky.

At 0.37 miles, you'll arrive at a post marked Point of Interest 4, where you'll find remnants of a building foundation that likely dates to the 1800s. Not much farther along, at 0.47 miles is a split; turn right to take Collier Trail. (Note that this trail leads uphill to overlooks along a power line. If you wish to hike on a level surface, turn left and go to the Blacklick Trail, which this hike uses for the return.)

On the Collier Trail, pass the first right near the edge of the woods and continue straight at 0.54 miles. You'll see faded orange blazes and Point of Interest 8, where you may notice the wide array of vegetation. At 0.72 miles, come to a choice to turn left or continue straight; turn left (going straight leads to an overgrown path). Immediately after this left, the ascent to reach an overlook becomes steeper, gaining 100 feet in elevation when you've reached a T with an old road at 0.8 miles. Turn left, and at the Y take the right branch, following the orange blazes. Reach a clearing and the first view down the power line in about 400 feet. You can see a grove of planted trees that are marked Christmas Trees on the county map and are circled by a path called the Candlestick Trail. When you continue back into the woods, find shagbark hickory and red maple among other hardwoods, and walk through a patch of ferns. Keep your eyes peeled for the faded double orange blazes on a tree to the right, marking your right turn up the hillside at 1.14 miles.

Again make a steep climb, this time gaining 148 feet before reaching the next plateau at 1.27 miles. On the way up find American beech trees, more maples, some oaks, and even a few hemlocks. The trail becomes level again and leads to Point of Interest 9, which is a charcoal flat; I found tailings near the site. Iron-making was Blacklick Valley's first industry. Point of Interest 10 is a view north and west across the Blacklick Valley and is found just before the next power-line clearing at 1.48 miles. It appears that the hillside can continue to be climbed in this manner, using switchbacks and walking through the clearings for views; but this is where this hike turns around. Either way, retrace your steps back to the meadowlands, just be careful to look for the orange blazes so you don't miss the turns that lead from the old roads down through the woods.

Once you've reached Parker Lane again, walk straight until you reach the sign for Collier Trail and bear right. Pass the intersections with the Candlestick Trail at 2.58 and 2.63 miles (unless you wish to add this loop by turning right) to reach the Blacklick Trail, which leads to Blacklick Creek at 2.72 miles.

Blacklick Creek is more than 100 feet wide here. Clarke Run (not to be confused with Clark Run of the Charles F. Lewis Natural Area, a nearby hike also in this book; see hike 41) and Mardis Run are tributaries, running down from the north. The color of Blacklick Creek reflects the result of one of the biggest environmental problems Pennsylvania faces. Its water is a rusty orange-brown color; the rocks and boulders in it are stained the same, showing the amount of acid mine drainage that affects this creek. Various communities have programs that try to address the problem, but overall it remains a toxic pollutant in too many of our waterways. Just across the creek is the Ghost Town Trail; it uses the railroad bed that once supported the Blacklick and Ebensburg railroads, which operated in part to support the mining towns of the area. The trail is named for five mining towns that once existed along its corridor but are now lost to history. You can hear voices floating over the water at times, as users of the trail bike, walk, run, horseback ride, or cross-country ski over its flat, packed limestone surface.

Reach Point of Interest 2 at 2.93 miles. A wetland now, this was once a sharp bend, or "oxbow" in the creek. The trail continues to parallel the creek, making for a scenic hike, despite the unnatural color of the water. Pass the two connector trails coming from the left and continue along Blacklick Creek, where you'll find white and pin oak, wild ginger, and an abundance of plant life. In spring, there are likely many wildflowers sprouting up.

Pass Point of Interest 1 (the county guide discusses acid mine drainage) at 3.3 miles. Continue straight past the left turn for the Wetlands Trail at 3.46 miles before reaching the parking lot and the hike's end at 3.5 miles.

▶ NEARBY ATTRACTIONS

The 16-mile Ghost Town Trail can be accessed from five different locations; the Eliza Furnace is accessed at a picnic area near its midpoint. Buttermilk Falls is also nearby (2 miles south of US 22 at Clyde). Directions can be found at **www.indianacounty parks.org.** The Charles F. Lewis Natural Area (hike 41) has a beautiful hike with views of cascading Clark Run and the Conemaugh Gap.

CHARLES F. LEWIS NATURAL AREA: RAGER MOUNTAIN TRAIL LOOP

KEY AT-A-GLANCE INFORMATION

LENGTH: 4.8 miles

CONFIGURATION: Loop

DIFFICULTY: Moderate to difficult (due to steep ascent and descent)

SCENERY: Clark Run, views of Conemaugh Gap and Laurel Ridge, charcoal beehive oven, rhododendron

EXPOSURE: Mostly shaded

TRAFFIC: Light to moderate

TRAIL SURFACE: Dirt and rock

HIKING TIME: 3–3.5 hours

ACCESS: Open year-round, 5 a.m.– a half hour after sunset

MAPS: Available by visiting the Gallitzin Forest District office in Ebensburg or calling (814) 472-1862; also at the trailhead; USGS Vintondale

FACILITIES: Picnic area near trailhead, no toilets

SPECIAL COMMENTS: Wear good hiking boots or trail shoes. Also, be careful; bears live in this area (though they've harmed no one in reports I've seen).

Charles F. Lewis Natural Area: Rager Mountain Trail Loop

UTM Zone (WGS84) 17T

Easting 670946

Northing 4475334

▶ IN BRIEF

A steep initial hike affords views of waterfalls cascading down Clark Run and leads to a ridgeline walk through pretty forest. The final leg, a somewhat steep descent, includes some rock-to-rock stepping through a lovely boulder field.

▶ DESCRIPTION

This 384-acre natural area was named to honor Dr. Charles Fletcher Lewis for his extensive efforts in conservation. During his lifetime, Lewis was a teacher, newspaper editorial writer, first director of the Buhl Foundation, and president of the Western Pennsylvania Conservancy. Among the achievements the Buhl Foundation counted during Lewis's time were the former Buhl Planetarium, Chatham Village, and the acquisition of many education and conservation grants.

Following his retirement from practice, he began a 13-year tenure with the Western Pennsylvania Conservancy (most of which he served without accepting salary), during which he guided the organization into becoming an action-oriented group whose methods have received regional and national recognition. Under his direction, the conservancy initiated, planned, and assisted in acquiring land for five major state parks; acquired other lands totaling 38,000 acres for parks and natural areas in western Pennsylvania; and established the Kaufmann Conservation on Bear Run, including Fallingwater. (See the Bear Run Nature Reserve hike—hike 46—in this book.)

Begin the hike with a stop at the information board near the trailhead, immediately in front of the parking area. There you'll find booklets with

▶ DIRECTIONS

From Pittsburgh, take US 22 East to PA 403 (Dilltown–Johnstown exit). Drive south on PA 403 for 3.5 miles; turn left into the parking area.

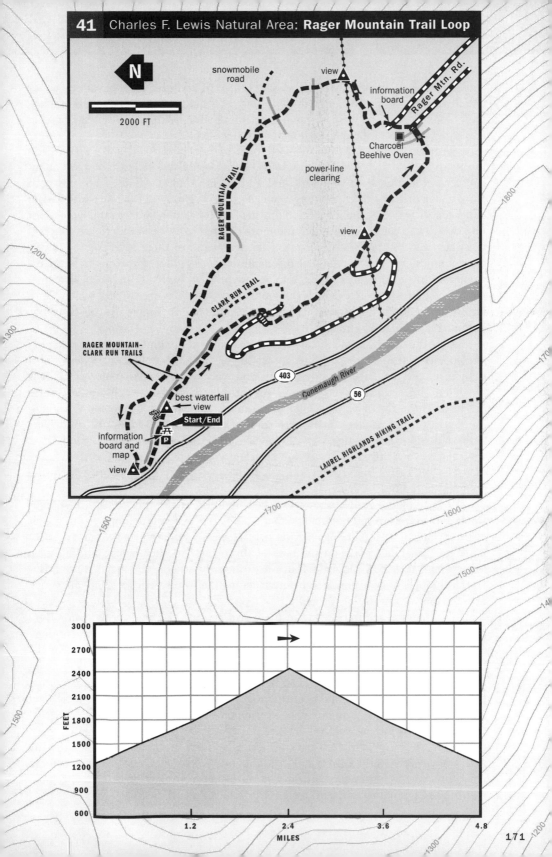

41 Charles F. Lewis Natural Area: **Rager Mountain Trail Loop**

background information about Charles F. Lewis, in addition to publications about the area's geology, history, and natural resources; a rough map can be found in a box there, too. The best map is the one on the information board itself, but the booklet is worth reading and the map in this book will suffice.

To begin the hike, follow the wide path straight ahead and make a right, following the yellow blazes up the trail steps found beyond the split-rail fence at about 452 feet. Note that both the Clark Run and Rager Mountain trails share this path along the southern side of the gorge, and it is the beginning of the steepest part of either trail. The rapid gain in elevation provides the landscape for the fast flow of Clark Run, which cascades over boulders and moss-covered rocks on your left, creating scenic waterfalls. You are afforded one of the best views of them at 900 feet. As you ascend this steep section, you'll also see tall hemlocks growing to your right. Hardwoods in this area include tulip trees (yellow poplar), basswood, and sugar maple. After the climb's intensity decreases, you can see large flat sheets over which Clark Run flows before the trail travels farther away up the hillside and eventually turns out onto an old road at 0.77 miles.

Here the Rager Mountain and Clark Run trails split, with Clark Run turning left and following the old road before descending (where the trails later rejoin). Turn right to follow the Rager Mountain Trail and walk about 30 feet before making a quick left up a set of trail steps; the blazes for this trail are orange. The trail continues its ascent to the narrow ridgeline between the Conemaugh Gorge and Clark Run but it is not nearly as steep as the climb along the run. At 1.29 miles, the trail meets with an access road. Turn left and follow the road and its orange blazes uphill. At 1.45 miles, you'll reach a power-line clearing where you have views of the Conemaugh River Gorge and Laurel Ridge, and also of power plants from which one assumes these lines are fed.

When you are ready to move on, be mindful that the trail continues straight through the clearing and not down either side. (Note that you do not want to go left at the pylon; the red markings are the natural area boundaries and are not a trail.) Look for the orange blaze on the base of the pylon. Another orange blaze can be found on a flat rock as you make your way toward the woods. You may have to bushwhack through some overgrowth before reaching the wood's edge and opening back into the forest.

Back among the trees, you are treated to a variety of hardwoods, some large boulders, and a patch of ferns. Walk over a bridge and some logs that lie where there are a few water runoffs, and cross an old road at 2 miles. Look for an old charcoal beehive oven to the left of the trail not long after this road crossing and before you reach the larger Rager Mountain Road at 2.14 miles, where there is another information board with map. Not long after entering the woods on the other side, you'll find a perfect log on which to sit and have a snack on the left side of the trail.

The trail is not difficult to follow; still, look for the double blaze on a tree soon to be sure and turn right with the trail. Cross another bridge and then recross the power-line clearing at 2.44 miles. The trail continues straight and you may have to navigate some overgrowth again (and cross over the somewhat discernable grass road) to reach its other side and reenter the woods.

This section of the woods is very pretty, but there is a patch of greenbrier between two water runoffs at about 2.72 miles. Watch your legs if any of the vines reach out from the sides of the trail. After the second runoff, the vines give way to ferns. In this area, you'll see witch hazel, sassafras, and a variety of maples and oaks. At 2.85 miles, cross a snowmobile trail blazed with orange triangles, and quickly reach an old road. More triangular blazes suggest snowmobilers may use this road as well. Do not continue straight here but turn left, following the orange rectangular blazes. The trail then leaves the road very quickly with a right turn; follow the orange blazes into the woods. Continue the slow descent and cross another road at 3.31 miles.

The Rager Mountain Trail rejoins the Clark Run Trail at 3.86 miles, where you reach a T with the old road. Go straight and descend through rock outcroppings. This is a very pretty section of the hike. Stepping from rock to rock, notice how the green hues of the moss covering some of the rocks combine with that of the rhododendron to contrast the gray. Look up and to the right periodically to see the large rock band that begins at about 3.95 miles. After a stone mileage marker found at 4 miles, the boulder field thins out and the trail is more level for awhile, traveling through thin forest with more rhododendrons before making one more steep descent toward the river. At 4.46 miles, after one such descent, the trail veers sharply left, but you can walk right to get one more view of the Conemaugh Gap before turning left to continue downward. Enjoy a few more small boulders to navigate on the trail, and some very large ones to admire off the trail on your left.

At 4.66 miles, come to a T and turn left. Here you are walking on an old roadway once called Locust Street used before PA 403 was built; you may notice its remaining asphalt underneath your feet. Continue straight past a trail going off to the left shortly after; veer right with the trail and cross the stream. This leads you to the trail you came in on. Turn right to return to your car.

▶ NEARBY ATTRACTIONS

The Blacklick Valley Natural Area has some beautiful and diverse hiking; directions and suggested hikes can be found in this book. Buttermilk Falls is also nearby (2 miles south of PA 22 at Clyde), as are the Eliza Furnace and the Ghost Town Trail; directions can be found at **www.indianacountyparks.org.**

JENNINGS ENVIRONMENTAL EDUCATION CENTER TRAIL LOOP

ⓘ KEY AT-A-GLANCE INFORMATION

LENGTH: 4.5 miles

CONFIGURATION: Loop

DIFFICULTY: Easy to moderate

SCENERY: Prairie, deciduous and coniferous forest, sawmill ruins, historic ore pits, wetland restoration project, and an interpretive kiosk

EXPOSURE: Sunny in meadows, shaded in wooded areas

TRAFFIC: Light

TRAIL SURFACE: Grass and dirt

HIKING TIME: 2–2.5 hours

ACCESS: Trailhead never closes

MAPS: Available by visiting the Jennings Environmental Education Center or calling (724) 794-6011; also available via the Pennsylvania Department of Conservation and Natural Resources Web site, **www.dcnr.state.pa.us**; USGS Slippery Rock

FACILITIES: Restrooms and first aid at the Jennings Environmental Education Center, pit toilets and recycling area at the prairie area parking lot, picnic groves around the education center

SPECIAL COMMENTS: This route combines several trails. If you don't have much time, you can hike the trails on one side of the road and return another day to complete those on the other.

▶ IN BRIEF

Jennings provides a unique combination of prairie and forestlands. The relict 20-acre prairie ecosystem is rare in Pennsylvania. It has survived the climatic changes that transformed other prairies into forests, due to its 20-foot-thick layer of impermeable clay that dissuades the growth of trees. Visitors should try to visit in late July or early August when the prairie is in full bloom. The late bloom time is common for prairie plants, which prefer the hot, dry weather of midsummer.

▶ DESCRIPTION

Begin the hike at the obvious trailhead, which is marked by two stone pillars dedicated to Dr. Otto Emery Jennings, one of Pennsylvania's most renowned botanists; he was influential in protecting the prairie.

The hike begins on the park's Blazing Star Trail, through a 40-foot-long canopy before breaking onto the prairie, where interpretive signs mark the way. In summer you are treated to a spectacular array of color as you begin this leg of the hike. Common growers in this area include goldenrod, lady slipper, yellow and white daisies, along with others plants found mainly in prairie lands or open woods, like coneflower, mountain mint, and culver's root. In July or August, the bright purple flowers of the trail's namesake will dominate the scene, clustering on four- to six-foot stalks.

When you reach the intersection with the Prairie Loop, make a right. The interpretive signs

---

Jennings Environmental Education Center Trail Loop

UTM Zone (WGS84) 17T

Easting 583676

Northing 4540367

▶ DIRECTIONS

From Pittsburgh, take Interstate 79 North to PA 422 West to PA 528 North. The center is approximately 12 miles north of Butler. The parking area from which the hike starts is on the left off of PA 528, before the parking area for the environmental education center.

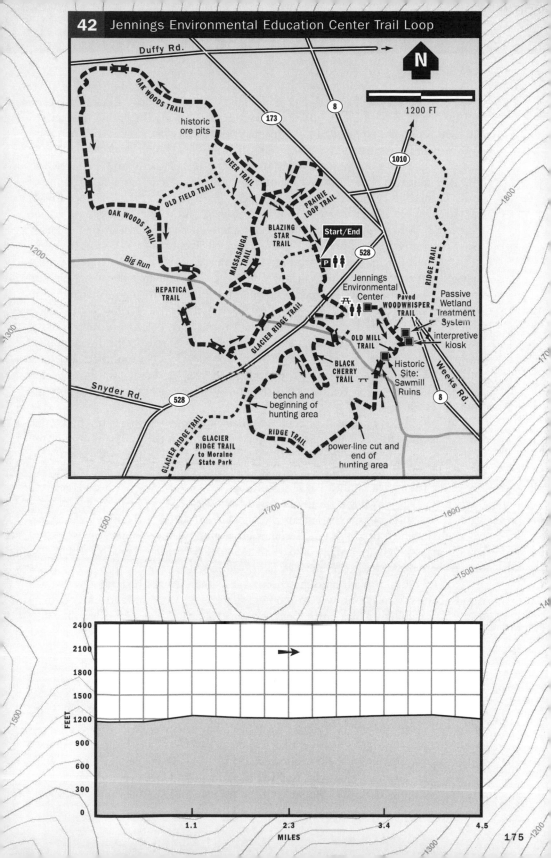

Duffy Rd.

N

1200 FT

OAK WOODS TRAIL

historic ore pits

173

8

1010

DEER TRAIL

OLD FIELD TRAIL

PRAIRIE LOOP TRAIL

OAK WOODS TRAIL

BLAZING STAR TRAIL

Start/End

Big Run

MASSASAUGA TRAIL

528

HEPATICA TRAIL

Jennings Environmental Center

WOODWHISPER TRAIL
Paved

RIDGE TRAIL

Passive Wetland Treatment System

interpretive kiosk

GLACIER RIDGE TRAIL

OLD MILL TRAIL

Snyder Rd.

BLACK CHERRY TRAIL

Historic Site: Sawmill Ruins

Weeks Rd.

528

bench and beginning of hunting area

8

GLACIER RIDGE TRAIL

GLACIER RIDGE TRAIL to Moraine State Park

RIDGE TRAIL

power-line cut and end of hunting area

2400
2100
1800
1500
1200
900
600
300
0

FEET

1.1   2.3   3.4   4.5
MILES

continue and there is evidence of pioneer trees (discussed on one of the signs), so called because they will try to pioneer the land and convert it to forest; they soon find they cannot penetrate the thick clay and die off, leaving the prairie unchanged. Hundreds of aspen, poplar, and black locust trees may briefly populate a square yard and you will likely see these beginners in multifarious stages of growth before they've died off, since their attempts are continual. At the top of the prairie loop, reached after 0.25 miles, look to the most distant ridge. This is a lateral moraine, a mound of gravel pushed up against the side of a glacier, a leftover from the glacial age that is now tree-covered. Don't forget to look for the birds and other wildlife that pervade the prairie. You may spot a goldfinch, bog lemming, hawk moth, or one of many species of butterflies that prefer the open prairie environment.

At about 0.3 miles turn right onto Deer Trail, a mixed dirt and grass trail that changes to typical Pennsylvania rockiness in spots. This stream valley along Big Run was once filled with majestic American elms. Most of these trees have succumbed to Dutch elm disease, a fungus introduced to North America in the 1930s. Other common bottomland trees that prefer the rich, moist soils and cooler temperatures of Big Run Valley, including yellow birch and basswood, now stand where the elms once grew. If you've visited in spring, the delicate woodland wildflowers that carpet the valley will make up for the not yet fully bloomed prairie. *Hepatica* spring beauties, and other flowers race to come out before the tree canopy closes and blocks sunlight from the forest floor.

At 0.48 miles exit the Deer Trail, and make a right onto Oakwoods Trail. Look for the historic ore pits believed to have been excavated in the 19th century for ore-bearing clay before you begin the gentle climb out of the valley. The mild ascent leads to drier hardwood forest consisting primarily of oak, maple, hickory, and cherry. The size of the trees are an indication of the economic value of these hardwoods realized by the colonists, which they nearly depleted by 1820.

At 1.4 miles bypass the left for the Old Field Trail and continue on the Oakwoods Trail, which descends and becomes fairly muddy. At 1.5 miles leave the Oakwoods Trail by making a right onto Hepatica Trail, which can be a bit difficult to discern here because it sometimes washes out during heavy rains.

At 1.8 miles turn left onto the Glacier Ridge Trail. Do not turn right or you will travel about 14 miles one way to Moraine State Park. Descend and cross a small bridge that is followed by a much longer bridge at almost 2 miles. Shortly you will be able to see Big Run as it passes close to the trail. You may spot a frog or hear geese flying overhead. In just about 0.1 mile make a sharp left onto the Massasauga Trail. (If you make a right here you quickly return to the parking area.) This trail is named after the massasauga rattlesnake, now endangered in Pennsylvania due to the loss of its wet meadow habitat.

At 2.2 miles you again encounter an intersection with the Oakwoods Trail. Make the right to continue on the Massasauga Trail and at 2.4 miles, where the trail intersects with Deer Trail, go straight on Deer Trail. (Going left on Deer Trail takes you back to the historic ore pits on the Oakwoods Trail.) At 2.5 miles you are back to the Blazing Star Trail. Backtrack along this trail to the parking lot. Once in the parking lot, go right and cross PA 528. Take the path up the wooden steps to the trails on the west side of the park. You will pass by a picnic area on your left and can also see the Jennings Environmental Education Center. You can visit there now or wait until you end the hike there.

To continue hiking, turn right where you see the sign for Old Elm Trail. Follow the trail and cross a bridge over Big Run. At the end of the bridge, make a right onto Black Cherry Trail. This portion of the trail system runs close to PA 528. You will notice the noise for a brief time until you intersect and make a right onto the Ridge Trail, where you begin to leave the road noise behind. The trail becomes narrower and is lined with boulders. At about 3.5 miles you will find a bench to break your steady ascent. Note that this section of the trail is open to hunting; it is posted directly above the bench.

You will descend for about 0.25 miles when you cross a power-line cut and exit the hunting area. Descend a pair of steps and walk straight toward a bench placed to provide comfort. From it you'll have a view of two small waterfalls coming together and the sawmill ruins on the opposite bank. Go left from the bench, walking over the bridge and make a right onto Old Mill Trail. You will ascend slightly and come to an unmarked meadow; turn left to reach an interpretive kiosk (at 4.4 miles). There are placards describing the mining history and legacy of the area; the passive wetland treatment system; a more active wetland treatment system using underground piping and tanks; and the wildlife, flora, and fauna of the area. The wetlands and information are worth the short jaunt to the kiosk.

When you walk down the steps from the kiosk take the path to the right and arrive at the unmarked but paved Woodwhisper Trail. The trail is accessible to those pushing strollers or wheelchairs and is dotted with benches along the way. This trail takes you to the Jennings Environmental Education Center and the end of the hike. When you have finished at the center, just walk back across PA 528 to the parking area and your car.

▶ NEARBY ATTRACTIONS

Jennings Environmental Education Center provides educational programs for all ages; call them at (724) 794-6011 for information. Moraine State Park is not far; see hikes 43 and 44 in this book.

MORAINE STATE PARK: NORTH SHORE HIKE OR HIKE AND BIKE

KEY AT-A-GLANCE INFORMATION

LENGTH: 9.6 miles (4.8 miles if using car shuttle; 11.8 if using bike path)

CONFIGURATION: Out-and-back or loop using bike path

DIFFICULTY: Easy

SCENERY: Mixed deciduous and conifer forest, wildflowers, meadows, pond, headquarters for the Pennsylvania chapter of the North Country Scenic Trail

EXPOSURE: Mostly shaded

TRAFFIC: Light

TRAIL SURFACE: Dirt

HIKING TIME: 5 hours (2–2.5 hours if car shuttling)

ACCESS: Park open sunrise–sunset

MAPS: Available at the park office, (724) 368-8811; maps are also available in PDF format online via the Pennsylvania Department of Conservation and Natural Resources Web site **www.dcnr.state.pa.us;** USGS Portersville and Prospect

FACILITIES: Restrooms, vending machines, and bike rental at trailhead; picnic areas, restrooms and vending machines at Davis Hollow Marina; boat rental and launches

SPECIAL COMMENTS: To avoid bringing two cars or hiking back, drop and lock up a bicycle at the Davis Hollow Outdoors Center and take the bike trail back. The Center is also called the North Country Trail Pennsylvania Headquarters. The first on park signs and the latter on the park map.

Moraine State Park:
North Shore Hike or Hike and Bike

UTM Zone (WGS84)   17T

Easting   573380

Northing   4536259

▶ IN BRIEF

This hike travels the Glacier Ridge Trail, which is also a part of the North Country Scenic Trail. It offers solitude with easy hiking and plenty of chances to see wildflowers. You can loop back via the 7-mile Bicycle Trail (access at lower marina parking lot) for views of the lake on the return.

▶ DESCRIPTION

The 16,725-acre Moraine State Park, like many of our treasured state parks, has a legacy in early resource extraction. Today, enjoying the greenery and lake, one would be pressed to imagine that this land was once leveled and pitted with both deep and strip mining for bituminous coal and wells for extracting oil and gas. The Western Allegheny Railroad was built to haul these minerals along with mined sand and gravel deposited by earlier glaciers (giving both park and trail names), and clay, limestone, and shale mined for ceramics and bricks.

▶ DIRECTIONS

From Pittsburgh, take Interstate 279 North to Interstate 79 North. Take Exit 96, Prospect–Portersville, and turn left on US 488 West. In 0.7 miles, turn right on US 19 North and follow 0.3 miles, veering right onto West Park Road. Follow 2.4 miles and turn right at the sign that indicates the South Shore (do not follow the sign for North Shore straight ahead). Pass the sign for the North Country Scenic Trail. Make a right at the T and drive 0.6 miles, following the signs for bicycle rentals. Turn right and right again to drive to the back of the parking lot to find the trailhead. If dropping off a bike or setting up a car shuttle, pass the bicycle rental facility and follow North Shore Drive 5.8 miles to the Davis Hollow Marina. Drive straight at the sign for the Davis Hollow Visitor's Center. Park in one of the eight spots designated on the near end of the lot for the center.

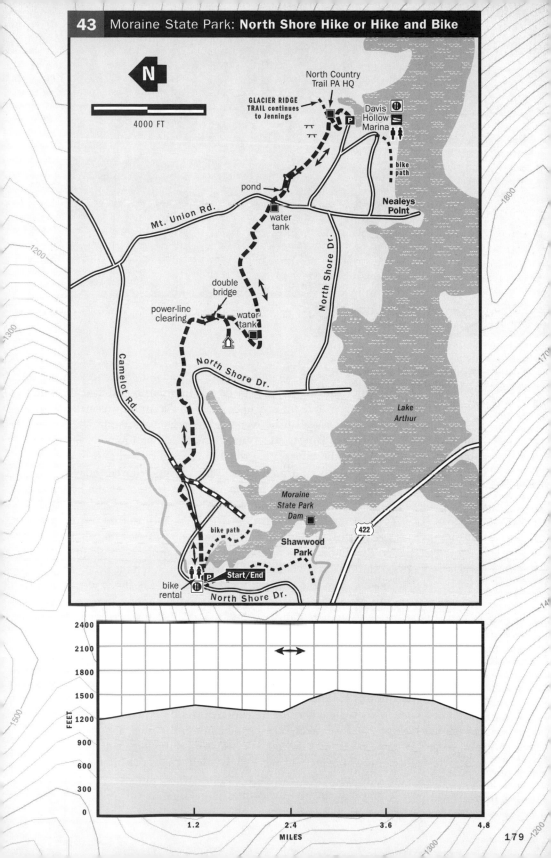

N

4000 FT

North Country
Trail PA HQ

**GLACIER RIDGE
TRAIL** continues
to Jennings

Davis
Hollow
Marina

P

bike
path

pond

water
tank

Mt. Union Rd.

North Shore Dr.

Nealeys
Point

double
bridge

power-line
clearing

water
tank

Camelot Rd.

North Shore Dr.

Lake
Arthur

Moraine
State Park
Dam

422

bike path

Shawwood
Park

bike
rental

P

Start/End

North Shore Dr.

FEET

2400
2100
1800
1500
1200
900
600
300
0

1.2   2.4   3.6   4.8
MILES

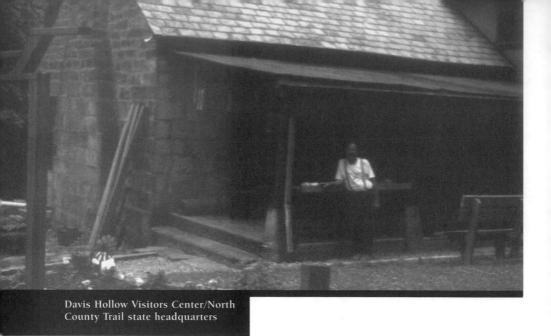

Davis Hollow Visitors Center/North
County Trail state headquarters

Fortunately, Frank W. Preston, an immigrant from England, formed the Western Pennsylvania Conservancy with the support of friends in order to purchase the land, recreate the glacial landscape, and preserve open space. Lake Arthur was created with the building of a damn to form a smaller version of glacial Lake Watts. The former Pennsylvania Departments of Forests and Waters, and mines and mineral industries cooperated to seal and backfill mines, plug the 422 gas and oil wells, treat the soil, and plant the thousands of trees, shrubs, grasses, and clovers enjoyed today.

To begin this hike, walk to the trailhead marked with an information board and sign at the far end of the parking lot. There are two signs there for the North Country Scenic Trail. The grass trail quickly gives way to dirt, and in just a few hundred feet there is a stagnant stream down the hillside on the left. Pass a bench and turn left to cross Hidden River Bridge. Along the way, see mayapple, blooming trees and shrubs, and moss with tiny white wildflowers growing from it. On the other side, just beyond a second bench, cross the bike path and continue back into the woods. In 0.36 miles, the trail turns into a wide, mowed path. You are approaching a crossing of North Shore Drive; a sign here indicates the distance. When you reenter the trail, you'll see oxeye daisies and more blooming trees and shrubs as you walk along another brief mowed section. Once in the wooded area again, the trail begins to head uphill through lush green forest and up some rocks. Pass through a mixed conifer and deciduous forest, and perhaps spot yellow cinquefoil growing here. Then go down stone stairs to a gravel road (Camelot Road) at 0.81 miles.

Stone stairs lead up the other side. In this area you'll find fan club moss, ferns, and sassafras, maple, and oak trees. You are walking on the ridge and can still hear road noise. Fortunately, this dies down soon. Don't miss the large oak at 1.3 miles, located just at a point where the trail veers slightly left. Here, during the early summer, you may also find the lovely spotted touch-me-nots, yellow flowers that hang delicately down from a thin stem off the plant.

The trail winds down and leads over a bridge fording a small stream. Almost immediately after the bridge, a trail veers off to the right. Head left following the main trail. There are many old oaks, shagbark hickory, and a mixed section with conifers. When you cross a small water runoff at 1.74 miles, be sure to look at the moss-covered rocks that cascade down its center. A stream runs alongside the trail briefly at about 2 miles and after crossing it, walk though a power-line clearing and over a small bridge. Conifers in this area include the eastern white pine, and deciduous trees include the tulip tree and American beech.

Cross the set of bridges over a stream at 2.2 miles, and you'll see a yellow-blazed trail on the right that leads to a shelter for North Country Scenic Trail through-hiker camping. Continue left. Narrow-leafed hawksbeard, a branched dandelion-like flower, and lots of ferns can be found here. I also saw what looked like evidence of a porcupine. The trail begins a steady incline and at 2.5 miles, it becomes wide and grassy, as if it used to be an old road. Find purple thistle and oxeye daisies. The trail horseshoes left around a water tank and double blazes on both posts and tree mark the way back into the woods.

At 3.67 miles you'll notice another water tank, this one off the right of the trail. Look through the woods carefully or take a walk back to admire the painting on the tank. It looks like Paul McCartney of the Beatles. Just beyond, a set of trail steps leads down to Mount Union Road. Across the road, the entrance back into the woods is just a little to the right and is marked with a large sign.

Back into the woods, cross a power-line clearing and you'll see a pond to the left. I was fortunate enough to see a snake curled up in the middle of the trail. Just as I was about to get a great picture of it, my dog came back and stepped on it and the harmless snake slithered off into the water. Cross a bridge and make the sharp right away from the pond to cross another bridge over a water runoff. Shortly after this crossing, at 3.94 miles, you'll come to a junction with a yellow-blazed trail to the left. This appears to be the former main path for the Glacier Ridge Trail per the Moraine State Park map. To reach the cabin, continue straight, following the blue blazes and sign for the marina.

After crossing another small water runoff at 4 miles, find white beardtongue, daisy fleabane, and more oxeye daisies. There's also some whorled loosestrife; you'll be able to recognize this delicate beauty by noticing that the yellow flowers and the leaves are whorled around the stem, usually in groups of four, and that the center of the flower is dotted with red. When you reach the post with double blue blazes, turn left with the trail to go to the cabin rather than using the old trail, which has been rerouted. (Going straight on that trail leads to the parking lot.) There are pin and black oak trees in this section.

There are two nicely built benches to the left of the trail that have been dedicated by the North Country Trail Association volunteers. At 4.58 miles, you'll reach a junction. The trail continues straight; make the sharp right turn to walk down to the cabin. The beautifully restored historic cabin is worth a visit, and talking to Joe Burton, the cabin's caretaker, is an additional pleasure.

The original construction of this cabin, using hand-hewn logs and hand-carved stone, took place before the American Revolution. The cabin was once the summer home of Mrs. Katherine Davis (thus the name) and her sister Miss Eleanor Holt. The walls are made of wormy American chestnut and there is even a safe built within a stone wall. Now, the cabin houses the Pennsylvania headquarters of the North Country Scenic Trail and is a haven for through-hikers or those who would like to rent it for a getaway. The cabin's caretaker notes that there is no phone or e-mail access there, but the cabin comfortably sleeps 8 to 10 guests and is able to hold 15. (See Nearby Attractions following this description for contact information.) There is a shared common area, a fully equipped kitchen, nice bunkrooms, and even a couple's room in the attic. Camping is also allowed outside of the cabin and showers are available to cabin dwellers and campers alike at the Davis Hollow Marina.

At the time of my visit, volunteers from the American Hiking Society were hammering away, building a tent platform; they had already built benches for the bike trail and a 200-foot walkway for another trail. Kudos to them and all of the volunteers of the North Country Trail Association as well.

Turn around and hike out via the same trail. If you've shuttled cars or dropped a bike, walk down the path in front of the cabin and follow the gravel road to the parking area. To reach the bike path, go to the lower parking area for the Davis Hollow Marina and turn right on the paved path. This 7-mile path provides views of Lake Arthur along the way.

▶ NEARBY ATTRACTIONS

To make reservations or check for Davis Hollow Visitor's Center cabin availability, contact Linda Matchett at (724) 779-6235 or lmatchett@zoominternet.net. For information on the North Country Scenic Trail, go to www.northcountrytrail.org. For information about Moraine State Park's boat rental, facilities, or interpretive environmental programs and activities, contact the park office at (724) 368-8811 or e-mail: morainesp@state.pa.us. Other park cabins are available to rent; go to **www.dcnr .state.pa.us.** Also, see the Moraine State Park South Shore Trails Loop (hike 44) in this book.

MORAINE STATE PARK: SOUTH SHORE TRAILS LOOP

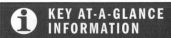

▶ IN BRIEF

This hike could be considered a tour of the South Shore of the 16,725-acre Moraine State Park. Combining three existing loops, the hiker weaves from wooded trails to the shoreline of Lake Arthur and back.

▶ DESCRIPTION

From the park office, head toward the obvious intersection, crossing Pleasant Valley Road and making a left on Big Run Road. Turn right onto the trail. There is no sign here to indicate it, but this is the Sunken Garden Trail. The trail starts off by showing some of the variety you will experience throughout the hike, passing under both deciduous and coniferous trees and through a meadow. About 800 feet along this grassy trail you will pass by one of the park's recycling centers. The trail will widen through some pines and when you've hiked about a third of a mile, there is a choice to turn right or left. Go left, turning right only leads to the road. You will soon walk back into tree cover and, after crossing a short bridge, through what is essentially a small pine forest. The trail will change from grassy, dirt-mixed mud to a carpet of pine needles as you pass through. The pleasant walk in the conifers doesn't last long. Shortly begin a slow climb for about a half mile during which you might notice Jacob's ladder afoot and berry trees beside and above you. After a very brief descent, ascend again but this time for only about 0.2 miles to reach approximately 1,370 feet, the

① KEY AT-A-GLANCE INFORMATION

LENGTH: 5.9 miles

CONFIGURATION: Combined loop

DIFFICULTY: Easy to moderate

SCENERY: Deciduous and coniferous forest, meadows, Lake Arthur

EXPOSURE: Mostly shaded

TRAFFIC: Light

TRAIL SURFACE: Grass and dirt

HIKING TIME: 3–3.5 hours

ACCESS: Park is open from sunrise to sunset

MAPS: Available at the park office at the trailhead or at **www.dcnr.state.pa.us/ stateparks/parks/moraine_maps.aspx;** USGS Prospect

FACILITIES: Park office, restrooms, picnic areas, boat rental and launches

SPECIAL COMMENTS: Moraine State Park conducts a variety of interpretive environmental programs, including guided walks, campfire talks, and hands-on activities; contact the park office at (724) 368-8811 or e-mail morainesp@ state.pa.us. Volunteer organizations develop projects and offer interpretive boat tours based out of McDaniel's Boat Launch; contact the Moraine Preservation Fund at (724) 368-9185. Also, see the Moraine State Park North Shore Tour (hike 43) in this book.

▶ DIRECTIONS

From Pittsburgh, take Interstate 279 North to Interstate 79 North. Take the Prospect–Portersville exit and turn left following PA 422 and signs for Moraine State Park, South Shore. Make a left onto Pleasant Valley Road and park in the parking lot for the park office.

Moraine State Park: South Shore Trails Loop

UTM Zone (WGS84)   17T

Easting   576032

Northing   4532341

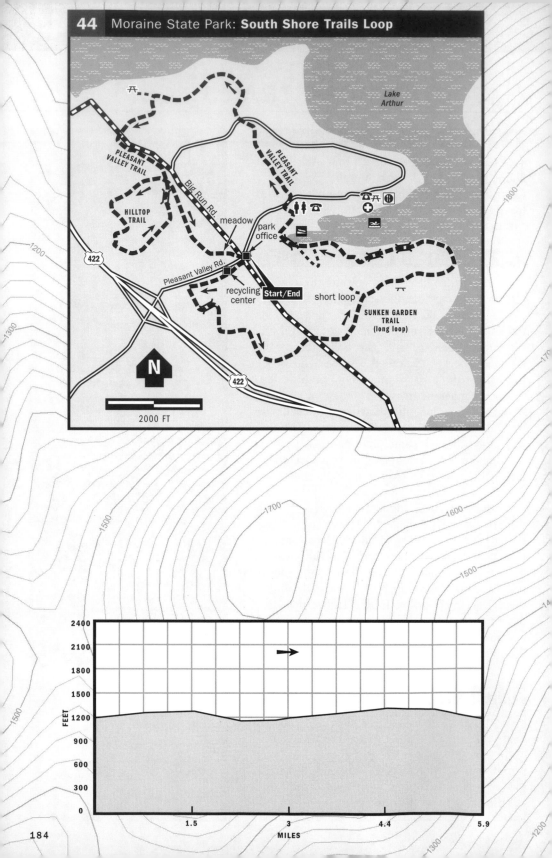

Lake
Arthur

PLEASANT
VALLEY
TRAIL

PLEASANT
VALLEY TRAIL

Big Run Rd.

HILLTOP
TRAIL

meadow

park
office

422

Pleasant Valley Rd.

recycling
center

Start/End

short loop

SUNKEN GARDEN
TRAIL
(long loop)

N

422

2000 FT

second highest point on this lakeside trail. If you are hungry, start looking for the apple trees; you may get lucky and find a ripe one. Watch out for the hawthorns, though.

At 1.1 miles, cross the gravel road and continue on the wide path back into a more forested area. At 1.4 miles, turn right for the long loop of the Sunken Garden Trail. If you make a left here the remainder of the hike is cut short and does not lead to the lake. You'll find wild roses and more apple trees before you descend for about a half mile. At the end of the noticeable descent (1.5 miles) take time to enjoy the peacefulness in this beautiful setting by sitting on a bench; it's roofed by a pine tree and provides a soft place for your boots on its needles. The break is followed by another descent; watch your step down the grassy, muddy path. You come out to a lakeside view, but unfortunately there is nowhere to sit here. After enjoying the breezes off the lake and the site and smell of the water, follow the trail back into the woods. At 2.24 miles you'll cross the first of two 20-foot-long bridges. Continue and be taken aback by a beautiful field packed with goldenrod and butterflies. Your other senses receive a treat as well thanks to the sounds of the water and children's laughter, the feel of light breezes, and the softness of pine needles beneath your feet as you pass through another pine forest.

At 2.5 miles turn right at an unmarked T and head back toward the lake. You may see a family of ducks here amid the lily pads and perhaps some gaiter-clad anglers out in the water. You will shortly find yourself at another unmarked T; turn right, cross a bridge, and look over the wetland. Soon, you'll emerge from the woods to the Pleasant Valley picnic area. If you wish, you can stroll down to the water; swimming and boating are permitted in the bay. Restrooms, a concession area, first aid, and a phone are available.

When you are ready to leave the area, go left up the access road and right on the main road. Look left for the reentry point and enter the Pleasant Valley Trail; there is a sign posted at the trailhead. The narrow trail starts with grass and turns to dirt where you are again surrounded by young deciduous forest. At about 3.2 miles the trail will break out into a meadow and then to a road crossing. Head straight across the road to pick the trail up on the other side. At 3.9 miles, make a left at the unmarked branch in the trail. (Going straight will lead you to another parking and picnic area by the water.) After passing through more mixed forest along a fairly level section of the trail, cross Big Run Road and begin an ascent that continues for about a quarter mile. At the intersection found at 4.5 miles, make a right to tour the Hill Top Trail. (You may skip this 1-mile short loop by going straight.)

You will trade between small inclines and declines as you hike along this loop. When you see signs indicating trails for the short loop and long loop, take the short-loop branch (unless you want the long loop, adding 2 miles to your hike). A steep descent delivers you to another pine forest section and then an unmarked intersection; go right and walk over the single-track bridge. Return to the intersection with Pleasant Valley Trail and make a right. When you have reached another meadow there is a house off to the right. You are almost finished. The trail ends across from the parking lot at the park office.

(See Special Comments for nearby attractions.)

TODD SANCTUARY LOOP

KEY AT-A-GLANCE INFORMATION

LENGTH: 2.2 miles

CONFIGURATION: Loop

DIFFICULTY: Easy

SCENERY: Watson's Run, wake robin trillium, smaller white trillium, hemlocks, mayapples, pond

EXPOSURE: Mostly shaded

TRAFFIC: Light

TRAIL SURFACE: Dirt

HIKING TIME: 1.5 hours

ACCESS: Open year-round, dawn–dusk, except during the Pennsylvania buck and doe season. (Hunting is not allowed, but there is heavy hunting activity on neighboring properties.)

MAPS: Available at the trailhead or online at www.aswp.org (neither is entirely in agreement with the posts and trail names at the sanctuary, though); USGS Freeport

FACILITIES: None

SPECIAL COMMENTS: The directions go around the Monroe Bridge as it is in repair. Check the Web site included in Maps for current status. Sign in at the informational kiosk. Dogs are not permitted.

Todd Sanctuary Loop

UTM Zone (WGS84) 17T

Easting 609591

Northing 4509906

IN BRIEF

Definition of *sanctuary*: A place of refuge for birds, wild animals, et cetera. Sanctuary is the perfect descriptor for this remote-feeling gem. Consider yourself part of the "et cetera" and relax for a peaceful hike.

DESCRIPTION

The Todd Sanctuary came into being when, in 1942, W. E. Clyde Todd, noted ornithologist at Carnegie Mellon University, donated a parcel of land that today has been expanded to 176 acres to the Audubon Society of Western Pennsylvania.

After signing in at the kiosk, walk down the stone and wood stairs to the gravel path. If you are here during spring, look over the hillside for wake robin trillium, a deep purple large-flowered trillium I've not found to be nearly as abundant as the smaller white variety. The waterway you'll notice at the bottom of the hill is Watson's Run and the hike travels over it several times. Turn right and follow the hemlock-lined gravel path to reach a post, which may have a sign indicating that the cabin and trails are to the left. The name "Ravine" for the Ravine Trail is also carved in it and painted purple, trailside of the post. This begins the loop; walk straight ahead to follow the Ravine Trail.

In about another 250 feet, notice a sign that says "Old Mill" pointing left. I didn't see an old mill, but a quick walk (about 30 feet) in that direction provides a nice view of the run's waters

DIRECTIONS

From Pittsburgh, take PA 28 North to Butler–Freeport (Exit 17). Turn right onto PA 356 North and go 3.6 miles. Turn right onto Sarver Road; travel 3.5 miles. Turn right on Kepple Road and drive 1.2 miles to the sanctuary parking lot on left (a sign marks the property coming from the opposite direction).

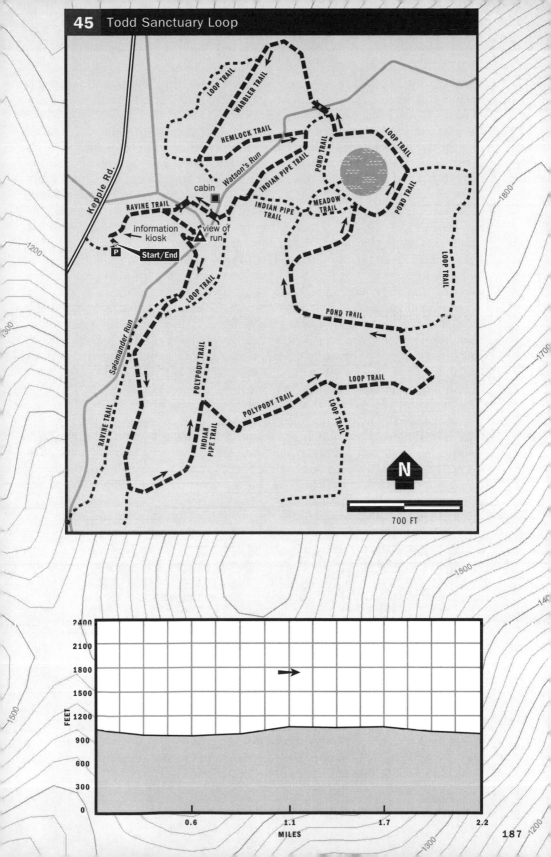

LOOP TRAIL
WARBLER TRAIL
HEMLOCK TRAIL
Watson's Run
cabin
Kepple Rd.
RAVINE TRAIL
information kiosk
view of run
P
Start/End
INDIAN PIPE TRAIL
INDIAN PIPE TRAIL
POND TRAIL
MEADOW TRAIL
LOOP TRAIL
POND TRAIL
LOOP TRAIL
Salamander Run
LOOP TRAIL
POND TRAIL
LOOP TRAIL
POLYPODY TRAIL
INDIAN PIPE TRAIL
POLYPODY TRAIL
LOOP TRAIL
RAVINE TRAIL
LOOP TRAIL

N

700 FT

2400
2100
1800
1500
1200
900
600
300
0
FEET
0.6   1.1   1.7   2.2
MILES

cascading down shelved rock. As you hike, it's likely that the constant birdsong is becoming noticeable. It will accompany you throughout the hike in this sanctuary. Come to Watson's Run and use the large rocks to cross it, or perhaps stop awhile to enjoy its soothing sound; this is a great spot for lunch on a warm day.

At the junction for Loop and Ravine trails, turn left onto Loop Trail, which is blazed in red. Soon come to a T with a post showing Loop Trail running in both directions. Turn right. The trail here is rocky, but the grade is very easy. At 0.32 miles turn left at the post for Loop Trail. The Ravine Trail and Watson's Run are below to the right. Heading up the easy grade, jack-in-the-pulpits and hemlocks stand out. The trail becomes narrower and then soon opens where there is a lot of deadfall. Look closely to follow the trail around fallen trees. At almost 0.5 miles there is a directional sign for the trail, and shortly after another to turn left to follow the Loop Trail. (The trail appears to go straight here but it has been rerouted.) Turn left. Jacob's ladder, wild rose, and mayapples can be found along this section.

At 0.5 miles, you'll come to an intersection for Indian Pipe Trail. Go straight, following its white blazes. Upon entering this trail it is as if someone drew a line against heavy use. The trail is narrow and green, with ground cover growing close and over it. This doesn't impede one's ability to see the trail; it just appears as though few shoes have tread upon it. Many wildflowers grow along its sides as well as fields of mayapples. In early July, the plant for which this trail is named blooms its smoking pipe–like white blossoms. In early May, other white and purple wildflowers are flourishing.

Arrive at 0.63 miles at an intersection with the orange-blazed Polypody Trail; turn right. This eastern segment of the Polypody Trail begins with dainty purple wildflowers, and in another 250 feet opens wide through a young forest of black birch and red maples. The trail is named for the small, evergreen polypody fern that grows on the western section of the trail. Here, fan club moss is found in abundance, as are patches of mayapples. This is an inner trail of the sanctuary and no sound can be heard except bird calls and songs, and the occasional scattering of small animals.

At 0.82 miles, you'll reach the end of the Polypody Trail and a choice of going straight ahead or turning right on the Loop Trail. There is a sign here, currently supported only by a fallen tree. Go straight (turning right would loop you back in the direction from which you hiked). More mayapples and the tiny white flowers that had blanketed the Indian Pipe Trail are found along this section of the Loop Trail.

A sign for Pond Trail is found at 1 mile. (Note that the map on the Web site calls this the Meadow Trail, but the kiosk map name matches the sign and calls it Pond Trail. There actually is both a Meadow Trail and a Pond Trail; they later split. The trail is blazed in yellow and the color is consistent among all resources.)

Turn left to follow the level Pond Trail, which meanders through open meadows that were once farm fields. The absence of rocks on or along this Pennsylvania trail seems evidence of the area's past. Now, very young red maples and crab apple thickets grow. Turn right at the double yellow blazes at 1.13 miles. At 1.18 miles, where the sign indicates straight for the Indian Pipe Trail, turn right on Pond Trail. Walking next to some crab apple trees, notice the "thorns" that grow from their twigs; these are actually modified branches known as spur branches.

You'll arrive at another sign at 1.3 miles indicating a hard left to follow the

Meadow Trail. Take the Pond Trail, keeping the pond to your left. Notice a Y where the left goes directly to the edge of the pond. Continuing to the right on the trail and under more crab apple trees, you may see deer tracks and perhaps raccoon tracks, too. The trail travels closely to the pond on the far side and here I startled a couple of bullfrogs. They responded by jumping into the pond and poking their metallic green heads above the water for a look at me too.

At 1.4 miles, find a sign for a connection to the Loop Trail. The sign only points to the right; but this is where Pond Trail ends, so both directions are for the Loop Trail. Stay straight. (Going right would take you back to where you departed from the Loop Trail 0.4 miles prior.) Soon the trail travels farther from the pond and back into the woods. Pass by what appears to be the remains of an old rock wall and at 1.5 miles come to a juncture with another branch of Pond Trail. Go right to stay on Loop Trail and head away from the pond. A juncture with Indian Pipe Trail comes up quickly; bypass it and continue on the Loop Trail.

After a short, smooth descent through some hemlocks, cross a small stone bridge over Watson's Run, where you'll find skunk cabbage. The trail is fairly easy and level after a small rise away from the run. Leave the Loop Trail at 1.68 miles and travel straight on the Warbler Trail, which is blazed in blue. This trail follows an old logging road built in the 1950s. Although the map from the kiosk states that many hemlocks were killed by a looper moth outbreak, there are still some to enjoy throughout this beautiful section.

At 1.8 miles the Warbler Trail ends with a choice to take the Loop Trail or Hemlock Trail. Make a left onto the green-blazed Hemlock Trail to complete an exploration of every trail within the sanctuary. Huge skunk cabbage and many mayapples mark its beginning, which leads to some soggy steps to streamside groves of hemlocks hugging the sides of the trail. Cross over Watson's Run again, using the rocks, and reach a junction with Indian Pipe Trail. Turn right on Indian Pipe Trail, where you may spot a few white trilliums. At 2 miles there is another post oriented in a bit of a confusing way. Turn right to continue on Indian Pipe to where it meets Loop Trail. Come to another post and walk to the right over a well-constructed bridge above scenic Watson's Run. This leads to the cabin. Surrounding it is a couple of benches that make a nice resting spot. Cross the bridge for the final trip over the run to return to your car.

▶ NEARBY ATTRACTIONS

There are restaurants and markets along PA 356. Nature walks and tours of the small cabin located near the sanctuary entrance are conducted. More information can be found at the **www.aswp.org** or by calling Beechwood Farms at (724) 963-6100.

SOMERSET AND FAYETTE COUNTIES

BEAR RUN NATURE RESERVE: SOUTHEAST LOOP

KEY AT-A-GLANCE INFORMATION

LENGTH: 8.1 miles

CONFIGURATION: Loop

DIFFICULTY: Moderate to difficult due to elevation gain and distance

SCENERY: Ancient hemlock stand, pine grove, deciduous trees, Bear Run, and Beaver Run

EXPOSURE: Mostly shaded

TRAFFIC: Light away from front trails

TRAIL SURFACE: Dirt path, sometimes rocky with roots

HIKING TIME: 4–5 hours

ACCESS: Open year-round

MAPS: Bear Run Nature Reserve map available at trailhead or by contacting the Western Pennsylvania Conservancy at (724) 329-8501 or (412) 288-2777; USGS Mill Run

FACILITIES: No restroom facilities; camping available for backpackers (no registration required)

SPECIAL COMMENTS: Pets are not permitted on the reserve. Hunting is also not permitted but occasionally has been reported within the reserve's outer boundaries.

Bear Run Nature Reserve:
Southeast Loop

UTM Zone (WGS84)   17S

Easting   631620

Northing   4418420

IN BRIEF

The Western Pennsylvania Conservancy owns and protects this 5,000-acre reserve located on the western slope of Laurel Ridge. The trails and terrain are diverse and notably beautiful and peaceful. This hike includes passing through a stand of virgin hemlocks, dense woods, and many views of the clear waters of Bear Run.

DESCRIPTION

There is something about stepping between the information sign and registration and comment box onto the trail in this particular reserve that signifies almost instantly that this is going to be a special place. The beauty of the trail and woods ahead immediately draws one in, making the hiker feel as though he or she is walking into the world the way it should be.

The hike begins on the Wagon Trail, through a grove of pines and on a bed of their long, fallen needles. Just a few hundred feet in, make a right on Arbutus Trail. If it's muddy, use the large flat stones placed to assist visitors in keeping their boots dry and the trail from becoming a mess. Follow this to a post for Pine Trail, which leads to the left. Continue straight on Arbutus and do the same at the following intersection with Ridge Trail. As you walk through the mix of pine and deciduous trees you may still hear a little road

DIRECTIONS

From Pittsburgh, take I-376 East and enter the Pennsylvania Turnpike I-76 East (toll road). Take Exit 91, Ligonier-Uniontown. Turn left onto PA 31 East. Go straight for 2.1 miles and then right onto PA 711–PA 381 South and follow for 10 miles to Normalville. Make a left at the T, continuing on PA 381 South, and follow it about 7.5 miles. Bear Run Nature Reserve is on the left. Drive up past the Bear Run Center building to the parking area.

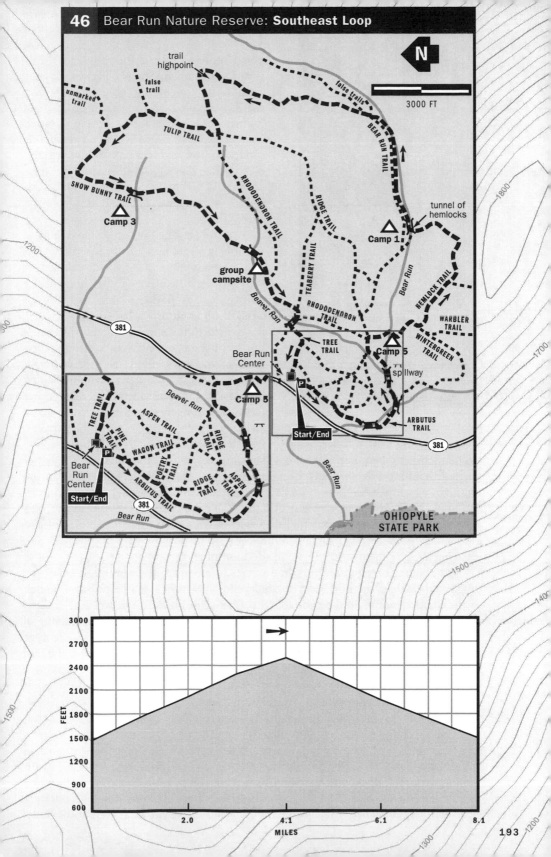

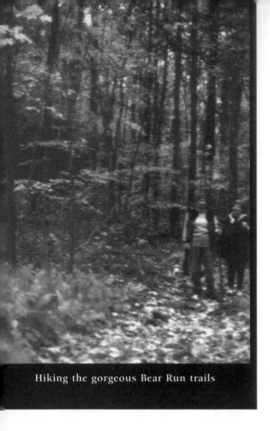

Hiking the gorgeous Bear Run trails

noise until you hike farther inward. PA 381 is not a busy road, though, and the passing cars are infrequent. Stepping carefully over rocks, a couple of boulders, and roots, and following a walk on a long section of raised wooden planks, you will find you are among rhododendrons tall enough to give a sense of entering the wild and leaving the trappings of humankind behind. Only the sounds of the wind, water, and birdsong are audible now.

You'll see the source of the sound of running water when you reach a 25-foot-long wooden bridge that provides a fine first view of scenic Bear Run. Continuing, at 0.5 miles you may notice a wide trail, but go straight on Arbutus. In less than 0.2 miles, cross Bear Run again via another charming bridge; this one has a flat seat along the left side, providing a comfortable place to sit and admire a small waterfall complemented by mosses and overhanging rhododendron. Once you leave this spot and reenter dense walls of rhododendrons the trail narrows. Pass by a left for Aspen Trail and continue straight, crossing Bear Run once more. The run will be traveling close on the left of the trail briefly before the bank rises up. Once you pass Wintergreen Trail on the right, however, the bank drops prior to a spillway and another bridge. Over the bridge and around a bend is a bench across from a second spillway. If you want to rest, this is a good spot. Next ascend the trail up a pair of stone steps heading to the left and away from the water. If you are an admirer of rhododendrons you will love this trail; it is chock-full of them, and you are headed for more.

At about 1 mile the Arbutus Trail comes to an end with an intersection of the Ridge Trail. Make a right on Ridge (blazed yellow). Within 0.1 mile pass the branch to the Rhododendron Trail on the left and turn right on the Hemlock Trail (blazed white). Mainly deciduous trees and a sea of rhododendron occupy the beginning of the Hemlock Trail but a stand of virgin hemlocks will soon be visible. Pass the large boulder high on the trail on the left and Camp 5 on your right. As you follow the trail to the right, the hemlocks for which the trail was named come into view, making a pretty sight as you cross Bear Run once again. The trail begins to ascend, becomes rockier, and leaves the hemlocks for deciduous trees.

At 1.5 miles, pass the turn for the Wintergreen Trail and continue the consistent climb, passing the turn for Warbler Trail at 1.8 miles. The trail twists and turns and becomes rather steep for the next 0.3 miles. Look carefully for the white blazes and double blazes for turns. Shortly after the trail levels it becomes a steep descent through a tunnel of small hemlocks. This part of the trail is especially tranquil and picturesque. Cross the small bridge over Bear Run and delight in walking under the eight-foot-long branches of the ancient hemlocks. Finally, you've arrived at the trail's feature, and it is worth the hike up to reach it. The trail opens out very wide and towering hemlocks line each side for about 200 feet.

You'll come to a campfire ring in the center of the trail, indicating you've reached Campsite 1. Looking up the hill to the right reveals another site included in this camping area. Go straight to avoid disturbing someone's camp, and shortly, at 2.5 miles, you'll reach a point where the trail opens wide on the right. Turn right (up grass) and look up to the right—you are making a U-turn around the camps to take the Bear Run Trail (blazed orange).

The Bear Run Trail does indeed follow Bear Run, but it is high above it and leaves it behind and out of sight because this trail leads higher and closer to the ridge than does the Ridge Trail. You immediately begin to ascend, heading up to a high point of 2,478 feet. The trail is wide for awhile and offers a variety of nut trees; you may find some to munch along the way. Do not take the unmarked, false trails found at almost 3.5 miles; just keep heading upward, and at 4 miles notice that the trail begins bearing right and becoming narrower as you hike around the knoll that marks the high point. You'll know you are almost to the high point when the trail veers left around it. There is no marker or a grand view here, but there is a sense of serenity, solitude, and peace that makes the trek worth every step. This is a nice spot for lunch, and there is a rock and a log just around the bend.

Quickly descend a few hundred feet and, at 4.8 miles, reach a three-way intersection where the Rhododendron Trail is straight ahead, the Ridge Trail is on the left, and the Tulip Trail is on the right. Make a right on Tulip Trail (blazed yellow), which begins with a fairly level walk through some older hardwoods on a narrower and rockier trail. Pass by another unmarked false trail at 5.3 miles, heading left instead where you descend about 400 feet before reaching an intersection. The Laurel Trail is straight ahead and the Snow Bunny Trail is to the left (the Tulip Trail ends here). Turn left on Snow Bunny (blazed orange). This widening trail then crosses a bridge over a feeder stream. If you are here in the autumn you will find yourself surrounded by every color of leaf imaginable. At about 6 miles Campsite 3 is on the right, and at 7 miles there is a group campsite.

At 7.25 miles, you'll reach an intersection with the Rhododendron Trail (Snow Bunny ends here); go straight, not left, on Rhododendron and pass the left for Teaberry Trail at 7.5 miles. In just 0.1 mile, take the right onto Tree Trail (blazed yellow). Pay attention when the trail begins to veer left after the bridge to avoid taking either of the two false trails on the right. Go straight when you reach the Aspen Trail branch on the left to walk through the silent and serene long-needled pine grove to the trail start. When the silence ends with familiar road noise, the hike is almost over. Eight miles marks the end of the Tree Trail. Make the left around the meadow. Bear Run Center and the parking lot come into view, and you finish at 8.12 miles where you began.

▶ NEARBY ATTRACTIONS

Fallingwater, which has a cafe, is just up PA 381 South on the right. There are small local restaurants on PA 381 North, too. Or you can head farther south for the many stores, cafes, and restaurants in Ohiopyle.

FORBES STATE FOREST: LICK HOLLOW INTERPRETIVE NATURE TRAIL

KEY AT-A-GLANCE INFORMATION

LENGTH: 0.8 miles (from car and return to car included)

CONFIGURATION: Loop

DIFFICULTY: Easy

SCENERY: Deciduous forest and Lick Run

EXPOSURE: Shaded

TRAFFIC: Light

TRAIL SURFACE: Dirt

HIKING TIME: 0.5–1 hour

ACCESS: Open Memorial Day–Labor Day, Thursday–Monday, 11 a.m.–dusk

MAPS: Available at the park office (lower-level parking area) and at the Forbes District Forest Office on US 30 in Laughlintown, (724) 238-1200, or via e-mail at fd04@state.pa.us; low-quality PDF maps are also available online via the Pennsylvania Department of Conservation and Natural Resources Web site, **www.dcnr.state.pa.us** (but there is not enough detail on these); USGS Brownfield

FACILITIES: Restrooms, picnic tables, charcoal grills, drinking water

SPECIAL COMMENTS: This short trail, in conjunction with this interpretive guide (and the one provided by the forester, if you'd like), is a great learning experience and perfect for any novice to the woodlands.

Forbes State Forest:
Lick Hollow Interpretive Nature Trail

UTM Zone (WGS84)   17S

Easting   613216

Northing   4412907

IN BRIEF

The Lick Hollow Area is really very beautiful. It has an abundance of picnic tables nicely spaced and most are shaded. In combination with Lick Run and the available hikes, this is a perfect place to have a family day.

DESCRIPTION

To reach the trailhead, follow the road you just drove in on back toward the information board. Look to the left for the trailhead, which is marked with a box on a post that contains the interpretive trail guides. Take a guide and walk straight onto the path.

Reach Post 1 right away. In the guide, the forest service notes the change in temperature that is felt immediately once within the forested area. This is due to the shade and the water vapor expelled from the undersides of the leaves; one of the larger trees in the forest can give off 50 to 100 gallons of water on a hot day. At Post 2 are native tulip trees, also called tulip poplar or yellow poplar. Look for green, cup-shaped flowers up in the branches or their petals, easily identified by the orange color at their bases, on the trail. One of the tallest and most beautiful of the eastern hardwoods, this tree typically grows 80 to 120 feet. According to the guide, the trees here are approximately 60 to 80 years old and likely began growing after the last timber harvest in the early 1900s. A tonic for heart ailments was once made from the tulip tree's bitter, aromatic roots.

DIRECTIONS

From Pittsburgh, take PA 51 South to US 40 East. Travel 8 miles to the Lick Hollow gate, or take US 40 East business route and travel about 6.5 miles to the Lick Hollow gate. Drive down the gravel road 0.3 miles and make the first right to park in the upper lot.

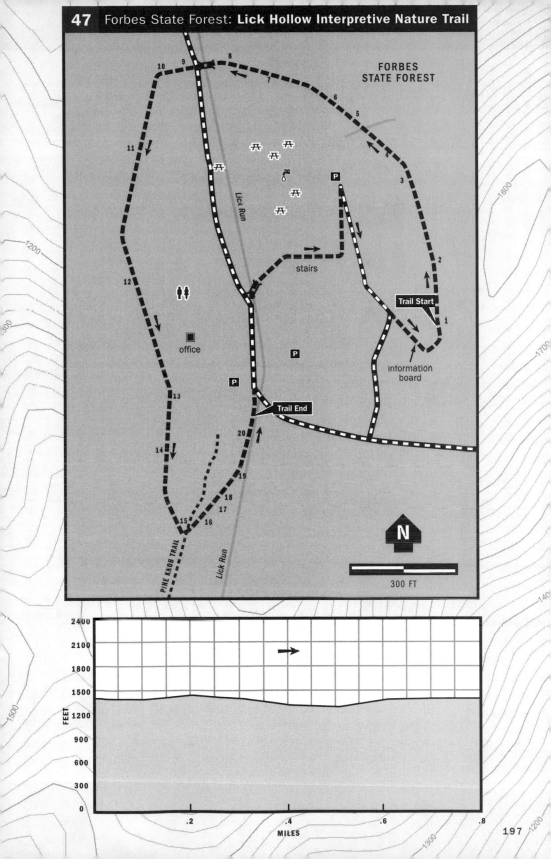

FORBES
STATE FOREST

Lick Run

stairs

Trail Start

information
board

office

Trail End

PINE KNOB TRAIL

Lick Run

N

300 FT

Post 3 is placed next to a black cherry tree. When in spring bloom, the small flowers of this tree are grouped at the ends of leafy branches in elongated clusters usually 4 to 6 inches long. The tart, edible cherries mature in late summer and provide an important food source for birds and wildlife. The bark and roots contain hydrocyanic acid, which has been used in cough medicines and for flavoring.

Post 4 is just a short walk. In the guide, the importance of leaving rotting logs, stumps, and branches is explained—they serve as a food source and nesting ground for insects and the insects serve as a food source for small animals. Bacteria and fungi attack the wood and turn it into new rich soil in which other trees and plant life grow.

Cross a small water runoff to reach Post 5. Here, you'll find the white ash tree; look for the diamond-shaped pattern of its bark. Its leaves are not lobed, and their white undersides give the tree its name; and it produces green, winged seeds. The straight, narrow-grained wood of this tree is used to make hockey sticks, baseball bats, tennis rackets, snowshoes, and furniture. The white ash is the tallest (about 40 to 60 feet) of all 16 ash-tree species in the United States.

At Post 6 arrive at a maple tree. This is a red maple, also known as a scarlet maple, soft maple, and swamp maple. The first two names are due to the brilliant red color of its leaves in spring and fall, reddish wing-shaped seeds, and the reddish flowers produced by both the male and female in late winter or early spring. Even though this tree is also called soft maple, its wood is hard and brittle. The red maple enjoys the greatest distribution of all tree species along the East Coast. Pioneers used bark extract for ink and cinnamon-brown and black dyes.

Walking to Post 7 takes you to a power-line clearing, or electric line right-of-way (as it's called in the book). The guide states that wildlife and birds find the meeting of two different habitats to be beneficial. I did notice quite a bit of birdsong as I approached. It also is nice to read in the guide that it is the policy of the Bureau of Forestry that herbicides are not used to clear or maintain electric line right-of-ways on state forestland. Notice the fenced-in area on the left. This area was used to plant saplings to be used for reforestation. Perhaps it will be used again for more new trees.

When reaching Post 8, you are in a riparian zone—the area along the water's edge. The trees and plant life here are very important to aquatic species living in the water because they provide shade to keep the water's temperature down. They are also being promoted for use along rivers and other waterways at the edges of farm fields and industrial zones to assist in filtering pesticides and other harmful substances before they reach the water.

The short walk to Post 9 leads to an American sycamore tree. This is one of the largest broadleaf trees in the state and can be easily identified by its often massive trunk and two-layer bark, the top one peeling to show its whitish, yellowish, or greenish inner layer. It is also known as an American plane, buttonwood, or button-ball tree, the last name after its nutlets, which look like small green balls.

Cross the wooden bridge over scenic Lick Run and notice the moss-covered rocks and boulders strewn along its length. Cross the service road, and continue to Post 10 where you find an area once used as a log landing during a timber harvesting in 1979. The area has since been seeded and several apple trees were also planted.

The trail heads uphill here and is lovely with fern and boulders. You are now walking on a retired logging road, which is what is discussed in the guide for Post 11. The old road follows the natural contours of the hillside. Walking up to Post 12 see if you can pick out any of the trees discussed so far, such as the American sycamore. There are also a variety of maples and birch. The birch trees can be identified by their distinct bark, with thin furrows or bark peeling horizontally. As you make your way to Posts 12 through 14, the guide discusses select harvesting (at Post 12) done in 1979 and thinning stands of trees (Posts 13 and 14).

About 100 feet after Post 14 the trail begins to travel back downhill. At Post 15 a large old American beech (smooth gray bark) that is lying beside the trail can be found. According to the guide, it was about 250 years old, and at least 32 kinds of birds and mammals in Pennsylvania who are cavity nesters make good use of hollow trunks such as this. Cross the trail junction with Pine Knob Trail to reach Post 16, which marks the red oak tree, a fast-growing tree whose wood is used for many products such as flooring, kitchen cabinets, and high-quality veneer. A field of ferns can be admired on the way to Post 17. At this point on the trail, the guide notes that you are standing on an old log-tram road that was probably used around the turn of the century. Temporary railroad tracks were laid so that logs could be hauled by small locomotives from the upper valley down to what is now the Lick Hollow picnic area.

Post 18 brings you to an eastern hemlock, the state tree. It is one of four species of hemlock in the United States and the only one native to Pennsylvania. The top, or terminal shoot, is flexible and tends to curve away from the direction of prevailing winds; it commonly leans in an easterly direction. The tannin (tannic acid) from its bark was once used to tan hides. The eastern hemlock can be extremely long-lived, some surviving up to 600 years, which is good because this tree does not reproduce well; young trees are fragile and often do not reach maturity. It also does not transplant well.

At Post 19 take a good look at the growths coming out of the pieces of the tree trunk, another interesting fact pointed out in the guide. These growths are called conks, and they are the external fruiting bodies of a fungus that caused decay inside the tree trunk while it was still standing. Also notice the many pretty rhododendrons in the area, along with more large red oaks and red (smooth) maple. The rhododendrons are commonly found along shaded streams in the Appalachian Mountains and are gorgeous in bloom in late June and early July. Their impenetrable thickets provide refuge from predators of deer and other wildlife; these are discussed in the guide at Post 20.

Walk down to the road, past the park office and make a right over the bridge crossing Lick Run. If returning to your car, walk through the picnic area and up the stairs. If you are fortunate enough to be enjoying a picnic here, it's a beautiful place. For a longer hike, see Nearby Attractions below.

▶ NEARBY ATTRACTIONS

For another hike without traveling, go to the Lick Hollow Pine Knob Overlook Trail (hike 48) in this book. There are many other attractions in this area, including Laurel Caverns, and places to eat are located by continuing west a little way on US 40. Other hikes or tours can be found in this book for nearby Quebec Run (hike 50), Fort Necessity National Battlefield (hike 51), and Friendship Hill National Historic Site (hike 52).

FORBES STATE FOREST: LICK HOLLOW PINE KNOB OVERLOOK TRAIL

 KEY AT-A-GLANCE INFORMATION

LENGTH: 4.2 miles

CONFIGURATION: Out-and-back

DIFFICULTY: Moderate

SCENERY: Expansive overlook view, deciduous forest, mountain laurel, abandoned gristmill stone

EXPOSURE: Shaded except at overlook

TRAFFIC: Moderate

TRAIL SURFACE: Dirt

HIKING TIME: 2.5 hours

ACCESS: Open Memorial Day–Labor Day, Thursday–Monday, 11 a.m.–dusk

MAPS: Available at the park office (lower-level parking area) and at the Forbes District Forest Office on US 30 in Laughlintown, (724) 238-1200, or via e-mail at fd04@state.pa.us; low-quality PDF maps are also available online via the Pennsylvania Department of Conservation and Natural Resources Web site, **www.dcnr.state.pa.us** (but there is not enough detail on these); USGS Brownfield

FACILITIES: Restrooms, picnic tables, charcoal grills, drinking water

SPECIAL COMMENTS: If interested in learning a little about the history and flora of the area, you might consider doing the Interpretive Nature Trail (hike 47 in this book) first.

Forbes State Forest:
Lick Hollow Pine Knob Overlook Trail

UTM Zone (WGS84)   17S

Easting   613067

Northing   4412827

▶ IN BRIEF

The Lick Hollow Area is beautiful. It has an abundance of picnic tables nicely spaced and most are shaded. In combination with Lick Run and the available hikes, this is a perfect place to have a family day. This hike also provides an outstanding view from a rocky outcropping overlook, so bring your binoculars.

▶ DESCRIPTION

To reach the trailhead, simply turn 180 degrees from facing the parking area and Lick Run and look for the trailhead sign across the gravel road. Follow the direction of the sign, away from the park office building. About 100 feet in, pass the trail veering off to the right and follow the blue blazes. At this point, the trail appears to be an old road and may be a former tram road. These thoroughfares were set up for temporary train tracks to haul logs from the upper reaches of the valley when these mountains were logged around the turn of the century.

Cross over the intersection with the Nature Trail and continue straight. There is a well-stocked map box just beyond the intersection. The environment around the trail is lush and green with ferns and moss; boulders dot the area everywhere. There are a couple of eastern hemlocks in the beginning, although deciduous hardwoods prevail in the woody landscape. Watch your footing, as the trail becomes rocky. Cross over the first of several small water runoffs that seep across the trail down to Lick Run.

▶ DIRECTIONS

From Pittsburgh, take PA 51 South to US 40 East. Travel 8 miles to the Lick Hollow gate, or take the US 40 East business route and travel about 6.5 miles to the Lick Hollow gate. Drive down the gravel road 0.4 miles and make the second right to park in the lower lot.

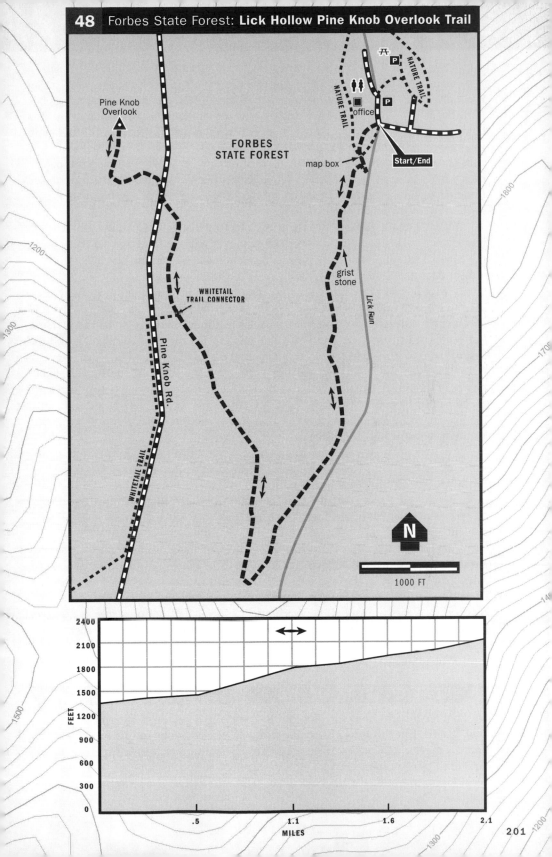

Pine Knob
Overlook

FORBES
STATE FOREST

office

P

P

NATURE TRAIL

NATURE TRAIL

Start/End

map box

grist
stone

Lick Run

WHITETAIL
TRAIL CONNECTOR

Pine Knob Rd.

WHITETAIL TRAIL

N

1000 FT

2400

2100

1800

1500

1200

900

600

300

0

FEET

.5   1.1   1.6   2.1

MILES

At just 0.3 miles is a sign directing you to turn left to see a large gristmill stone; it is only about 20 feet off of the trail. There was once a gristmill at nearby Quebec Run, but it is unknown whether this particular stone (which was found here) was being made for it. After checking it out, return to the trail, where you'll find tulip trees, white ash, and pin oak as you hike. Tulip trees are one of the tallest and most beautiful eastern hardwoods, producing a cup-shaped flower with long green petals, each with an orange base. If you've arrived after they've bloomed, you're sure to see these petals lining the trail. You are likely to be looking down, anyway, as there are also many chaotic small boulders to negotiate.

At 0.63 miles, you'll notice the trunk of a tree that is being hollowed out while it is standing. This could be the work of carpenter ants, termites, or perhaps conks, the external fruiting bodies of a fungus. A peek inside offered me no clues, though I did see deer mushrooms in this area.

Cross several more water runoffs around 0.84 miles. At 1 mile, you'll reach a section where mountain laurel can be seen along the trail and the grade of the trail becomes a bit steeper. There are young maples and huge boulders, some of which the trail winds directly around. For these, blue paint marks the way. Once you round the first of these to turn right for the switchback, the grade is reduced.

Traversing the hillside, you'll find enormous blackjack and chestnut oaks and plenty of mountain laurel. You'll also hear a lot of birdsong that, unfortunately, is accompanied by road noise from US 40 the entire way. I can't say I found it disturbing enough to be very distracting. At 1.38 miles, the forest has thinned noticeably and ferns grow down the hillside as far as you can see.

At 1.64 miles, you'll come to a connector to the White Tail Trail, which runs south along Pine Knob Road to your east for awhile. White Tail Trail goes all the way to the Quebec Wild Area. Continue straight; you are getting very close to the overlook. Reach Pine Knob Road at 1.9 miles and turn right, looking for the blue blazes. As you round the bend left, leave the main road to reach the overlook. Do not go straight and downhill.

You'll reach a group of boulders across this dirt road. Follow the blue blazes to a rocky outcropping. Walking past the initial set, the blazes indicate the clearest and safest place to walk up the boulders. Pass through a tunnel of fragrant mountain laurel and take in the view. Enjoy a break on the boulders and pick some of the wild blueberries if they are ripe. If you've brought binoculars, the forester says that you can see the buildings of downtown Pittsburgh on a clear day Alas, it wasn't clear enough during my visit.

When finished, just turn around and retrace your steps.

▶ NEARBY ATTRACTIONS

For another hike without traveling, go to the Lick Hollow Area Interpretive Nature Trail (hike 47) in this book. There are many other attractions in this area, including Laurel Caverns, and places to eat are located by continuing west a little way on US 40. Other hikes or tours can be found in this book for nearby Quebec Run (hike 50), Fort Necessity National Battlefield (hike 51), and Friendship Hill National Historic Site (hike 52).

FORBES STATE FOREST: MOUNT DAVIS NATURAL AREA

▶ IN BRIEF

The Mount Davis overlook tower offers a spectacular 360-degree view. The trails are pretty, especially in spring and fall. You can make this hike shorter or longer, as you wish.

▶ DESCRIPTION

Mount Davis, at 3,213 feet, is the highest point in Pennsylvania. It is not a pinnacle but a broad flat plateau, and it's surrounded by 5,685 acres of state forest land. Although not high by many standards, wind in the area keeps some of the trees stunted and frost can be present any month of the year. The mountain is named after John Nelson Davis (1835–1913), an early settler who was an active community leader, teacher, and ordained minister, among his many occupations. He was also one of the oldest Civil War veterans of his time, and an avid naturalist fascinated with the environment of Mount Davis.

From the parking lot, walk south of the information board, uphill to the edge of the picnic area (opposite end from the restrooms and picnic shelter) and find a post with a High Point Trail sign. Walk into the woods along the wide dirt path. The abundance of mountain laurel seen will accompany you for much of this hike, as will ferns, sassafras, and witch hazel trees. In 700 feet

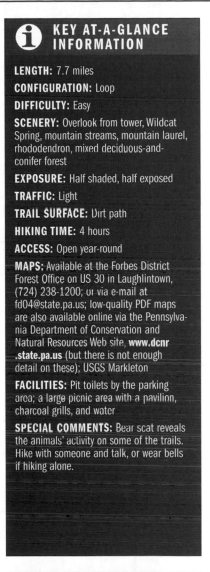

▶ KEY AT-A-GLANCE INFORMATION

LENGTH: 7.7 miles

CONFIGURATION: Loop

DIFFICULTY: Easy

SCENERY: Overlook from tower, Wildcat Spring, mountain streams, mountain laurel, rhododendron, mixed deciduous-and-conifer forest

EXPOSURE: Half shaded, half exposed

TRAFFIC: Light

TRAIL SURFACE: Dirt path

HIKING TIME: 4 hours

ACCESS: Open year-round

MAPS: Available at the Forbes District Forest Office on US 30 in Laughlintown, (724) 238-1200; or via e-mail at fd04@state.pa.us; low-quality PDF maps are also available online via the Pennsylvania Department of Conservation and Natural Resources Web site, **www.dcnr.state.pa.us** (but there is not enough detail on these); USGS Markleton

FACILITIES: Pit toilets by the parking area; a large picnic area with a pavilion, charcoal grills, and water

SPECIAL COMMENTS: Bear scat reveals the animals' activity on some of the trails. Hike with someone and talk, or wear bells if hiking alone.

▶ DIRECTIONS

From Pittsburgh, take Interstate 376 East and enter Pennsylvania Turnpike I-76 East (toll road). Take Exit 110, Somerset. Follow PA 281 South 18.8 miles and turn left on Fort Hill Road. Follow 3.5 miles and turn left on High Point Road (Township Road T 330). Follow 3.8 miles and turn left on Mount Davis Road (SR 2004). Drive 3.8 miles (past the Mount Davis Monument, unless you wish to skip the hike and go straight to the tower) and turn right into the picnic area parking lot.

Forbes State Forest: Mount Davis Natural Area

UTM Zone (WGS84)   17S

Easting   656847

Northing   4406443

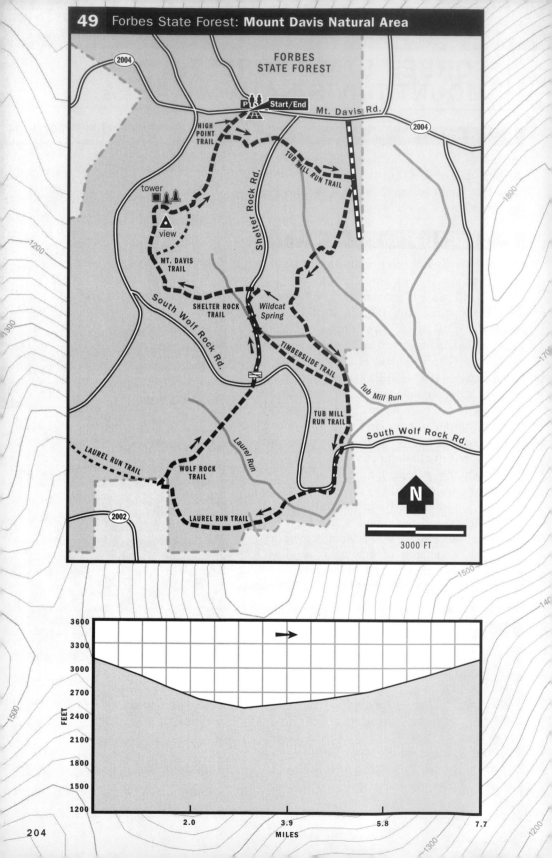

FORBES
STATE FOREST

2004

2004

Start/End   Mt. Davis Rd.

HIGH
POINT
TRAIL

tower

Shelter Rock Rd.

TUB MILL RUN TRAIL

view

MT. DAVIS
TRAIL

SHELTER ROCK
TRAIL

Wildcat
Spring

South Wolf Rock Rd.

TIMBERSLIDE TRAIL

Tub Mill Run

LAUREL RUN TRAIL

Laurel Run

TUB MILL
RUN TRAIL

WOLF ROCK
TRAIL

South Wolf Rock Rd.

N

2002

LAUREL RUN TRAIL

3000 FT

1800

1700

1500

1200

1300

1300

1200

1500

1400

3600
3300
3000
2700
2400
2100
1800
1500
1200

FEET

2.0   3.9   5.8   7.7
MILES

(0.13 miles) turn left onto the Tub Mill Run Trail (there is a sign on a tree). This trail winds along the eastern slope of Negro Mountain and, as are all of the Mount Davis Trails, is blazed with blue rectangles. This trail narrows and is soft with moss, cushioning the hiker's steps in many places and helping to make up for the rocky bits, as does the scenery.

At 0.46 miles, reach Shelter Rock Road (not marked here). Turn left, then make a quick right to reenter the woods on the other side. Along this section you'll find rhododendrons mixed in with the mountain laurel. By 0.70 miles, you'll step rock-to-rock for a ways. It won't take long to notice that you are heading downhill for much of the length of this trail. Don't worry about going up to Mount Davis, however. None of the grades on this hike are steep; it is relatively flat, considering that this is the highest point in the state. The side growth is dense until about 0.97 miles, where you make a sharp right (if you reach an old nameless road, you've missed the turn) into a more open area. At

Autumn hiking on Laurel Run Trail

1.32 miles, the trail veers right; look for the blue blazes. (There is not another trail here; it just looks as though the trail could go straight.)

Soon you'll see some rocks off to the left and shortly after make your first water crossing of a tributary to Tub Mill Run; use rocks to cross its 10- to 12-foot expanse. The trail then travels through a field of ferns as far as the eyes can see. Another section of sandstone boulders keeps the scenery interesting and at 2.12 miles, the trail winds down through many of them. You'll see lots of sassafras growing here, as well as a mixture of oaks and maples, including striped maple, and come upon a grove of hemlocks at 2.25 miles. Shortly, Tub Mill Run parallels the trail and is quite a sight as it flows over moss-covered rocks in the streambed, under the branches of hemlocks, rhododendrons, and mountain laurels. There are berry bushes growing here as well, and bear scat warns to make your presence known. Bears generally leave people alone; they just don't like to be surprised.

At 2.52 miles, follow the obvious sharp right and steep descent to cross Tub Mill Run and walk through walls of rhododendron. After the crossing, you'll see huge sandstone boulders on the left of the trail and come to a T at 2.58 miles. The unsigned trail coming from the right is the Timberslide Trail. Turn left and continue on Tub Mill Run Trail. (You can shortcut the hike by turning right and following Timberslide Trail up to Shelter Rock Road if you wish. If you follow that route, turn left on Shelter Rock Trail to reach the tower.) On this lowest elevation of the hike, the environment changes for a bit, the forest is young, and early-growth hemlocks soon accompany greenbrier and small deciduous trees.

You'll reach South Wolf Rock Road (unsigned) at 2.96 miles; turn right to walk along it and relish the towering hemlocks that parallel its sides. Pass the two roads on the right and veer left onto Laurel Run Trail when you see it branching off on the left side of the road at 3.36 miles. This trail is lovely, and begins a low-grade gain in elevation. In fall, it is picturesque with colorful leaves scattered underfoot. Cross a couple of tributaries to Laurel Run and then the run itself at 3.5 miles. Cross another tributary and at about 4 miles, it parallels the trail for a while.

At 4.42 miles, leave the Laurel Run Trail by turning right onto the signed Wolf Rock Trail. Moss-covered rocks once again cushion your steps for more than 100 feet. Wolf Rock Trail ends when it meets South Wolf Rock Road (unsigned). Cross the road and continue straight ahead and around the gate to pick up the grassy Shelter Rock Road. This road is closed to vehicles and serves as a wide hiking path. After following it almost 0.25 miles, turn right and take the few steps to see Wildcat Spring (it is well marked with a sign). Look closely in the clear spring to see where water comes bubbling up through the sand. Back on the road, cross an old wooden plank bridge over Tub Mill Run. From here, begin a slow, steady uphill climb, spotting goldenrod and black cherry trees along the way. Keep an eye to the left to see the signed post for Shelter Rock Trail at 5.82 miles.

Turn left onto it and continue the low-grade climb. Make the final crossing of Tub Mill Run at 5.96 miles. At 6.5 miles, you may notice the three oaks that horizontally band out from one trunk on the left side of the trail. You are pretty much walking along the top of Mount Davis and, for a ways along this section, in between walls of sassafras, oaks, tall ferns, and mountain laurel. At 6.76 miles, pass the Mount Davis Trail (not on the park map) on the right and reach the road that loops the tower.

Once on the road, turn right and then left for the exhibits, which tell of the physiology of the area, flora and fauna, former industry, and other interesting tidbits of local history. When finished, continue walking through the exhibit area and veer right to reach the tower. Climb the stairs to reach the top of the tower for a spectacular 360-degree view. When you've come down, walk back through the exhibits to pick up the High Point Trail, which is not labeled with a sign using its name but one that says "To Picnic Area."

Follow this level trail, passing the right for the Mount Davis Trail (unsigned) and later the Tub Mill Run Trail. From there, follow the High Point Trail back out to the picnic area and to your vehicle.

▶ NEARBY ATTRACTIONS

Enjoy a meal, some ice cream, pleasant people, and a gorgeous view at the Shepherd's Farm Restaurant and Ice Cream Shoppe (call [814] 395-3448) on PA 281, where you can also buy local preserves and honey. They are located just a mile or so farther south on PA 281 than the turn for Fort Hill Road. Other eating establishments can be found by continuing farther south to Confluence or by heading north to Somerset.

FORBES STATE FOREST: QUEBEC RUN WILD AREA

▶ IN BRIEF

The Quebec Run Wild Area is a special treat. The entire hike is pretty any time of year. But if you go during late June or July, you will walk through bowers of rhododendron and mountain laurel in bloom.

▶ DESCRIPTION

The Quebec Run Wild Area is on the eastern slope of Chestnut Ridge, which is part of the Appalachian Mountain chain. Chestnut Ridge is the westernmost principal anticline of the chain in Pennsylvania. Anticlines are basically the tops of layers of rock that have folded due to geologic forces to form an arch; we commonly call anticlines ridges or mountains.

The Quebec Run Wild Area encompasses 7,441 acres of the 58,000-acre Forbes State Forest. Its Pottsville sandstone provides the acidity needed to nourish the abundant rhododendron and mountain laurel. Its heavily forested confines include almost all of the Quebec Run and Tebolt Run watersheds. The forest is mostly third-growth, as its valuable timber was harvested around 1938 or 1940. The moist environs of the bottomlands near creeks are where most of the hemlocks and rhododendron thickets thrive.

The hike begins on Hess Trail. The trailhead is opposite the parking area (there is a sign). Start on the blue-blazed trail, which has a very low uphill grade. This turns into a slightly rolling grade for the first half mile. In the beginning of the hike, find sugar maples and English and scarlet oaks

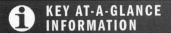

ℹ KEY AT-A-GLANCE INFORMATION

LENGTH: 3.8 miles

CONFIGURATION: Loop

DIFFICULTY: Easy

SCENERY: Quebec Run, rhododendron, mountain laurel, deciduous forest, old surface gold mine

EXPOSURE: Mostly shaded

TRAFFIC: Light

TRAIL SURFACE: Dirt and rock

HIKING TIME: 2 hours

ACCESS: Open year-round

MAPS: Available at the Forbes District Forest Office on US 30 in Laughlintown, (724) 238-1200, via e-mail at fd04@state.pa.us, or at the forest office at Ponderfield Tower (located off Skyline Drive, past the Laurel Cavern turnoff); low-quality PDF maps are available online at **www.dcnr.state.pa.us** (there is not enough detail on these, though); USGS Brownfield

FACILITIES: None

SPECIAL COMMENTS: The dirt road in the final leg to the trailhead can be a little rough in spots but is fine for passenger vehicles. If you don't want to drive upward, turn downward and exit to US 381 North to US 40.

Backcountry camping is permitted, but you should obtain a permit from one of the forest offices.

▶ DIRECTIONS

From Pittsburgh, take PA 51 South to US 40 East. Travel about 9.3 miles and turn right onto Skyline Drive (SR 2001), immediately after the Laurel Summit Inn. Drive 6.4 miles and turn left on Quebec Road. Drive down this dirt road 1.3 miles and turn right to park for the trailhead.

Forbes State Forest: Quebec Run Wild Area

UTM Zone (WGS84)   17S

Easting   612943

Northing   4402758

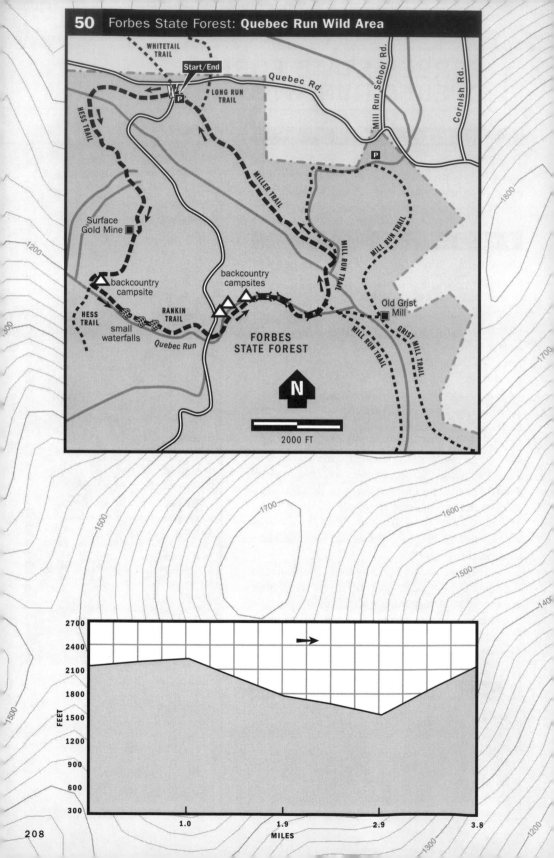

WHITETAIL
TRAIL

Start/End

Quebec Rd.

P

LONG RUN
TRAIL

Mill Run School Rd.

Cornish Rd.

HESS TRAIL

MILLER TRAIL

P

1800

MILL RUN TRAIL

MILL RUN TRAIL

Surface
Gold Mine

backcountry
campsites

1200

backcountry
campsite

Old Grist
Mill

HESS
TRAIL

RANKIN
TRAIL

small
waterfalls

Quebec Run

FORBES
STATE FOREST

GRIST MILL TRAIL

MILL RUN TRAIL

1300

1700

N

2000 FT

1500

1700

1600

1500

1500

1400

1200

2700
2400
2100
1800
1500
1200
900
600
300

FEET

1.0   1.9   2.9   3.8
MILES

1300

1200

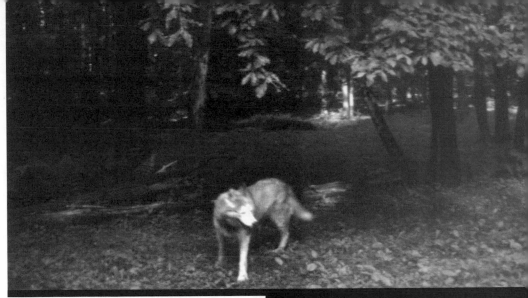
End of Miller Trail

among the deciduous trees. Moss covering rocks and the base of many of the trees are a preview to the enchanting environment to come. The solitude enhances the experience. The only sound I was able to hear in this isolated section of Forbes State Forest was a titmouse and other birds singing.

In 0.35 miles the woods open out more, especially on the left side of the trail, where ferns are flourishing and tulip trees are growing. Soon, you'll see many huge boulders lying about all around the trail. You are coming up on 0.5 miles, and the trail then takes a long, slow descent toward Quebec Run. Continue past the signposts indicating that you are on Hess Trail. As the trail veers toward the left, huge rhododendrons line the sides of the trail; these give way to tunnels of mountain laurel. Deciduous trees such as blackjack oak, yellow buckeye, elms, and maples are also found here.

Cross a small water runoff and find yourself in rhododendron again and then, once you're heading uphill, more mountain laurel. These two beauties will alternately appear in groups or mixed throughout the hike. They are often confused, and although they look similar, a couple of facts will make them easy to distinguish. The leaves of the mountain laurel are shorter and narrower than those of the rhododendron, whose leaves are typically 3 to 6 inches long. Their flowers also give them away. Those of the mountain laurel are small and cup-shaped and are usually white or light pink with pink spotting the bottoms of the petals and the tips of the stamens. The flowers of the rhododendron each have five obviously separated petals, can be white, pink, or purple, but are much more uniform in color. Both sets of flowers grow in clusters and are quite beautiful to see.

Look for a small circular depression at 1.07 miles to the right of the trail. This was once a surface gold mine. At 1.18 miles the drop toward Quebec Run becomes steeper and turns toward the right and through walls of rhododendron. Following this, the forest thins again and you reach a junction with the Rankin Trail at 1.39 miles, just after passing a backcountry campsite. Hess Trail continues straight. Turn left on Rankin Trail to walk beside Quebec Run.

Along the Rankin Trail, find conifers and fan club and hair cap mosses. There are many tunnels of rhododendron and mountain laurel, but deciduous trees and hemlocks are interspersed throughout, as are giant boulders. However, by 1.55 miles, the hemlocks line the trail on both sides for a bit. The mix of beauty here, accompanied by the gurgling of Quebec Run and eventually the sight of it, gives this wild area a feeling of magic. It is truly a wonderland for the nature lover.

The first real look at the run is a beauty. A small waterfall cascades down the run over moss-covered boulders. You'll walk over several small water runoffs and pass what appears to be a road access at 1.91 miles before reaching Quebec Road at 2 miles. Head slightly left to see the post showing Rankin Trail continuing. The mixed forest includes a variety of maples, oaks, and tulip trees. Soon you are walking under the branches of hemlocks and there are few backcountry campsites. The setting for these campsites is so perfect that I wished I'd been carrying a full backpack, prepared to stay the night.

At 2.27 miles, you'll reach a bridge crossing Quebec Run and finally get a clear view from the trail. The bridges you are crossing were constructed by the Pennsylvania Conservation Corps. After this bridge you cross another over a runoff, into mixed forest and make a sharp left over another bridge fording Quebec Run. Walking under hemlocks again, the conifer forest you are in soon changes to mixed forest, then thins more until you walk through another open area covered with ferns.

You reach the end of the Rankin Trail and a T with Mill Run Trail at 2.61 miles. Turn left on Mill Run Trail. Just after this junction I saw a black snake that slithered into the woods as I was trying to capture it on film. In this muddy section, find skunk cabbage and lots of ferns. At 2.75 miles, use rocks to cross Mill Run and then meet up with Miller Trail. Mill Run Trail continues to the right. Take Miller Trail uphill. Along this section, find yellow common cinquefoil and pink partridgeberry; the latter is recognized by its tiny, delicate, four-petal flowers, which rise up from the end of a creeping stem.

By 3.1 miles the trail begins to climb a little more steeply. Along the way the gradient changes, but it is a continuous uphill climb from here until you get close to the trail terminus. I saw not-yet-ripe wild blueberries and a fungus that looks like destroying angel, a white, somewhat flat-topped fungus that is deadly if eaten. Come to a juncture with Long Run Trail when you've almost finished at 3.7 miles. This new trail is not currently shown on the Bureau of Forestry map but heads northeast to cross Quebec Road and later connects to the Whitetail Trail to form an additional 2.5-mile circuit. (Whitetail Trail travels all the way to Pine Knob at Lick Hollow.) Continue straight on Miller Trail to the parking area.

▶ NEARBY ATTRACTIONS

There are other hikes within the Quebec Run Wild Area (not shown on this map) and many other attractions in this area, including Laurel Caverns. Places to eat are located on US 40. Other hikes or tours can be found in this book for nearby Lick Hollow (hikes 47 and 48), Fort Necessity National Battlefield (hike 51), and Friendship Hill National Historic Site (hike 52).

FORT NECESSITY TOUR AND WOODS WALK

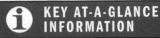

IN BRIEF

You can make a day of it by combining history, walking, and driving if you like by beginning at the Fort Necessity–National Road Interpretive and Education and Visitor Center; tour Washington's Tavern; and take the walk, which incorporates visiting the reconstructed Fort Necessity, the former French Camp, and traces of Braddock's Road. Continue by driving to the park's other historic sites, and perhaps along more of our country's first national road.

DESCRIPTION

Fort Necessity National Battlefield is a national park comprising approximately 900 acres in three separate sites. Start with the visitor's center at the main site, where Fort Necessity is located. Here, watch the slide presentation, talk to the rangers, and visit the museum to learn about the reason for the battle and construction of Fort Necessity. This is where George Washington, young and inexperienced in 1754, led and lost his first battle of the French and Indian War.

If you can, take a tour of Washington's Tavern next. The tavern was one of many that were built along the first national road to accommodate the steady stream of travelers who were heading for new opportunity through the Allegheny Mountains and into the Ohio River Valley. Built around 1828, the tavern is filled with period furniture, cookware, and clothing, and its former hustle and bustle is brought to life by the ranger's description of its history.

The walk described here is a tour of the battlefield where you can read interpretive signs, tour

KEY AT-A-GLANCE INFORMATION

LENGTH: 1.2 miles

CONFIGURATION: Loop

DIFFICULTY: Easy

SCENERY: Fort Necessity, Washington's Tavern, Braddock's Road trace, French Camp, meadow flowers, mixed deciduous-and-conifer forest

EXPOSURE: Half shaded, half exposed

TRAFFIC: Moderate

TRAIL SURFACE: Pavement and dirt

HIKING TIME: 1 hour, including fort and reading information plaques

ACCESS: Park is open year-round, sunrise–sunset; visitor center is open daily, 9 a.m.–5 p.m.

MAPS: Available at the visitor's center or online at **www.nps.gov/fone;** USGS Fort Necessity

FACILITIES: Restrooms at the visitor's center; picnic area

SPECIAL COMMENTS: Plan ahead and go during visitor center hours. Ask for the tour times for Washington's Tavern (on site), and time your tours of the center, tavern, and battlefield for the fullest experience. Fee: $3 for persons age 17 and older; National Park memberships are recognized.

Fort Necessity Tour and Woods Walk

UTM Zone (WGS84)   17S

Easting   620906

Northing   4408313

DIRECTIONS

From Pittsburgh, take PA 51 South to Uniontown. Take US 40 East 10 miles and turn right into the parking area.

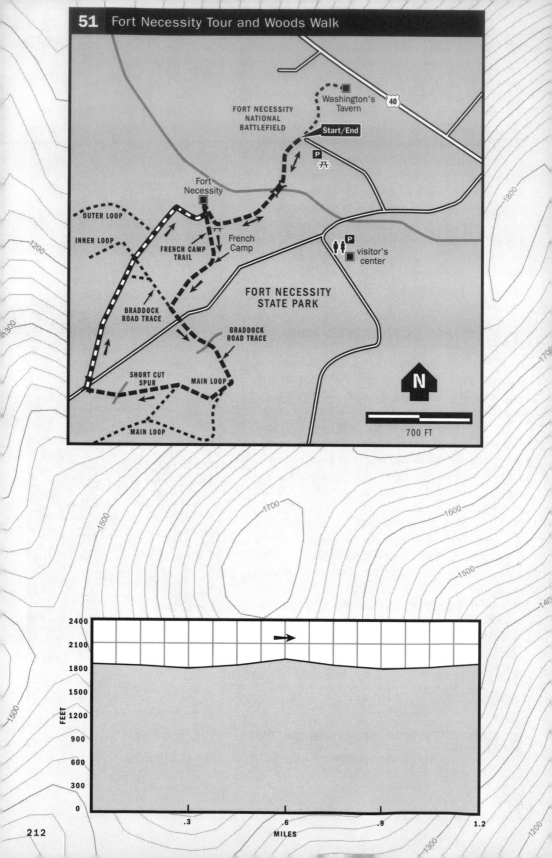

FORT NECESSITY
NATIONAL
BATTLEFIELD

Washington's
Tavern

40

Start/End

P

Fort
Necessity

OUTER LOOP

INNER LOOP

FRENCH CAMP
TRAIL

French
Camp

P

visitor's
center

FORT NECESSITY
STATE PARK

BRADDOCK
ROAD TRACE

BRADDOCK
ROAD TRACE

SHORT CUT
SPUR

MAIN LOOP

N

MAIN LOOP

700 FT

FEET

2400
2100
1800
1500
1200
900
600
300
0

.3   .6   .9   1.2
MILES

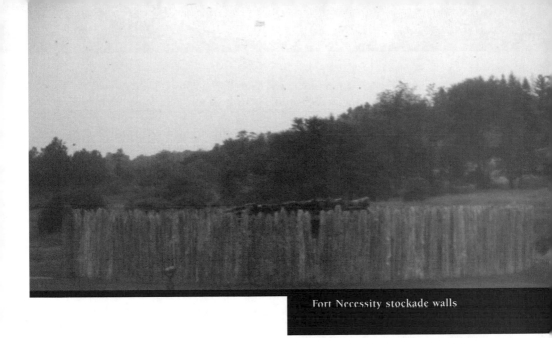

the reconstructed Fort Necessity, see the area where the French soldiers camped, stroll along tracings of Braddock's Road, and finish with a pleasant short hike back through the woods and meadow.

The walk begins at the bottom of the walkway from Washington's Tavern. From there, walk straight ahead along the paved path that passes beside the picnic tables. Look around as you approach the fort. From the early to mid-1800s, the widowed Rebecca Sampey ran Washington's Tavern with her seven children and used this area as an orchard.

Over the wooden bridges are information plaques from which you can learn more about the battle and Washington's surrender negotiations before proceeding to the fort. In the summer of 1754, when George Washington and the British troops were here, this was known as the Great Meadows. Washington chose the area for his camp because it was open and water was available.

Read on once you have reached the fort. That summer was Washington's second visit. During his first, he was sent from Virginia as a British emissary to ask the French, who had been building forts in the area, to leave. They refused and Washington returned to tell the governor the news. In response, the governor ordered Washington back here to build a road to the fort he was having constructed at the Forks of the Ohio. Washington returned in late May 1754 and, having learned that the new fort at the forks had fallen to the French, eventually set up camp in the Great Meadows to continue the road and await orders. The events, instead, led to what is felt to be the true marker in a series that began the war fought between England and France for control of the North American continent.

Soon after Washington and his men set up camp, he learned of a French camp about 4 miles west and traveled with his men through the night to meet them. They arrived, surrounded the camp (now known as Jumonville after the slain French leader), and a shot was fired—no one knows from which side. A skirmish ensued from which one French soldier escaped, leading Washington to construct a "fort of necessity" for fear that the French would return in force. In Washington's favor, the remainder of the Virginia regiment arrived, as did more reinforcements, along with nine swivel guns (the type of miniature cannon found outside of the fort). However, the 293 men were not enough to overcome the 600 French soldiers and 100 Native American warriors who arrived July 3.

They fought that day. The ground in this meadow was already very wet, though, and it rained during the battle, turning the trenches you see surrounding the fort to traps of mud and water, and making it almost impossible for the British soldiers to use their flintlock muskets. The slits you see between the lengthwise split-log walls of the fort not only let the men fire out, but also allowed the bullets coming from the nearby forest to penetrate the barrier.

Walk inside the fort and you'll find a storehouse, built in the fashion and with the materials that reflect how it may have been constructed at the time. Archeological digs provided the evidence and guidelines for the reconstruction of the fort.

When you have finished at the fort, continue by backtracking briefly along the walk, crossing the last bridge, then cutting straight through the grass, past the three-quarter-cut split-log benches and to the opening in the woods. There is a post that identifies this as the French Camp Trail. Just around the bend find the clear area deemed to be where the French must have camped during their brief encounter. Pass through the camp and reach the tracing of the Braddock's Road at 0.37 miles; turn left here. As you walk through this section of woods, admiring the tulip trees, red maples, hemlocks, and oaks, and crossing the paved road with a marker showing you are on historic Braddock's Road, realize that you are walking along a path that helped change the history of the nation.

Almost a year after the battle at Fort Necessity, General Edward Braddock and more British troops were sent to seize Fort Duquesne, which had been built by the French at the Forks of the Ohio. With an army assembled at Will's Creek (Cumberland), Maryland, they led the front thrust using the road Washington had blazed through the wilderness, with Washington as Braddock's aide-de-camp and expert on the terrain. The trail was not adequate for the army's artillery and wagons; they had to blow and cut their way through.

As you walk upward and through these woods, imagine the thick virgin forest they would have been facing at the time. General Braddock and his men were unfamiliar with the rough terrain and the wilderness-fighting tactics that would have been needed to succeed against the French and their Native American allies. He drilled his men in British-style open volleys that proved disastrous. He was unwilling to learn the warfare methods of the Native Americans and as a result, General Braddock and his troops were completely beaten near their objective in what became known as the Battle of the Monongahela, where the general suffered a wound that proved fatal. Although General Braddock failed at his ultimate assignment, the road you are walking on became the first major east–west route through Pennsylvania. It is known as Braddock's Road and the first national road (US 40) parallels much of it.

Today, a lovely second-growth forest surrounds the old road as well as a stand of pines built by the Civilian Conservation Corps in the mid-1930s. The pines are found near the intersection where the Main Loop Trail veers right and the Braddock

Road trace appears to continue uphill and left into the woods at 0.5 miles. Veer right on the Main Loop and reach another Y just after the trail begins to lead downhill. Here, the Main Loop branches off to the left. For a longer hike through these lovely woods, you can take the Main Loop but this hike continues straight on the Shortcut Spur, for which you will see a post ahead. Heading straight, the trail travels downhill, over a couple of water runoffs and back across the paved road.

Across the road, the path changes to a dirt road. Follow it straight, past the intersection with Braddock's Road and the Inner Loop Trail at 0.86 miles, and then past the left turn onto the Outer Loop Trail at 0.9 miles, from where you can see the fort and meadow.

Following the path through the meadow, find thistle, swamp milkweed, sneeze-weed, and many butterflies. If you are here in the early or later parts of the day, you will probably see plenty of birds and deer, as a flattened area in the tall grasses gave evidence of comfortable bedding. Follow the path along the meadow and past the fort, turning right to retrace your steps to your vehicle.

▶ NEARBY ATTRACTIONS

For more hiking take the Main Loop or Inner Loop trails or hike at Jumonville Glen. To see the rest of the park, pick up the park fact sheets and drive to Braddock's Grave, which is approximately 1.5 miles west on US 40. From there, drive to Jumonville Glen. To reach it, continue on US 40 West and turn right on Jumonville Road (SR 2021).

FRIENDSHIP HILL TOUR AND HIKE

KEY AT-A-GLANCE INFORMATION

LENGTH: 4 miles

CONFIGURATION: Loop

DIFFICULTY: Easy

SCENERY: Gallatin House (former home of Albert Gallatin), Monongahela River, wildflowers, deciduous woods, some hemlocks

EXPOSURE: Mostly shaded

TRAFFIC: Light

TRAIL SURFACE: Dirt and grass, short time on pavement

HIKING TIME: 3 hours (including tour)

ACCESS: Park is open year-round, sunrise–sunset; Gallatin House and visitor's center open daily, 9 a.m.–5 p.m. Call ahead for winter hours October–April at (724) 725-9190, or visit **www.nps.gov/frhi.**

MAPS: Available at the visitor's center; USGS Masontown

FACILITIES: Restrooms at the far end of the parking lot near the picnic pavilion; picnic area with grill

SPECIAL COMMENTS: Plan ahead and go during visitor's center hours. Small to large groups can call ahead to arrange a tour with the park ranger. Otherwise, self-guided audio tours are available; no fee. There is also a bookshop within the house.

Friendship Hill Tour and Hike

UTM Zone (WGS84) 17S

Easting 591525

Northing 4403616

▶ IN BRIEF

Friendship Hill National Historic Site is a lesser-known gem in the National Park Service system as is its former owner, Albert Gallatin, in our familiar history. A visit is worth taking to amend that fact. A tour and hike on the beautiful grounds offer a truly educational and enjoyable time.

▶ DESCRIPTION

The Gallatin House has been well preserved and boasts a most interesting history of a man who played a largely influential role in the forming of our country's republic. Begin the tour and hike from the parking lot by walking up the paved path where you'll find an information board and, up around the bend, a metal casting of Albert Gallatin in his surveying days.

Born in 1761 in Geneva, Switzerland, Albert Gallatin was drawn to the American Revolution and the New World. After traveling to and around this country, Gallatin tutored French at Harvard College, surveyed, and speculated and with a partner, purchased 120,000 acres in Virginia and the Ohio River Valley. Continue up the path and turn right at the top to reach the house; don't miss the information board on the way.

Once inside the house, you can learn about both its history and that of its original owner. At the time Albert Gallatin purchased Friendship Hill in 1786, he had visions for building industry in the wilderness and thought that the Monongahela River would play a key role in commerce. He began building this home after marrying Sophia

▶ DIRECTIONS

From Pittsburgh, take PA 51 South 40.8 miles (near Uniontown) to US 119 South and follow 17 miles. Turn right onto PA 166 North. Follow 2.7 miles and turn left into Friendship Hill. Follow the tree-lined park road to the parking area.

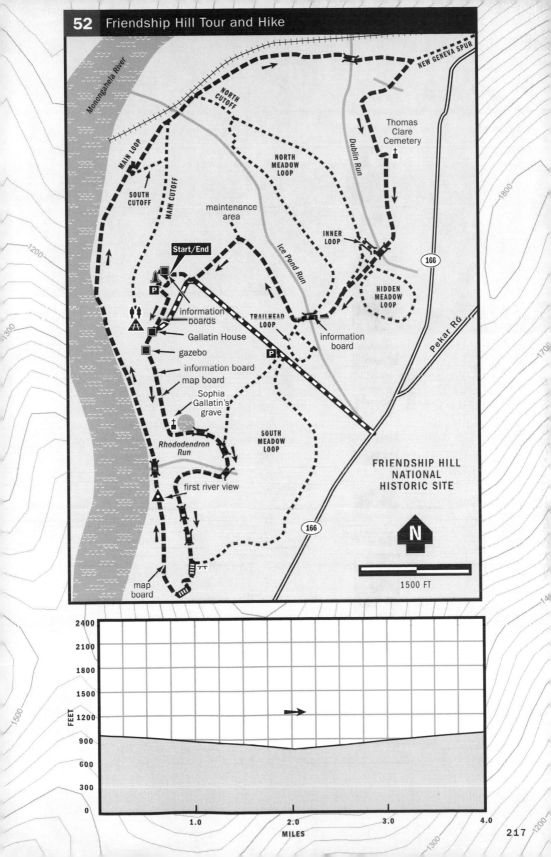

Mononahela River

NEW GENEVA SPUR

NORTH CUTOFF

Thomas Clare Cemetery

MAIN LOOP

Dublin Run

SOUTH CUTOFF

NORTH MEADOW LOOP

MAIN CUTOFF

maintenance area

Start/End

166

INNER LOOP

Ice Pond Run

information boards

Gallatin House

gazebo

information board

map board

Sophia Gallatin's grave

HIDDEN MEADOW LOOP

TRAILHEAD LOOP

information board

Pekar Rd

Rhododendron Run

first river view

SOUTH MEADOW LOOP

FRIENDSHIP HILL NATIONAL HISTORIC SITE

166

N

map board

1500 FT

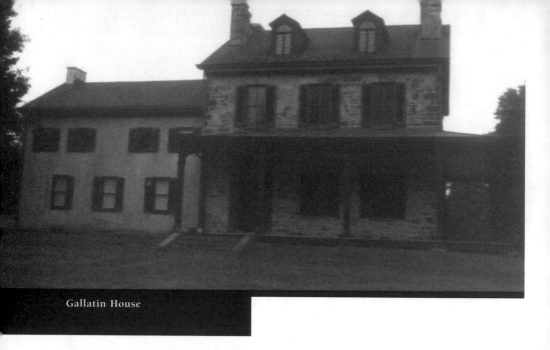

Gallatin House

Allegre in 1789. Sadly, their marriage lasted only six months, ending with Sophia's death. During that year of emotional extremes, Gallatin delved into politics by playing a role in the delegate to the Pennsylvania convention on the state's constitution. In the years that followed he went on to become a Pennsylvania state assemblyman, a U.S. senator (later disqualified due to citizenship), a U.S. representative, and an advocate of the people during the Whiskey Rebellion. He also remarried and started a family.

A growing family led to eventual additions to the house, which you can learn about during the tour. Gallatin will probably be best remembered for his time served as U.S. secretary of the treasury, from 1801 to 1814, (the longest term held in this position), under presidents Thomas Jefferson and James Madison. As secretary of the treasury, Gallatin devised the plan that financed the Louisiana Purchase and the exploration of those lands by Lewis and Clark (Missouri River Basin) and Freeman and Curtis (the Red River area in Louisiana). He submitted to Congress a plan for a road and canal system linking the country that, although rejected, was the seed that began the first national road (US 40). Gallatin also fathered the idea that federal expenditures should be kept in check to lift the country from debt. To this end, he started the House of Ways and Means Committee.

In the meantime, Gallatin had bought 650 additional acres in this area on George's Creek to found New Geneva. He later built a school, boat landing, gristmill, store, glassworks, and a gun factory. His grand ideas ultimately did not succeed in his absence as he served in his government positions. The exhibit inside the house provides much more information on his accomplishments, including the years after he left the position of secretary of the treasury, which expound on his myriad talents. Many are notable but perhaps most exemplary of his diverse abilities was the study he published on Native American tribes that is still considered to be among the most comprehensive records of their history.

When you have finished touring the home, you will have a much better knowledge base about the land, the changes to the home that occurred over time with different building materials and practices, and the man that sparked the area's development.

When you leave the house, walk left under the archway and to the stone gazebo. This was built after Gallatin's time in the 1890s and, much later, saved from sliding over the hillside by the National Park Service. It overlooks the industry that he once envisioned but never realized.

Continuing south of the gazebo, you'll find another information board; this one provides background about Gallatin's first wife, Sophia. Her grave is found past the map board at the bottom of the hill, after entering the woods, at 0.45 miles. It is thought she asked that her grave overlook the Monongahela. It may have been moved, as later owners of the property expanded the home; the walls were added to protect the site.

As you walk through Sophia's Woods, you'll see maples, oaks, and beech. Soon you'll arrive at a small pond where turtles are known to sun themselves on the rocks and our footsteps caused many frogs to leap into the water. Walk over the small bridge; pass the cutoff trail to the left (it leads to the upper half of the South Meadow Loop), and continue over a second small bridge. The third bridge crosses Rhododendron Run just before the trail veers west toward the river. This is a pleasant walk through moss-covered rocks, patches of ferns, and a variety of deciduous trees including hickory, witch hazel, and very old and large American beech trees.

Cross another couple of bridges over water runoffs and pass the left turn for the South Meadow Trail near the map board found at 0.93 miles. This hike follows the Main Loop, which is color-coded green on the map board and contains posts found along the way. Shortly after, the trail curves right and toward the river for a steep descent. Pass a bench and follow the long set of trail steps down. Another shorter set leads to a turn through some boulders with a slate outcropping. Follow the path and next three sets of trail steps down, passing another bench, and reach another map board at 1.07 miles. Here the trail is wide and level and appears to be a former road. Reach better views of the river beginning at 1.25 miles.

There are places along the trail where it would be easy to access narrow beach areas and dip your feet in while having a snack or just enjoying the sun. One comes up just after the first bridge on this section of the trail. When you reach it, take a look up to the right at the large slabs of rock caught in a still cascade in the ravine the water has carved. At 1.53 miles there is an opportunity to wind through a couple of larger boulders (or walk above them on the right). A huge slab of shale, directly across from an enormous old oak, can be admired up close at 1.64 miles.

Pass the South Cutoff found at 2.03 miles and the Main Cutoff at 2.2 miles, and cross Ice Pond Run (there is a culvert beneath the trail directing the water flow) to reach the North Cutoff shortly after. Continue straight, walking now beside the railroad. Trees bank both sides of the trail and some large hemlocks grow in the area. Cross lovely Dublin Run at 2.67 miles and stop on the bridge to admire some of the flowers growing in the area.

After the bridge, the trail veers north slightly and there are some tall pines surrounding its sides, providing a bed of needles to walk on. Also find jewelweed before you reach the turn to follow the Main Loop. The trail straight ahead is the New

Geneva Spur (an out-and-back that almost reaches George's Creek). Turn right—almost a U-turn—to follow the Main Loop Trail south and uphill along the wide old scree-filled road. Cross a runoff and, shortly after reaching the top of the hill, come to the Thomas Clare Cemetery at 3.07 miles. If you walk inside it, watch your step, there are sunken spots and small boulders that appear to be rough headstones. The headstone of Thomas Clare, who died in 1814 and had been the owner of this tract of land, is legible. Gallatin purchased this land after his initial acquisition of Friendship Hill; it was known as Dublin Farm.

At 3.3 miles, pass the path on the right called Inner Loop (marked School Spur on the park map and must lead to the North Meadow Loop) and continue straight over the bridge, recrossing Dublin Run. Walk straight through the intersection with the Meadow Loop to the right and Hidden Meadow Loop to the left. Continue straight again, past the second right for North Meadow Loop at 3.53 miles, and find an information board at Ice Pond Run that provides background on past and present effects of local industry. Friendship Hill is among the many parks in the national system that struggles with acidic mine drainage, which is caused when iron pyrite (fool's gold) is mixed with oxygen and water, and left to seep from abandoned mines.

When finished, turn right at the intersection. At 3.77 miles reach a junction and turn left (there's no post); straight leads to the maintenance area. This section of the trail borders the woods on the right and provides a nice walk with a meadow to the left. Here, you may spot meadowlarks, warblers, chickadees, or titmice in spring. Many butterflies are also flitting about. Pass the trail that meets this one at 3.85 miles and reach the road on which you entered the park at 3.92 miles. Turn right to reach your vehicle.

▶ NEARBY ATTRACTIONS

Eating establishments can be found in Port Marion (go to Apple Annie's in the alley behind Foodland if you are looking for great desserts), Uniontown, and Morgantown.

KOOSER STATE PARK LOOP

▶ IN BRIEF

Kooser State Park is quieter and serenely beautiful during the winter months when snow bends the branches of evergreens over icy Kooser Run. Summer, however, offers swimming and fishing in Kooser Lake. Pick your preference or visit more than once.

▶ DESCRIPTION

To begin the hike (or ski), walk to the far end of the parking lot, in the direction away from the park office, and turn right down the gravel road. Cross over the intersecting Tree Army Road and walk through the gated opening. This section is earmarked for cross-country skiing and is blazed with blue triangles. You are walking through the cabin area on Cabin Loop Road. The cabins here are well constructed and designed to complement the scenery. At 0.17 miles, veer right at the Y; the left leads to a group of cabins.

Come to the first in a series of quaint, split-rail wooden bridges. The trail crosses over feeders to Kooser Run and the run itself in several places. Skiing atop foot-and-a-half-high snow, with snow piled on the rails is fun in winter. Walk over the gravel drive and veer right, keeping the cabins to your left. If you are here during a season other than winter, the road noise may be bothersome along this section; this is the only downfall of this otherwise peaceful place. Walking over the second of the bridges takes you out of the cabin area. There are many hemlocks and evergreens mixed

ⓘ KEY AT-A-GLANCE INFORMATION

LENGTH: 2.4 miles

CONFIGURATION: Loop

DIFFICULTY: Moderate

SCENERY: Kooser Run, Kooser Lake, rhododendrons, mountain laurel, conifers and mixed deciduous forest

EXPOSURE: Mostly shaded, exposed around lake

TRAFFIC: Light

TRAIL SURFACE: Mainly dirt, some gravel and cement

HIKING TIME: 1.25 hours

ACCESS: Open year-round

MAPS: Available at the visitor's center or by calling (814) 445-8673; maps in PDF format are available online via the Pennsylvania Department of Conservation and Natural Resources Web site, **www.dcnr .state.pa.us;** USGS Bakersville

FACILITIES: Swimming, beach, concession (in summer), shower house at Kooser Lake, public phone at park office, picnic pavilions and tables, drinking water in camping areas and some picnic areas, restrooms available in various spots except in the upper woodland section of the hike

SPECIAL COMMENTS: You can cross-country ski or hike here; just note in the description where to change the hike to accommodate your needs.

▶ DIRECTIONS

From Pittsburgh, take Interstate 376 East and enter Pennsylvania Turnpike I-76 East (toll road). Take Exit 91, Ligonier–Uniontown. Turn left on PA 31 East, follow it 8.9 miles, and turn right into Kooser State Park. Drive up the road past the park office (on left) to the upper parking lot.

Kooser State Park Loop

UTM Zone (WGS84)   17T

Easting   651006

Northing   4435924

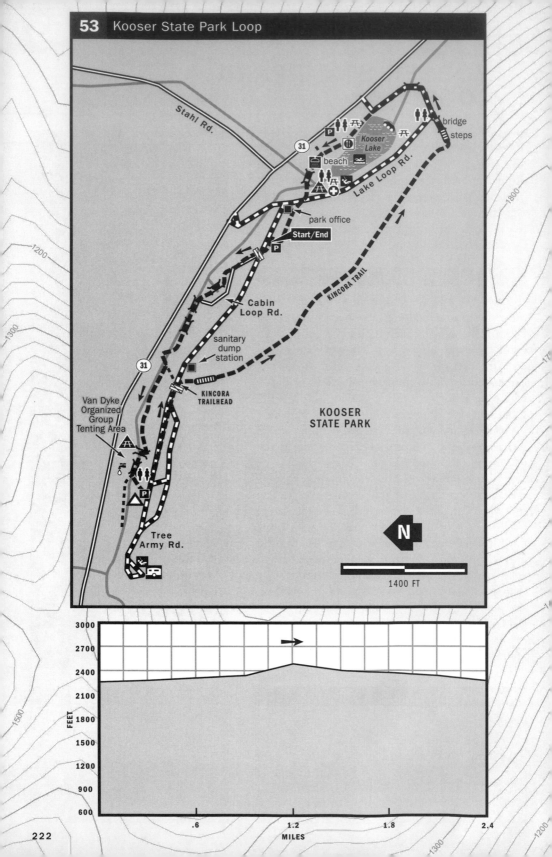

Stahl Rd.

31

Kooser
Lake

beach

bridge
steps

Lake Loop Rd.

park office

Start/End

Cabin
Loop Rd.

KINCORA TRAIL

sanitary
dump
station

31

KINCORA
TRAILHEAD

Van Dyke
Organized
Group
Tenting Area

KOOSER
STATE PARK

Tree
Army Rd.

N

1400 FT

FEET

3000
2700
2400
2100
1800
1500
1200
900
600

.6   1.2   1.8   2.4
MILES

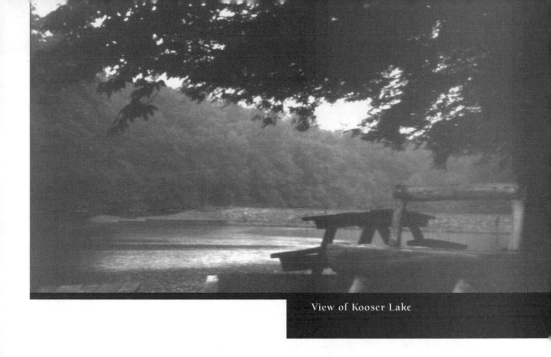

in with a few deciduous trees. Ferns fill in much of the undergrowth and mosses add to the greenery. Cross another small bridge and soon the path turns from dirt and small rocks to grass. Here you may find wildflowers in bloom.

At 0.4 miles, notice the sanitary dump station up to the left of the trail. You can turn left here to begin a trail up and into the woods immediately if you wish to cut a little distance. This hike continues straight and then loops back to pick up that trailhead. (If you are skiing, the woodlands trail is too steep and rocky, continue straight). Ahead, you'll find mountain laurel; it was in bloom in late July. The trail surface changes from grass to gravel to pine needles as you enter an enchanting grove of hemlocks and other conifers. Cross another short bridge to an open section that is occupied by a circular picnic pavilion and many single picnic tables, some underneath small shelters. The shelters are wonderful for protection from any weather. A small stove, soup, sandwiches, and hot chocolate in a daypack make for a great break on a brisk winter day.

There is also a water pump if you are in need of some liquid refreshment, and restrooms can be found after crossing the wide bridge ahead.

After crossing the bridge, you'll reach an open camping area with tent sites and picnic tables to the west and parking indicated by a sign to the east. If you are skiing, you can get more mileage by continuing straight and then turning around to either ski back on this path or on the park road above. Once you reach the parking area again, you can continue through it to loop the lake. If you are hiking, turn left and walk to the road, where you turn left again. (Continuing straight leads to RV sites and more tent camping. In summer, this may be crowded, in winter it is deserted.)

Fun to ski with groups in winter, the park road is scenic in summer as well. Rhododendrons, mayapples, ferns, and a variety of deciduous trees line its sides. Pass by the turn to a gravel road on the right, and walk around the gate to reach the Kincora Trail trailhead on the right (there is a sign).

The Kincora Trail is blazed with blue rectangles and begins with a steep climb up the hillside. Two sets of trail steps assist your climb and keep trail erosion under control. This part of the hike is more heavily wooded and allows you to enjoy more solitude. The path is narrower and in this section surrounded by mountain maples, hickory trees, mayapples, ferns, clovers, moss-covered rocks, and various undergrowth. At 1.1 miles, you've climbed about 146 feet and the grade lessons. Birdsong becomes more predominant than the sound of the fast-moving trucks and cars on PA 31, although they are still audible. If the road noise were not present, this trail would be among my favorites. Visually, it is outstanding.

At 1.27 miles, you've reached the highest point of the trail and begin a very gradual descent as the trail veers left and becomes quite rocky in sections. Step over, around, and through large rocks and small boulders. By 1.71 miles you are nearing the bottom of the descent. Walk down a short set of trail steps and over a series of plank bridges. Beech, oak, and hemlock trees are noticeable in this section. The trail ends on Lake Loop Road, which it meets at 1.87 miles. There are restrooms, picnic tables, and grills across and to the left of the road. Turn right to circle Kooser Lake and see the beach area. (Turning left will also get you back.)

Rhododendrons are thick and beautiful along the roadside and at the wide bridge crossing Kooser Run. After crossing, the road veers left and you pass a cabin on your right. At 2.03 miles, veer left to pick up a path and leave the road. The dam on your left and Kooser Lake were built by the Civilian Conservation Corps in the 1930s, as were most of the park's structures. You may notice that the trail markers have changed to blue triangles again. The road and path are used by cross-country skiers in winter. The path along Kooser Lake leads to a picnic area under hemlocks, restrooms, the beach, a concession, and a shower house. The picnic areas here are beautiful and this one is exceptional.

After passing through the picnic and beach areas, veer left following the path (right leads to the lake parking area). There is a sign pointing in the correct direction for the park office. Red maple, rhododendron, tulip trees, and daisies can be found as you approach and walk around the rustic stone and rough-sawn wood White Oak Pavilion. Rounding the pavilion on your left, cross another bridge over Kooser Run. There is a small path down to a bench next to the run. At 2.3 miles, cross Tree Army Road and walk through the grass. Pass the park office on your right and cross a tiny bridge. The parking area is visible ahead and toward the left.

▶ NEARBY ATTRACTIONS

You can swim or fish in Kooser Lake or, if looking for more hiking nearby, see the Laurel Hill State Park (hikes 54, 55, and 56) or the Forbes State Forest: Roaring Run Natural Area Loop (hike 29) entries in this book. You can find many eating and family-activity establishments on PA 31 or contact the Laurel Highlands Visitor's Bureau at (800) 333-5661 or **www.laurelhighlands.org.**

LAUREL HILL STATE PARK: HEMLOCK TRAIL

▶ IN BRIEF

The Hemlock Trail runs for the first part of the loop along the beautiful Laurel Hill Creek. The scenery here is spectacular with moss carpeting small rocks and boulders, the creek running wide and clear, and virgin hemlocks providing the final magic touch.

▶ DESCRIPTION

The Hemlock Natural Area at the center of the Hemlock Trail loop contains the only virgin trees remaining in this park. The eastern hemlock was officially made Pennsylvania's state tree in 1931 with the signature of Governor Gifford Pinchot.

To reach the trailhead of the scenic Hemlock Trail, cross the bridge and turn right at the Hemlock Trail sign. The yellow-blazed trail begins with tree branches drooping down and lining its sides like sentries; flat rocks support you across runoffs as your welcoming carpet. Note that mixed deciduous trees soon dominate the left-hand side of the trail, while hemlocks line Laurel Hill Creek on the right. At 0.11 miles, continue straight at the Y; you will come down this left branch on the return.

This trail leads closer to the creek, which it parallels for awhile. Enjoy the ferns and bright mosses against the backdrop of the dark, acidic

▶ DIRECTIONS

From Pittsburgh, take Interstate 376 East and enter the Pennsylvania Turnpike I-76 East (toll road). Take Exit 91, Ligonier–Uniontown. Turn left on PA 31 East, follow it 11.4 miles, and turn right on Trent Road (there is a state park sign at the turn). Drive 1.6 miles and turn right into Laurel Hill State Park. Drive 0.4 miles for the park office and visitor's center and 0.9 miles for the trailhead. For the trailhead, pull into the parking area on the right (before the bridge). Walk across the bridge to the trailhead on the right.

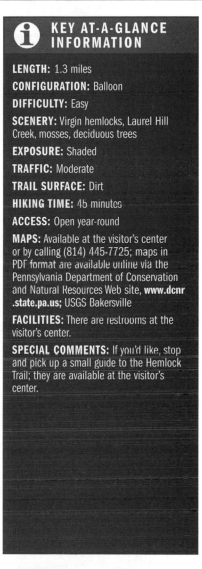

ℹ KEY AT-A-GLANCE INFORMATION

LENGTH: 1.3 miles

CONFIGURATION: Balloon

DIFFICULTY: Easy

SCENERY: Virgin hemlocks, Laurel Hill Creek, mosses, deciduous trees

EXPOSURE: Shaded

TRAFFIC: Moderate

TRAIL SURFACE: Dirt

HIKING TIME: 45 minutes

ACCESS: Open year-round

MAPS: Available at the visitor's center or by calling (814) 445-7725; maps in PDF format are available online via the Pennsylvania Department of Conservation and Natural Resources Web site, **www.dcnr .state.pa.us;** USGS Bakersville

FACILITIES: There are restrooms at the visitor's center.

SPECIAL COMMENTS: If you'd like, stop and pick up a small guide to the Hemlock Trail; they are available at the visitor's center.

Laurel Hill State Park: Hemlock Trail

UTM Zone (WGS84) 17T

Easting   650844

Northing   4430115

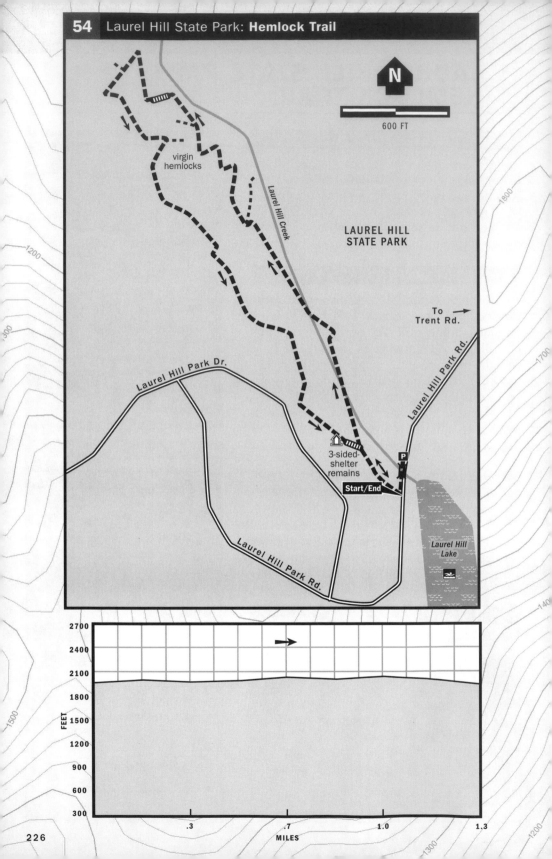

N

600 FT

virgin hemlocks

Laurel Hill Creek

LAUREL HILL STATE PARK

To Trent Rd.

Laurel Hill Park Rd.

Laurel Hill Park Dr.

3-sided-shelter remains

Start/End

P

Laurel Hill Lake

Laurel Hill Park Rd.

2700
2400
2100
1800
1500
1200
900
600
300

FEET

.3   .7   1.0   1.3
MILES

pine needles dropped by the hemlocks. Hemlocks, although evergreens, drop about one-third of their needles each year to allow new growth. The needles have collected over many years to create the thick mat of this forest floor. The tannin in the needles causes the soil to become acidic, and the great branches of the hemlocks allow only acidic soil-loving shade plants to grow in their company (notice which plants thrive in this environment).

At 0.23 miles, you can't miss the birch growing in the center of the trail and soon rhododendrons also dot the path. An outstanding mix, especially if you catch them in bloom. Rhododendrons are nurtured by the acidic soil, although they do require at least filtered sun to bloom. Notice a trail that runs down closer to the creek at 0.39 miles. You can head down to play awhile and rejoin the trail, which now leads uphill. Shortly the trail veers away from the creek.

At 0.5 miles, reach the beginning of the virgin stand of hemlocks. There are trunks here so wide that two people could not wrap their arms around and reach each other. As the park guide for this trail points out, there are not many stands of mature virgin trees remaining in Pennsylvania. These hemlocks grow slowly and take about 300 years to reach maturity. The record age for an eastern hemlock is 988 years. These giants grew from seeds so small that 200,000 of them would weigh just one pound. Being among trees of this size and age is always a magical and humbling, perspective-setting experience. I am thankful they escaped the ax although no one knows why. Their wood was considered inferior but thousands were cut and left to rot after being stripped of their bark, which was used to extract tannin for the nation's many leather tanneries.

When you are ready to move on, reach a Y with a branch to the left, and continue straight. The virgin hemlocks are interspersed with a few oaks, other deciduous trees, and boulders. The environment lifts the spirit and the feeling reminds me somewhat of walking among the virgin redwoods on the West Coast. Reach a set of dirt and cut-log trail stairs at 0.6 miles, taking you up the hill left, opposite Laurel Hill Creek. There is a bench at the top if you wish to sit and absorb this ancient area for a spell.

The creek stays in view as you continue up another, shorter set of stairs. Here the trees are mainly birch, oak, and hemlock. Stay to the left when you reach a spur on the right at 0.7 miles. (There is a sign to follow the self-guiding trail by staying left.) In this area you may notice the striped maples and tulip trees, and delicate wildflowers—depending on the time of the year. At 0.83 miles, come to a sign indicating to stay right for the interpretive trail. Going left heads straight downhill, cutting off some of the hike. If you prefer the lower trail, however, this will take you to it. Continue the upper loop of the trail by veering right and uphill. If you have the guide from the visitor's center, the posts with corresponding numbers continue along this path.

At almost 1 mile, you are near the top of the hill, and the section is carpeted with ferns in every direction. The trail begins to descend from this hillside traverse at 1.19 miles. Reach the remains of a three-sided shelter at 1.24 miles, just before a set of trail steps that lead down to the lower trail. Take these and rejoin the lower trail used to enter the loop. Turn right to return to the trailhead.

▶ NEARBY ATTRACTIONS

There are a variety of hikes in this park; see the Lake Trail and Pump House to Tram Road Trail hikes (55 and 56, respectively) in this book for descriptions. Swimming, fishing, and boating (rentals available) are also fun choices. For hiking in nearby locations, see the Forbes State Forest: Roaring Run Natural Area Loop and Kooser State Park Loop hikes (29 and 53, respectively) in this book. You can find many eating and family-activity establishments on PA 31 or contact the Laurel Highlands Visitor's Bureau at (800) 333-5661 or **www.laurelhighlands.org.**

LAUREL HILL STATE PARK: LAKE TRAIL

▶ IN BRIEF

The Lake Trail follows Laurel Hill Lake for more than a mile and then pretty Laurel Hill Creek for awhile before branching away for the final third of a mile, providing diverse and lovely scenery for the entire hike.

▶ DESCRIPTION

To reach the trailhead of the Lake Trail, stay on the parking lot side of the bridge and cross the road. Walk down the bank to see the trailhead and sign for the Lake Trail. Turn right and walk toward the lake, looking for the left that leads up onto the narrow, single-track trail. If you walk down closer to the lake first, you can find a side trail that comes up from the bank and joins the main in just 200 feet.

The trail follows this eastern shore of Laurel Hill Lake, not immediately at the water but close enough for good views along the way—and maybe to exchange a few friendly words with some anglers. It begins with a 420-foot elevation gain. Walk through mayapples, ferns, and a variety of shrubs and trees including Norway maples, and over a couple of small water runoffs. On your way up, in about 500 feet, you have a clear view of the lake through thin woods. The forest becomes a little thicker but the lake continues to be in view;

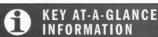

▶ KEY AT-A-GLANCE INFORMATION

LENGTH: 3.6 miles

CONFIGURATION: Out-and-back

DIFFICULTY: Moderate to difficult

SCENERY: Laurel Hill Lake, Laurel Hill Creek, deciduous trees, hemlocks, rhododendrons, wildflowers

EXPOSURE: Shaded

TRAFFIC: Light

TRAIL SURFACE: Dirt

HIKING TIME: 2 hours

ACCESS: Open year-round

MAPS: Available at the visitor's center or by calling (814) 445-7725; maps in PDF format are available online via the Pennsylvania Department of Conservation and Natural Resources Web site, **www.dcnr.state.pa.us**; USGS Bakersville and Rockwood

FACILITIES: There are restrooms at the visitor's center.

SPECIAL COMMENTS: The difficulty rating is higher due to the narrow, slippery, and steeper portions of the trail; wear good trail shoes or boots.

▶ DIRECTIONS

From Pittsburgh, take Interstate 376 East and enter the Pennsylvania Turnpike I-76 East (toll road). Take Exit 91, Ligonier–Uniontown. Turn left on PA 31 East, follow it 11.4 miles, and turn right on Trent Road (there is a state park sign at the turn). Drive 1.6 miles and turn right into Laurel Hill State Park. Drive 0.4 miles for the park office and visitor's center and 0.9 miles for the trailhead. For the trailhead, pull into the parking area on the right (before the bridge).

Laurel Hill State Park: Lake Trail

UTM Zone (WGS84)   17T

Easting   650870

Northing   4430165

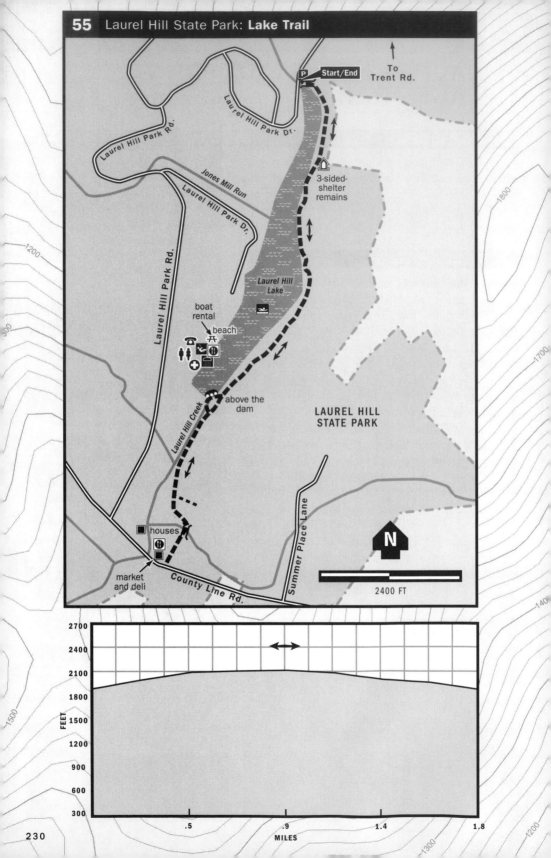

P **Start/End**

To
Trent Rd.

Laurel Hill Park Dr.

Laurel Hill Park Rd.

Jones Mill Run

Laurel Hill Park Dr.

Laurel Hill Park Rd.

3-sided-
shelter
remains

*Laurel Hill
Lake*

boat
rental

beach

Laurel Hill Creek

above the
dam

LAUREL HILL
STATE PARK

Summer Place Lane

houses

market
and deli

County Line Rd.

N

2400 FT

FEET

2700
2400
2100
1800
1500
1200
900
600
300

.5   .9   1.4   1.8
MILES

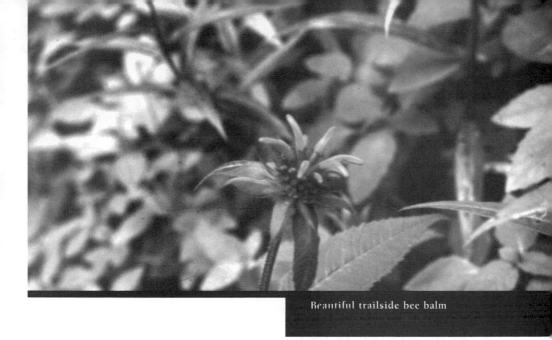

Beautiful trailside bee balm

find blackjack oak, shumard oak, rhododendron, and fan moss in the area.

Birdsong will likely fill the air. I heard many species including a catbird, a goose that must have been near or in the lake, and a woodpecker busy at work in the background. Just as you've crested this first gentle climb and have started down the other side, you'll see the remains of a three-sided shelter at 0.31 miles. I've seen another like this along the Hemlock Trail and wonder if it is left from the workers of the Civilian Conservation Corps (CCC), who, with the cooperation of several government organizations concerning public-use areas, restored this land. They also reforested, planting thousands of trees, after logging had devastated the area, turning it into a wasteland of stumps and brambles prone to forest fires and flooding. The forest around you had escaped the handsaw for longer than many other areas of the state due to the steep stream valleys and difficult hills. By 1886 though, technology made it possible to navigate it with specialized logging train engines and track that hauled the once majestic trees as cut logs to the mills.

The CCC also built the roads, trails, bridges, campsites, and buildings of the park, which has the largest concentration of their buildings in the state. When you look at the 63-acre Laurel Hill Lake during your hike, know that it was also their labor that created this pleasure.

Watch your footing on the short, steeper sections as you continue downhill to a section where many rhododendrons are growing lakeside. If you are fortunate, you'll be here in early July to see them in bloom. Walking at almost lake level, the familiar skunk cabbage also has taken root in this soggy ground. It is an area popular with a variety of fungi as well. The trail is narrow and crowded with tree roots and rocks. As you are looking down at where you are going, you may see yellow whorled loosestrife. Shores are a favorite habitat of these delicate, four-petal beauties. They are so named because they grow in whorls, usually four, around the stem, as do their leaves.

This section is relatively flat but you are beginning another slow, steady climb.

At 0.65 miles, as you reach your first sight of eastern hemlocks along this trail, the path becomes wide enough for two. Pass through a small grove of the hemlocks before coming to a bit of a steep climb that carries you through a larger grove that travels all the way down to the lake. Mountain maple and American basswood are among the deciduous trees. You may have to navigate a large tree lying across the trail as well as a rough section where some of the trail has slid away, pulled away by the great root masses of some other fallen giants.

After you've descended the hill some, at 1.04 miles, the beach is in sight, directly across the lake. The beach house you see was also built by the hands of the CCC. The trail flattens again down close to the lake. A colorful dragonfly or two may briefly accompany you. You are directly above the dam at 1.2 miles. Stay left and straight, unless you wish to walk along the fence close to the dam. If you do that, use the rocks at the creek's edge below and look left for a spur that brings you back to the main trail.

Now the trail travels along Laurel Hill Creek and is very flat with tall grasses and plants hugging it closely. Look for evidence of times when the creek rises over its banks. The trees are young and thin when you come to a choice to go left or straight at 1.58 miles. Although the left looks as though it leads into a refreshing pine forest, the trail travels straight ahead under juneberry and hawthorn trees. Also find oxeye daisies, yellow primrose, and Saint-John's-wort. Pass through a section where the underbrush is at least as tall as you and look for the tall, spectacular bee balm, with its ragged, scarlet pom-pom of tubular-shaped flowers, growing immediately before crossing a small bridge that fords a feeder stream of Laurel Hill Creek.

This leads to another unexpected grove of hemlocks. Pine needles carpet the trail, and the path is wide. Shortly after, at 1.72 miles, there is the beginning of a small neighborhood on the right. Walk through more conifers, including Norway spruce, Austrian pine, and eastern white pine as you are near the end of the trail. Also find yarrow, with its delicate, fernlike leaves, and common strawberries that ripen in July. If you like, stop at the market and deli, which serves lunch daily, by turning right when you reach the trail's end and walking 50 feet or so on the road. When finished, turn around and enjoy the walk back.

▶ NEARBY ATTRACTIONS

There is a market and deli that serves lunch daily at the end of the trail. If you're looking for more hiking, the park offers a variety. The Hemlock Trail (hike 54), which features the Hemlock Natural Area containing a virgin stand of hemlocks, and the Pump House to Tram Road Trail (hike 56) can be found in this book. Swimming, fishing, and boating (rentals available) are also fun choices. For hiking in nearby locations, see the Forbes State Forest: Roaring Run Natural Area Loop and Kooser State Park Loop hikes (29 and 53, respectively) in this book. You can find many eating and family-activity establishments on PA 31 or contact the Laurel Highlands Visitor's Bureau at (800) 333-5661 or **www.laurelhighlands.org.**

LAUREL HILL STATE PARK: PUMP HOUSE TO TRAM ROAD TRAIL

▶ IN BRIEF

This is a great hike for kids who enjoy splashing around in the creek below the small, scenic Jones Mill Dam and climbing the rocks at its side.

▶ DESCRIPTION

To reach the trailhead of the Pump House Trail, walk to the back of the parking area and around the wooden gate. The portion of the hike on the Pump House Trail is along this wide gravel path, obviously a former road. Its flat, wide surface makes it ideal for families with members of all ages to hike together.

Not far from the beginning, the Water Line Trail spurs off to the right. Stay on the orange-blazed Pump House Trail. Look for common straw-berries, sassafras, ferns, fungi, and a variety of maples and oaks, including mountain maple. Pass by the two lefts at 0.13 and 0.15 miles. You'll return from this direction if you loop using the Tram Road Trail on the return. Along this section, see cucumber trees, red-capped fungi, and more common strawberries. Kids love to find the fruit when it is in season (I found them ready for eating in early July).

At 0.57 miles, the Pump House Trail contin-ues right at the Y, heading toward the Martz Trail. Stay left to walk back to Jones Mill Dam. When

▶ DIRECTIONS

From Pittsburgh, take Interstate 376 East and enter the Pennsylvania Turnpike I-76 East (toll). Take Exit 91, Ligonier–Uniontown. Turn left on PA 31 East, follow it 11.4 miles, and turn right on Trent Road (there is a state park sign at the turn). Drive 1.6 miles and turn right into Laurel Hill State Park. Drive 0.4 miles for the park office and visitor's center and 0.9 miles for the trail-head. For the trailhead, pull into the parking area on the right (before the bridge).

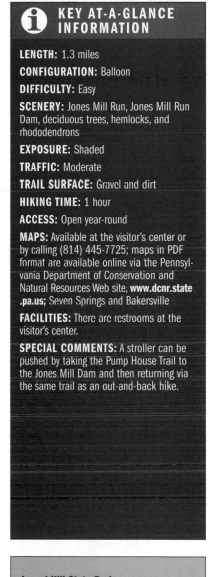

ⓘ KEY AT-A-GLANCE INFORMATION

LENGTH: 1.3 miles

CONFIGURATION: Balloon

DIFFICULTY: Easy

SCENERY: Jones Mill Run, Jones Mill Run Dam, deciduous trees, hemlocks, and rhododendrons

EXPOSURE: Shaded

TRAFFIC: Moderate

TRAIL SURFACE: Gravel and dirt

HIKING TIME: 1 hour

ACCESS: Open year-round

MAPS: Available at the visitor's center or by calling (814) 445-7725; maps in PDF format are available online via the Pennsylvania Department of Conservation and Natural Resources Web site, **www.dcnr.state.pa.us;** Seven Springs and Bakersville

FACILITIES: There are restrooms at the visitor's center.

SPECIAL COMMENTS: A stroller can be pushed by taking the Pump House Trail to the Jones Mill Dam and then returning via the same trail as an out-and-back hike.

**Laurel Hill State Park:
Pump House to Tram Road Trail**

UTM Zone (WGS84) 17T

Easting 649765

Northing 4429939

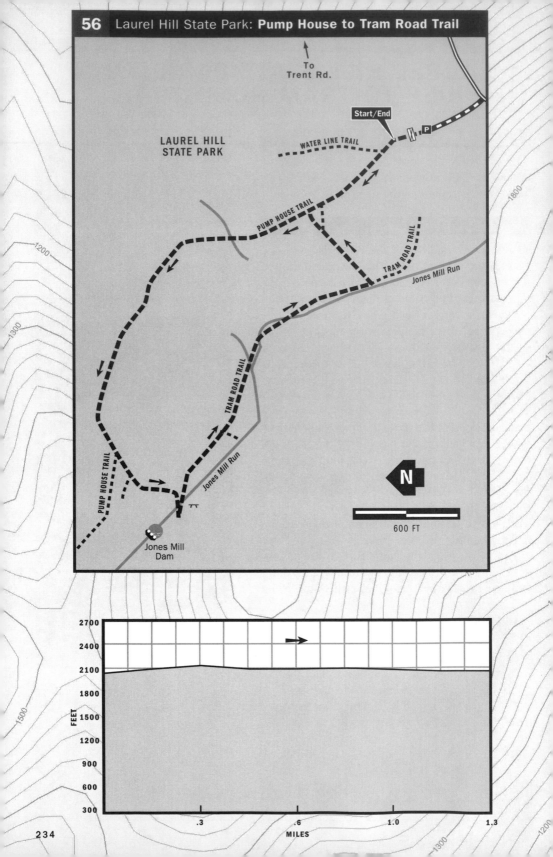

To
Trent Rd.

LAUREL HILL
STATE PARK

Start/End

WATER LINE TRAIL

PUMP HOUSE TRAIL

TRAM ROAD TRAIL

Jones Mill Run

TRAM ROAD TRAIL

PUMP HOUSE TRAIL

Jones Mill Run

Jones Mill
Dam

N

600 FT

FEET

2700
2400
2100
1800
1500
1200
900
600
300

.3   .6   1.0   1.3
MILES

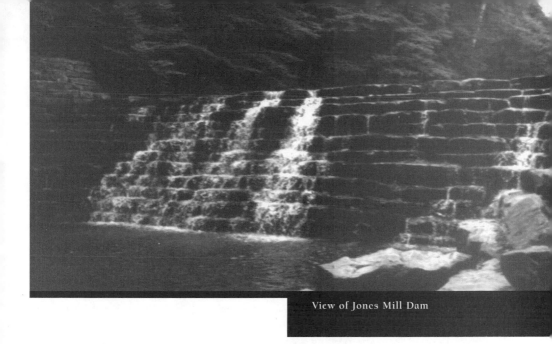

View of Jones Mill Dam

reaching the dam, staying right goes to the top, left to the bottom. You can walk up and down a path and rocks at the dam to go back and forth for a good look. The Jones Mill Dam is the handy work of the Civilian Conservation Corps who built almost all of the park's features and buildings. The park's roots were set in 1935, when 400 men arrived to restore and reforest this land through President Franklin D. Roosevelt's plan to put Americans back to work following the Great Depression. The park (then just a demonstration area) was a wasteland after near-complete logging. One virgin stand of hemlocks in the park survived and is worth the easy hike along the gorgeous Hemlock Trail to view it (see the trail's write-up in this book, hike 54). The CCC also built Laurel Hill Lake and many of the buildings, campsites, roads, and bridges throughout the park.

When you have finished at the dam, you can choose to return via the same way you came in, or to make a loop. If making the loop, be aware that this portion is on a rocky, dirt path with several crossings over Jones Mill Run. For some of these crossings, it takes pausing to look carefully for the correct trail and blazes to stay on track.

To make the loop, take the yellow-blazed Tram Road Trail by walking past the bench by Jones Mill Run and veering right onto the dirt path (there is not a sign). A short way in on this trail, at 0.73 miles, walk over a large fallen tree if it is still there. It looked as though it had been lying on the trail for a long while, so perhaps it is to become a part of the experience. Here, you'll find mountain laurel growing close to the rocky path and rhododendron populating the woods closer to the run.

The type of boulders and rocks you must navigate on this portion of the trail are why the Appalachian Trail through-hikers tend to curse Pennsylvania after a while; the state is famous for these rocky trails and outcroppings.

At 0.77 miles, a trail comes up from the run on the right; veer left, following the yellow blazes. At this point, the trail is very flat and navigating rocks is not required.

The Tram Road Trail follows what was once a railroad used to provide the rails upon which specialized trains ran to haul cut trees to the mills. Reach the first water crossing at 0.88 miles. Here is where the crossings can be a little difficult to find because other hikers have beaten narrow paths along the run, off of the main trail, and the run itself branches. This first crossing is of a branch of the main run. Look carefully for the yellow blazes and use the rocks to cross to the other side of this branch. Once you've crossed the water, the main branch of Jones Mill Run remains on your right. Cross again, this time going right over the main branch of the run so that once you've crossed, Jones Mill Run is on your left. The path is clear again after this crossing and the yellow blazes verify your choices.

In just another 106 feet, at 0.9 miles, cross the main branch of Jones Mill Run once more. There are many rocks here to make the crossing; just be careful if they are wet. Jones Mill Run is on your right after this last crossing. Once you've crossed, notice the large boulders to the right of the trail. The path is once again wide and resembles what one could think of as a former railroad bed. Reach a sign indicating the directions for various trails. The Tram Road Trail continues straight and returns down the road from the parking area. Turn left to return to the Pump House Trail. There is black oak growing here. At just 1.1 miles, the Pump House Trail is within view straight ahead and there is also a shortcut on the right. (This is the first left you saw on the way in on the Pump House Trail.) Either takes you back to the Pump House Trail, where you turn right to return to the parking area.

▶ NEARBY ATTRACTIONS

If you're looking for more hiking, the park offers a variety. The Hemlock Trail (hike 54), which features the Hemlock Natural Area containing a virgin stand of hemlocks, and the Lake Trail (hike 55) can be found in this book. Swimming, fishing, and boating (rentals available) are also fun choices. For hiking in nearby locations, see the Forbes State Forest: Roaring Run Natural Area Loop and Kooser State Park Loop hikes (29 and 53, respectively) in this book. You can find many eating and family-activity establishments on PA 31 or contact the Laurel Highlands Visitor's Bureau at (800) 333-5661 or **www.laurelhighlands.org.**

LAUREL RIDGE STATE PARK: LAUREL HIGHLANDS TRAIL—PA 653 ACCESS TO GRINDLE RIDGE

▶ IN BRIEF

This section of the 70-mile Laurel Highlands Trail travels Laurel Ridge, offering the unusual combination of a level hike and an overlook. This choice is a good one for beginning hikers (who can go as far as they wish and turn around) or beginning backpackers.

▶ DESCRIPTION

The parking area is circular. To reach the trailhead, park or walk to the northeast section, across from the picnic pavilion and cross-country ski concession, where you will find a sign. Just beyond it are an information board, map, and registration box. All hikers should register. You can sign out at the end of your hike, and park rangers will know you are out safely.

Since this section is not the beginning or end of the 70-mile Laurel Highlands Trail, the hike begins on an access spur that is blazed in blue, as are all parking and shelter access spurs of the main trail. Hike along this spur for 0.16 miles to reach the Laurel Highlands Trail, which is blazed in yellow. When you reach it, turn left at the T to travel north and cross PA 653 at 0.25 miles. Just after walking up the stone stairs on the opposite side of PA 653, you'll see an old cemetery to the right. This cemetery was used by Laurel Highland pioneers as indicated by the

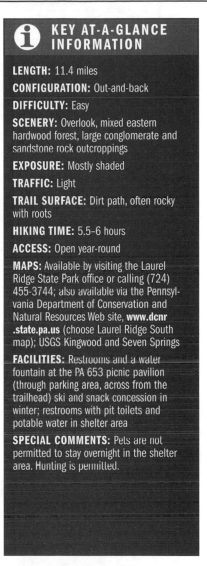

▶ KEY AT-A-GLANCE INFORMATION

LENGTH: 11.4 miles

CONFIGURATION: Out-and-back

DIFFICULTY: Easy

SCENERY: Overlook, mixed eastern hardwood forest, large conglomerate and sandstone rock outcroppings

EXPOSURE: Mostly shaded

TRAFFIC: Light

TRAIL SURFACE: Dirt path, often rocky with roots

HIKING TIME: 5.5–6 hours

ACCESS: Open year-round

MAPS: Available by visiting the Laurel Ridge State Park office or calling (724) 455-3744; also available via the Pennsylvania Department of Conservation and Natural Resources Web site, **www.dcnr.state.pa.us** (choose Laurel Ridge South map); USGS Kingwood and Seven Springs

FACILITIES: Restrooms and a water fountain at the PA 653 picnic pavilion (through parking area, across from the trailhead) ski and snack concession in winter; restrooms with pit toilets and potable water in shelter area

SPECIAL COMMENTS: Pets are not permitted to stay overnight in the shelter area. Hunting is permitted.

▶ DIRECTIONS

From Pittsburgh, take Interstate 376 East and enter the Pennsylvania Turnpike I-76 East (toll road). Take Exit 91, Ligonier–Uniontown. Turn left onto PA 31 East. Go straight for 2.1 miles and then right onto PA 711–PA 381 South and follow for 10 miles to Normalville. Make a left at the T, continuing on PA 381 South and follow 0.1 mile. Turn left on PA 653 East and follow it 5.5 miles. Turn right into the parking area.

Laurel Ridge State Park:
Laurel Highlands Trail–PA 653 Access to Grindle Ridge

UTM Zone (WGS84)   17S

Easting   639358

Northing   4424022

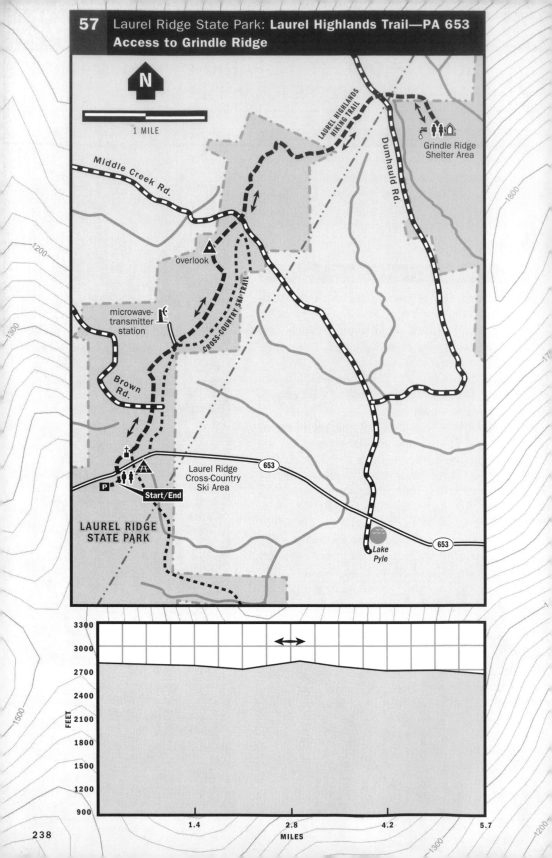

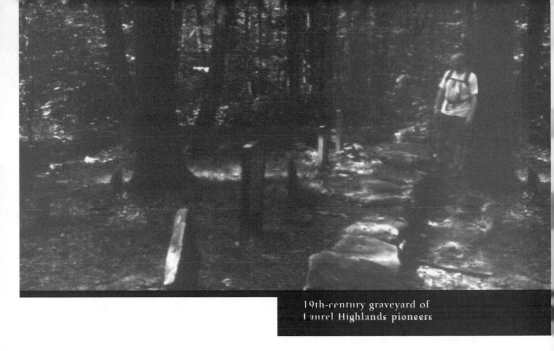

19th-century graveyard of
Laurel Highlands pioneers

headstones, which date to the mid-1800s. Take a walk over, as some of the head-stones are legible.

Back on the trail you'll notice that the easy, almost-level grade of this trail allows one to pay a little less attention to footing (although the trail does come complete with typical Laurel Highlands rocks) and more attention to the surrounding flora. Here, you'll find several black cherry trees, as well as a variety of maple, oak, and hickory trees. At 0.37 miles, enjoy walking among some shoulder-high boulders. Shortly after, pass Milepost 19. You are in approximately the center of the southern section of the Laurel Highlands Trail. The trail officially begins in Ohiopyle State Park with views of the Youghiogheny River and its northern terminus is located near Seward, Pennsylvania, with views of the Conemaugh River.

At 0.49 miles, walk over the first of many footbridges. Afterward, the trail becomes a bit rockier in some portions and you'll find your attention is periodically drawn to saving your ankles. Cross the access road (Brown Road) at 0.92 miles. You may notice the rocky outcropping on the left at 1.33 miles, just before Milepost 20. The scenery in this area includes many mosses and ferns, and some wildflowers. Daisy fleabane and Queen Anne's lace line some sunnier sections at breaks for access roads. The trail intersects the Orange Trail—one of the cross-country ski trails that circle through the area from the PA 653 ski concession near the parking area. Cross another access road at 1.56 miles, walk over flat stones and through a rocky section to cross over the Orange Trail once again. After this intersection, the trail leads through an open meadow where wild blackberries can be found. If you find them ripe as I did, you are in for a treat. Look west here (left when facing the northern direction you are traveling) to see the unmanned microwave-transmitter station (a tall conical-shaped white tower) that provides signals for aircraft navigation.

Witch hazel and American bladdernut are found growing in the area of Milepost 21 at 2.41 miles. When you reach this milepost, begin to look left for the short path to a large rocky outcropping. Turn left to walk out on the rocks when you see it. This is the only overlook of this section of the Laurel Highlands trail and provides a wonderful spot for both a break and a spectacular view. The near view is of the watershed of the middle fork of Laurel Run, which is a tributary to Indian Creek. On very clear days, the taller buildings of downtown Pittsburgh can be seen on the far horizon. Look for hawks flying above the valley as you have a snack or a drink.

After you've finished your break and continue along, you'll notice that flat rocks have been placed in various muddy sections to maintain the trail. Travel through a section where fern have dominated the undergrowth, spreading outward from both sides of the trail; pin cherry trees are also found here. Cross another dirt access road (Middle Creek Road) at 2.92 miles and bypass the trail to the right at 3 miles, which just leads to a pipeline access. Cross the pipeline just after Milepost 22. A narrow water run is forded by a short footbridge at 3.77 miles, just before reaching the second main feature of this hike: large conglomerate and sandstone boulders.

The trail weaves through several cottage-sized boulders, giving the hiker an opportunity to get a close-up view of these massive outcroppings. After meandering through the first short group, look for the trail split when you reach the second outcropping at 3.94 miles. This split allows you to walk straight ahead or make a left U-turn. Turn left and walk up the stone steps to wind through the rock walls, where you can easily see the dark iron deposits commonly found in rock here.

After the series of boulders ends, cross the third footbridge of this section, pass Milepost 23, which marks a pretty area featuring large beech trees—they are particularly nice in autumn when their leaves turn yellow. The trail leads over a series of footbridges that cross small feeder streams of Fall Run beginning at 4.34 miles. Through this section, find some larger oaks and a noticeable absence of rocks cluttering the trail. Cross Dumbauld Road, another dirt access road, and over another series of footbridges. Milepost 24 is found over the last of these at 5.15 miles. After it, at 5.3 miles, look for double yellow blazes, a blue blaze on the right, and a sign pointing right for the shelter area. Turn right and walk another 0.35 miles to reach the Grindle Ridge Shelter area.

The shelter area is a great spot to have some lunch, refresh your water supply, and use the facilities if you like before turning around. The rough-hewn Adirondack-style log shelters provide protection from weather if needed. When you've finished your break, turn around for the return hike.

▶ NEARBY ATTRACTIONS

You can use the picnic pavilion, picnic tables, and grills near the parking area in summer. In winter, temporary walls are restored on the pavilion, turning it into a ski concession where you can rent cross-country skis, obtain a ski pass, or just stop in to buy a snack or hot drink. There are many eating establishments on the way home along PA 31.

OHIOPYLE STATE PARK: CUCUMBER FALLS TO MEADOW RUN TRAIL LOOP

▶ IN BRIEF

Using the Cucumber Falls access allows easy viewing of the falls as a way to both begin and end the hike. This loop also features the Cascades Waterfall and an area called the Slides where water cascades over smooth boulders. It is a very beautiful hike.

▶ DESCRIPTION

The hike begins by walking down the gravel ramp and then stairs to an overlook of the bridal veil Cucumber Falls. The stairs continue but you can leave them at the dirt landing and go left to get closer for photos and perhaps a cooling spray. Return to the trail and continue down the remainder of the stairs, following the trail away from the falls. Step carefully, making your way over calf-high boulders. Once the trail levels out it will appear to head left toward Meadow Run. Look toward the right for the continuation of the true trail. It will be marked by a sign, which faces away from the water and says Meadow Run Trail End; you should pass with the sign on your left. Look up and inland for yellow trail blazes. A small waterfall over flat rocks can be seen here. You will walk beside a moss-covered, 100-foot-long

▶ DIRECTIONS

From Pittsburgh, take I-376 East, and enter the Pennsylvania Turnpike I-76 East (toll). Take Exit 91, Ligonier–Uniontown. Turn left onto PA 31 East. Go straight for 2.1 miles and then right onto PA 711–PA 381 South; follow for 10 miles to Normalville. Make a left at the T, continuing on PA 381 South, and follow 11 miles to Ohiopyle. Drive through the town and make a right on State Road 2019, Kentuck Road. There is a large brown park sign indicating a right for Cucumber Falls. A post for SR 2019 is not far from the turn. Make a right into the Cucumber Falls parking area.

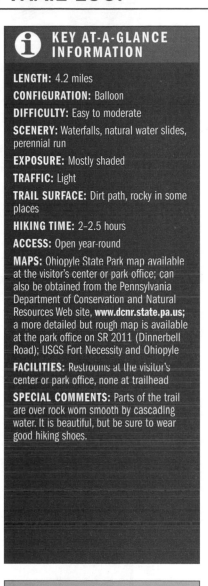

ⓘ KEY AT-A-GLANCE INFORMATION

LENGTH: 4.2 miles

CONFIGURATION: Balloon

DIFFICULTY: Easy to moderate

SCENERY: Waterfalls, natural water slides, perennial run

EXPOSURE: Mostly shaded

TRAFFIC: Light

TRAIL SURFACE: Dirt path, rocky in some places

HIKING TIME: 2–2.5 hours

ACCESS: Open year-round

MAPS: Ohiopyle State Park map available at the visitor's center or park office; can also be obtained from the Pennsylvania Department of Conservation and Natural Resources Web site, **www.dcnr.state.pa.us;** a more detailed but rough map is available at the park office on SR 2011 (Dinnerbell Road); USGS Fort Necessity and Ohiopyle

FACILITIES: Restrooms at the visitor's center or park office, none at trailhead

SPECIAL COMMENTS: Parts of the trail are over rock worn smooth by cascading water. It is beautiful, but be sure to wear good hiking shoes.

Ohiopyle State Park: Cucumber Falls to Meadow Run Trail Loop

UTM Zone (WGS84) 17S

Easting 628064

Northing 4413636

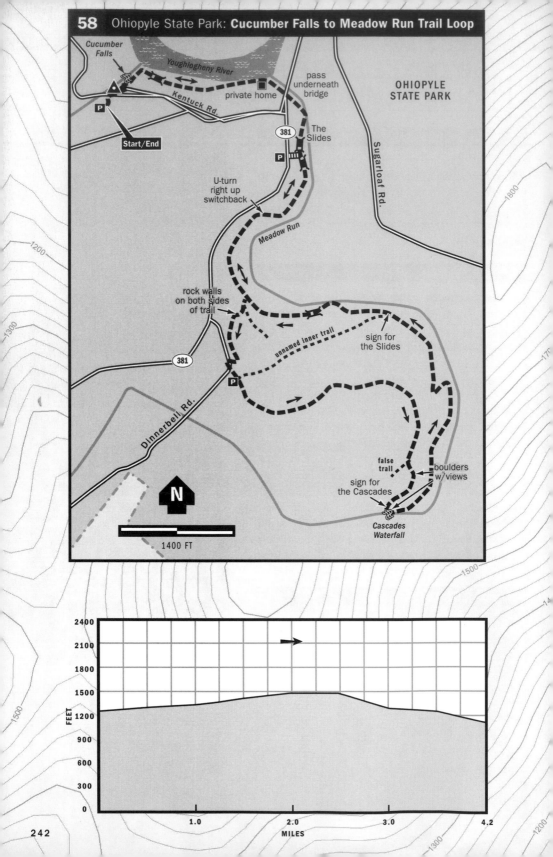

Cucumber Falls

Youghiogheny River

pass underneath bridge

OHIOPYLE STATE PARK

private home

Kentuck Rd.

P

Start/End

381

The Slides

P

Sugarloaf Rd.

U-turn right up switchback

Meadow Run

rock walls on both sides of trail

sign for the Slides

unnamed inner trail

381

P

Dinnerbell Rd.

N

1400 FT

false trail

boulders w/ views

sign for the Cascades

Cascades Waterfall

FEET

2400
2100
1800
1500
1200
900
600
300
0

1.0   2.0   3.0   4.2
MILES

boulder. Negotiate over rocks and tree roots while enjoying the view of water flowing over the boulders.

The trail heads left and over several more boulders, soon leveling out along the rapidly running water. At a little more than a half mile there is a private home to the right of the trail. Walking the trail to the left of the home leads under the bridge of PA 381 and immediately back into the woods. Large rocks, hemlocks, and the sound of the rushing water allow quick and complete immersion, as if the home and bridge hadn't been there at all. Shortly, you are walking along the Slides, a beautiful site of cascading water smoothing the rock in geologic time. Pass a set of stairs on the right that leads to a parking lot. Many people simply use this access to view the Slides and leave, but the hike is worth taking.

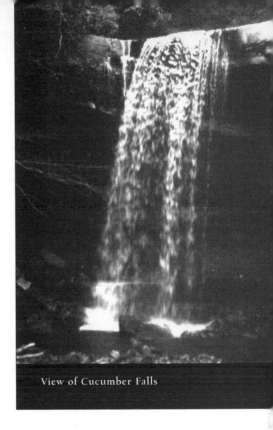

View of Cucumber Falls

Follow the yellow blazes beyond the Slides, walking up the wood-banked dirt stairs and over a small bridge. The rock continues as you pass underneath towering rhododendrons. One can't help but be swept away by the spectacular scenery. Soon the trail veers right again up away from the water. At about 0.75 miles be sure you are continuing up and to the right. You should be heading high away from the water; it is very easy to get off-trail here. Make a sharp right up the switchback. Step high over a log that has fallen across the trail and into which a wide notch has been cut for the hiker; it is blazed in yellow. The trail opens out, briefly allowing an open view of the tall hemlocks lining the left side of the trail. Beech and maple and many species of fern are also part of the makeup of these woodlands.

At 1.1 miles, make a right at the posted but unclearly marked intersection; shortly beyond that the trail passes in between a man-made, knee-high rock wall. A little road noise can be heard as you approach SR 2011 (Dinnerbell Road), which has a parking lot and access to the trail. There is a choice to continue straight or go left near the trail sign. Go straight to continue the loop. (Going left heads back down and cuts off most of the loop, reducing the hike by almost 1.5 miles. If you wish to do this—turn left, go down the hill, go straight at the Slides sign, and then left again before reaching the water.) Depending on the time of year, you'll have to watch your step to avoid stumbling over the many green apples lying about waiting for some critter to eat them and spread their seeds.

The trail ascends for a bit and alternates between being fairly smooth to sections with rocks and roots jutting up, but it is very manageable. At almost 2 miles watch out for the double blazes where you should turn left and avoid following the false trail across which some small logs have been placed. You should be descending and shortly after come to a boulder where you can step out for a nice view of the forest floor below.

Back on the trail another huge boulder rises up next to the trail. It is covered with moss and moist lichen, with rhododendron popping out of every opportune crack and a hemlock at its crest. Look up at the far end of the boulder to the underside of an overhang. The trail then veers left once more and you approach the Cascades Waterfall. Follow the direction of the sign's arrow straight back out onto the boulders to find yourself on top of the waterfall. Walk down the boulders for a beautiful view and then back to the trail the way you came. A few steps farther find another sign and access for a view of a smaller waterfall. When you have finished with the waterfalls here and return to the trail, it curves left and begins to ascend away from the water and then right, traveling next to a feeder stream to Meadow Run.

At 2.75 miles another intersection indicates a right for the Slides. To your left the trail goes uphill. Do not take that left; it is the connector trail that leads back to the SR 2011 access area. Turn right, toward the water and then left following the yellow blazes. The terrain is flat and closely following Meadow Run until you walk over a small wooden double-planked bridge and up another set of wood-banked dirt stairs.

At about 3.15 miles you'll reach the intersection where you originally turned up and right to begin the loop. Follow the sign for the Slides straight ahead. Don't forget to look for the sharp right back down the switchback. When you've reached the Slides again, step carefully on these smooth, water-worn rocks. They are usually wet and can be slippery. You will again pass by the stairs that give access to the Slides from the parking area. After negotiating your way for a bit more over the boulders, look left for the yellow blazes that lead back into the woods and Cucumber Falls. Go up the stairs to the parking lot.

▶ NEARBY ATTRACTIONS

There are many stores, cafes, and restaurants in Ohiopyle. There is also the Ohiopyle Riverfront Park area with restrooms, a snack bar, and great views of the cascading Youghiogheny River. For more hiking, see Ohiopyle State Park: Ferncliff Natural Area Loop (hike 59) or Ohiopyle State Park: Laurel Highlands Trail—Ohiopyle to First Shelter Area (hike 60).

OHIOPYLE STATE PARK: FERNCLIFF NATURAL AREA LOOP

▶ IN BRIEF

If you want a leisurely walk that is rather level and avoids the crowds, this trail provides an easily accessible escape into Pennsylvania's woods and is suitable for hikers of all ages.

▶ DESCRIPTION

Park in the parking lot at the trailhead for the Ferncliff Natural Area and walk over the bridge to the visitor's center. The bridge was rebuilt as part of the Rails-to-Trails system in the 19th-century style of the former train station. It is a pleasurable experience to walk along its length over the scenic Youghiogheny, letting the stresses of modern day melt away. The visitor's center has been maintained in much the same fashion of the time of its former operation. Inside you find friendly and helpful personnel, old photos and a bit about the area's past, restrooms, and many resources for local information.

Once you step back outside, look to the right at the beginning of the bridge for an informative sign about the history of the railroad companies who started and finished the train line into the heart of Ohiopyle. The train was in operation from 1914 to 1975. The walk from here marks the beginning of the trail described. Head back over to the bridge, pausing to take in the small rapids on your left, the wide view of the Youghiogheny to your right, and the scene of the curving bridge toward the woods into which you are about to venture.

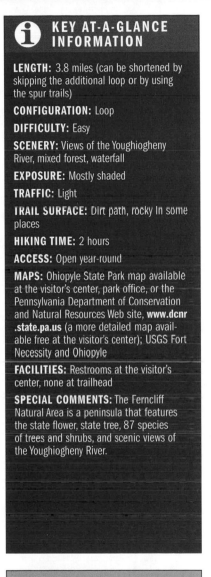

ℹ KEY AT-A-GLANCE INFORMATION

LENGTH: 3.8 miles (can be shortened by skipping the additional loop or by using the spur trails)

CONFIGURATION: Loop

DIFFICULTY: Easy

SCENERY: Views of the Youghiogheny River, mixed forest, waterfall

EXPOSURE: Mostly shaded

TRAFFIC: Light

TRAIL SURFACE: Dirt path, rocky in some places

HIKING TIME: 2 hours

ACCESS: Open year-round

MAPS: Ohiopyle State Park map available at the visitor's center, park office, or the Pennsylvania Department of Conservation and Natural Resources Web site, **www.dcnr.state.pa.us** (a more detailed map available free at the visitor's center); USGS Fort Necessity and Ohiopyle

FACILITIES: Restrooms at the visitor's center, none at trailhead

SPECIAL COMMENTS: The Ferncliff Natural Area is a peninsula that features the state flower, state tree, 87 species of trees and shrubs, and scenic views of the Youghiogheny River.

▶ DIRECTIONS

From Pittsburgh, take Interstate 376 East; enter Pennsylvania Turnpike I-76 East (toll). Take Exit 91, Ligonier–Uniontown. Go left onto PA 31 East. Go straight for 2.1 miles, then right onto PA 711–PA 381 South; go 10 miles to Normalville (first stop sign). Turn left at T onto PA 381 South; go 11 miles to Ohiopyle. Ferncliff parking is on right.

Ohiopyle State Park:
Ferncliff Natural Area Loop

UTM Zone (WGS84) **17S**

Easting **628700**

Northing **4414642**

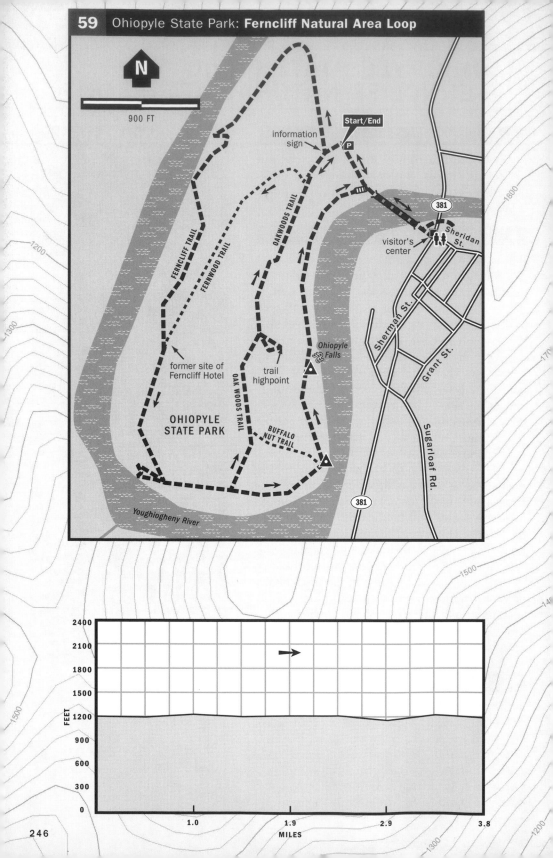

N

900 FT

information
sign

Start/End

P

381

visitor's
center

Sheridan
St.

Sherman St.

Grant St.

Ohiopyle
Falls

former site of
Ferncliff Hotel

trail
highpoint

FERNCLIFF TRAIL

FERNWOOD TRAIL

OAKWOODS TRAIL

OAK WOODS TRAIL

BUFFALO
NUT TRAIL

OHIOPYLE
STATE PARK

Sugarloaf Rd.

381

Youghiogheny River

1800

1200

1300

1700

1500

1500

FEET

2400

2100

1800

1500

1200

900

600

300

0

1.0

1.9

2.9

3.8

MILES

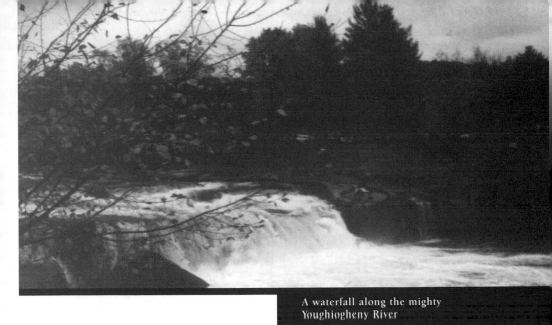

A waterfall along the mighty
Youghiogheny River

The peninsula upon which this trail system runs was formed when the mighty Youghiogheny was forced to carve its way around this resistant finger of sandstone. The site attracted the development of the former Ferncliff Hotel, which occupied the area in the neck of the peninsula from 1879 until the 1940s. The trails around the now protected peninsula were originally developed for the pleasure of the hotel guests.

There are information signs at both the trailhead and the first intersection following it. Make a right at the intersection onto the Ferncliff Trail. The long-needled eastern white pines are immediately prevalent, as is the tranquility that enfolds the entering hiker. The hike begins with a slight descent and at just about a third of a mile the Youghiogheny comes into sight between the trees. The trail begins to veer left and the tranquility becomes even more pronounced as boulders, then 15-foot-tall rhododendrons overtake the view. These soon give way to eastern hemlocks (the state tree). The moist environment allows for a variety of the water-dependent mosses to grow everywhere as well. Keep an eye out for a tree more than 100 feet tall growing straight up and on top of a triangular rock that juts out over the water. After it, the trail begins to rise slightly, and although it is relatively flat, careful steps are required to negotiate the many rocks and roots along the way. The river and its sounds will begin to fade as the trail curves away from the water. Black blazes become noticeable, marking this main outer loop of the peninsula trails. At the intersection of the Fernwood and Ferncliff trails, make a right to continue on the Ferncliff Trail, or to cut off a later loop and still see the former hotel site, turn left on Fernwood; you'll reach the site and information sign quickly.

Continuing on Ferncliff, the trail opens and becomes less rocky for a spell and a gray squirrel or two may be spotted crossing over it. A train might be heard in the distance, for a brief but fitting interruption of the natural sounds in the woods. Shortly after hiking about 1 mile, the long arms of an ancient hemlock extend over the trail, dwarfing those who pass underneath. These and the large white pines were saved from being harvested in 1911 and 1947 by the steep slopes that border the river.

At about 1.3 miles there is a short, steep path on the right that goes down to the

247

river. If you take it, go to the left around the large boulder. If you have a dog with you, be sure to have it on a leash. If you have a young child with you, don't venture down. Anyone who falls in the water here is not going to be able to escape being swept away in the rapids. The river is roaring in both sound and speed. If you've taken the path—and likely a picture of it—return to the trail, and continue on to more rhododendrons, hemlocks, and the state flower, the mountain laurel. There are also oak and other deciduous trees adding color and variety. Maple and beech are common while the tall, straight tulip poplar provides the highest layer of the forest canopy.

At 1.5 miles go straight, continuing on Ferncliff Trail at the sign indicating the Oakwoods Trail to the left. Soon after is a wide-open view of the river in a spot where it is calm and soothing. Here, there is a choice to take the Buffalo Nut spur trail left, which connects to the Oakwoods Trail. Go straight on Ferncliff. More open views continue as the trail closely follows the river. At about 1.8 miles take the stairs down to a rock overlook of small waterfalls. If children are present, keep them close. Cross the boulders following the black blazes on the rocks to return to the trail, which leads back out to the boulders once again. The park has provided lifesavers that may be cast out onto the water should someone accidentally fall in. This area is closed to swimming due to the waterfalls previously viewed downriver. Look left for the black-blazed tree to follow the trail leading up from the boulders back to the dirt path.

At just beyond 2 miles is a set of steps leading up to the Youghiogheny Bike Path. Take the stairs and turn left. Either end the hike or go back to the trailhead to take Fernwood Trail to the old hotel site.

To go to the site of the former hotel, walk back on the trail and take the Oak-woods Trail on the left and then make a right at the Fernwood Trail sign. The former site of the Ferncliff Hotel is about a one-third-of-a-mile walk back. It is difficult to imagine that a four-story, 50-guest room hotel and the accoutrements of a boardwalk to the train station, dance pavilion, tennis courts, a fountain, and a bowling alley once existed here. The protected woods have reclaimed the land and only the sign provides any indication of their existence. Here you are farther from the water and the trail is less rocky, widening enough for two people to walk side by side through a section banked with fields of ferns as far as the eye can see.

Once you reach the intersection with the Ferncliff Trail, explore the peninsula's inner trails by turning left on the Ferncliff Trail.

In about 0.4 miles, make a left and follow the Oakwoods Trail. There is a slight ascent as the river is left behind. At little more than 3 miles, there is an option to take a short hike up to the high point of the trail. If you take it, you'll find that there is not a very open view but the boulders on which you hiked earlier and the waterfalls are visible below. Once back on the Oakwoods Trail, follow it to the Fernwood Trail, and go straight to reach the trailhead. At the trailhead, go straight to the parking lot, or right if parked near the visitor's center.

▶ NEARBY ATTRACTIONS

There are many stores, cafes, and restaurants in Ohiopyle. There is also the Ohiopyle Riverfront Park area with restrooms, a snack bar, and great views of the cascading Youghiogheny River. For more hiking, see the other Ohiopyle State Park trails in this book (hikes 58 and 60).

OHIOPYLE STATE PARK: LAUREL HIGHLANDS TRAIL—OHIOPYLE TO FIRST SHELTER AREA

▶ IN BRIEF

This section of the 70-mile Laurel Highlands Trail is definitely the most spectacular. The steep climbs and descents afford many views of the Youghiogheny River and its beautiful valley, as well as scenic streams and the surrounding western Pennsylvania foliage. This out-and-back hike is one in which it is rewarding and worthwhile to see the sights from both directions.

▶ DESCRIPTION

If you have parked at the official trailhead, cross PA 381 and walk down the obvious street north of the general store, passing the alternative lot, to the registration box, which is located inside the gate at the end of the street. All hikers should register. You can sign out at the end of your hike, and park rangers will know you are out safely.

The trail will be dirt from here on, walk 200 feet or so, and make the sharp left up the steep dirt/log-banked stairs at the sign that says Hiking Trail. You'll go uphill about 200 feet, drop slightly, and rise again at a much gentler angle to reach a sign for Johnston–Ohiopyle, which has been placed there to point out the direction for anyone coming down the blue-blazed access trail on the left. You'll then settle into an easy pace on a relatively flat, albeit rocky, former road for approxi-

▶ DIRECTIONS

From Pittsburgh, take Interstate 376 East and enter Pennsylvania Turnpike I-76 East (toll). Take Exit 91, Ligonier–Uniontown. Turn left onto PA 31 East. Go straight for 2.1 miles, then right onto PA 711–PA 381 South; follow 10 miles to Normalville. Make a left at the T, continuing on PA 381 South; follow 11 miles to Ohiopyle. There is a parking lot on the right (official trailhead), or drive another hundred feet or so and turn left, pass the few businesses, and park in the lot on the right.

ⓘ KEY AT-A-GLANCE INFORMATION

LENGTH: 12.6 miles

CONFIGURATION: Out-and-back

DIFFICULTY: Difficult due to elevation gains and distance

SCENERY: Views of the Youghiogheny River and the river valley, several streams, and mixed eastern hardwood forest

EXPOSURE: Mostly shaded

TRAFFIC: Medium to heavy on weekends

TRAIL SURFACE: Dirt path, sometimes rocky with roots

HIKING TIME: 5.5–6 hours

ACCESS: Open year-round

MAPS: Available by visiting or calling the Laurel Ridge State Park office at (724) 455-3744 or via the Pennsylvania Department of Conservation and Natural Resources Web site, **www.dcnr.state.pa.us** (choose the Laurel Ridge South map); map is also available at the Ohiopyle Visitor's Center located in the former train station (walk there from the official trailhead parking lot by turning left on the bike path and crossing the bridge); USGS Ohiopyle

FACILITIES: Restrooms at the Ohiopyle Visitor's Center (see above), restrooms with pit toilets and potable water in shelter

SPECIAL COMMENTS: Pets are not permitted to stay overnight in the shelter area. Hunting is permitted.

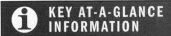

Ohiopyle State Park: Laurel Highlands Trail—Ohiopyle to First Shelter Area

UTM Zone (WGS84)   17S

Easting   629438

Northing   4414454

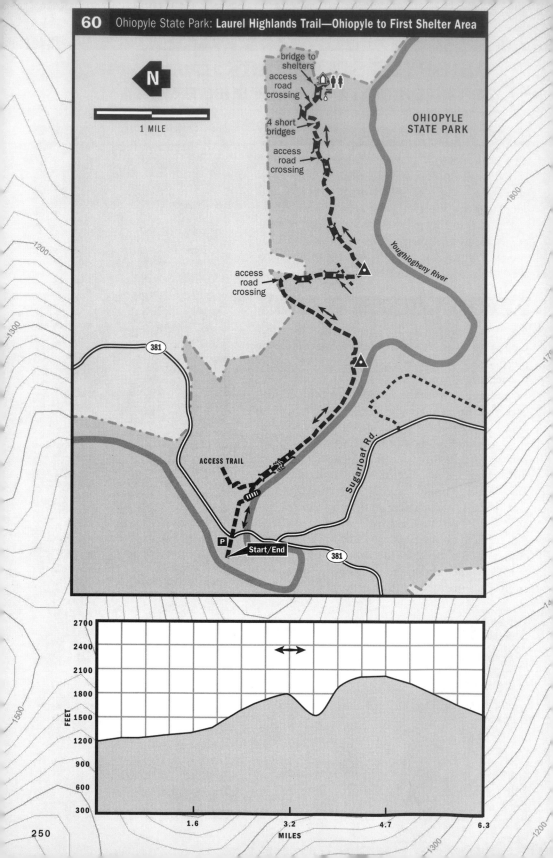

N

1 MILE

bridge to
shelters

access
road
crossing

OHIOPYLE
STATE PARK

4 short
bridges

access
road
crossing

access
road
crossing

Youghiogheny River

381

ACCESS TRAIL

Sugarloaf Rd.

P

Start/End

381

mately the next mile and begin to notice the yellow blazes that mark the remainder of the main trail about every 100 feet. Not long before the 1-mile marker, you cross two small half-cut log footbridges, the second over Sheepskin Run, a small stream prettily cascading down some rocks on the left.

Typical of the area, you will hike through maple, beech, oak, and other common deciduous trees, as well as mountain laurel and rhododendron. If it is autumn, the colors are fantastic; if it is spring or summer, the wildflowers and blooms of the mountain laurel and rhododendron will treat your visual and olfactory senses. Walk over the flat rocks that have been thoughtfully placed in boggier portions of this lower trail.

At 1.8 miles, the trail begins turning into and climbing up the mountain. You are pretty much climbing for the next 530 feet, during which time the views are becoming better and better. Past the 2-mile marker are a slight descent, another ascent, and views of the Youghiogheny River that can be enjoyed as you walk along. Don't miss the opportunity to take a break at the obvious outcropping in the middle of this ascent. The river makes a U-bend around the finger of the Virginia Flats below. Sugarloaf Knob is the high point directly across the river.

Carry on to the peak of this climb at 1,943 feet. There is another view here but it is not nearly as good since you are further back from the river and are looking through more trees. From here you begin a comparatively gentle descent until you reach 3.2 miles, where there is a sign indicating that the direction of the trail is to the right. This is the start of a steep descent via switchbacks, which lead down, away from the ridgeline and deeper into the woods. Cross an access road, and the descent continues on the other side until you reach the beautiful Rock Spring Run at 1,515 feet.

After crossing the bridge over this scenic water flow (the fullest along the entire length of the Laurel Highlands Trail), begin your way back up what starts out as a fairly gentle ascent. This soon changes. If ignorance is bliss for you, keep your eyes on the trail, otherwise, take a look up at the mountainside you are climbing toward the next ridge. It's steep and it's fun to have the workout. The angle lets off soon though and the ascent continues at a very reasonable level. Cross another small half-log cut bridge to the 4-mile marker and then over what appears to be an old access road that has grassed over since the days when it may have been actively used. Word has it that this was once a farmland with an orchard; if you are here in the proper season, you may find some apples along the way.

The ascent becomes even gentler as you follow the trail left around the mountain, putting the ridge on your left side and the river on your right. Here you ramble along for about a quarter mile, enjoying slight dips and rises and more views of the Youghiogheny River. Be careful though, the trail becomes quite narrow in places. You'll cross another of the now common footbridges shortly before you begin a descent that continues for little more than a half mile. Pass the 5-mile marker and know you have reached the bottom of this part of the descent when you cross another small bridge and over another old logging and access road.

Ascend slightly and then continue a gentle descent, passing the 6-mile marker and crossing a series of footbridges, including the 20-foot bridge over lovely Lick Run. After ascending up a short set of stone steps and over another old access road, you'll

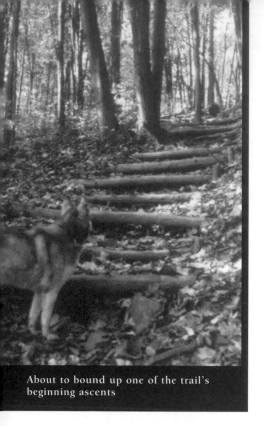

About to bound up one of the trail's beginning ascents

find, in about another 160 feet, that the woods open out and the entire feel of the environment changes. You are now away from the ridgeline again but this area in the heart of the woodlands is more open and gives an entirely different feel to your hike.

At about 6.1 miles, turn right at the sign for the shelters if you'd like to go down, have a look, and have some lunch before turning around. There is a water pump here that yields potable water, pit toilets, cut firewood, rough-hewn log Adirondack-style shelters, and space for tent camping.

When you've finished your break, turn around and expect just as pleasant a hike out as you enjoyed on the way in.

▶ NEARBY ATTRACTIONS

There are many stores, cafes, and restaurants in Ohiopyle. There is also the Ohiopyle Riverfront Park area with restrooms, a snack bar, and great views of the cascading Youghiogheny River. For more hiking options, see Ohiopyle State Park: Cucumber Falls to Meadow Run Trail Loop (hike 58) or Ohiopyle State Park: Ferncliff Natural Area Loop (hike 59).

60 Hikes within 60 MILES

PITTSBURGH
INCLUDING ALLEGHENY AND SURROUNDING COUNTIES

APPENDIXES
& INDEX

APPENDIX A: HIKING STORES

LOCATION/CITY

Eastern Mountain Sports, Pittsburgh
Ross Park Mall
1000 Ross Park Mall Drive
Pittsburgh, PA 15237
(412) 364-8078
www.ems.com

Exkursion, Monroeville
4037 William Penn Highway
Monroeville, PA 15146
(412) 372-7030
www.exkursion.com

REI, Pittsburgh
412 South 27th Street
Pittsburgh, PA 15203
(412) 488-9410
www.rei.com

APPENDIX B: PLACES TO BUY MAPS

LOCATION/CITY

Eastern Mountain Sports, Pittsburgh
Ross Park Mall
1000 Ross Park Mall Drive
Pittsburgh, PA 15237
(412) 364-8078
www.ems.com

Exkursion, Monroeville
4037 William Penn Highway
Monroeville, PA 15146
(412) 372-7030
www.exkursion.com

REI, Pittsburgh
412 South 27th Street
Pittsburgh, PA 15203
(412) 488-9410
www.rei.com

United States Geological Survey
(888) 275-8747
www.usgs.gov/pubprod/maps.html

Weldins, Pittsburgh
413 Wood Street
Pittsburgh, PA 15222
(412) 281-0123

APPENDIX C:
HIKING CLUBS

▶ NAME/LOCATION

Butler Outdoor Club
P.O. Box 243
Butler, PA 16003-0243
www.butleroutdoorclub.com

Explorers' Club of Pittsburgh
2005 Beechwood Boulevard
Pittsburgh, PA 15217-1726
www.pittecp.org

Keystone Trails Association
P.O. Box 129
Confluence, PA 15424-0129
www.kta-hike.org

North Country Trail Association,
Greater Pittsburgh Chapter
933 Norfolk Street
Pittsburgh, PA 15217
www.northcountrytrail.org/gpt/index.htm

Shenango Outing Club
Riverside Park Nature Center
P.O. Box 244
Greenville, PA 16125

Sierra Club–Allegheny Group
P.O. Box 824
Pittsburgh, PA 15217
(412) 561-0203
www.alleghenysc.org

Warrior Trail Association, Inc.
P.O. Box 103
Waynesburg, PA 15370-0103
www.greenepa.net/community/WarriorTrail

INDEX

INDEX

INDEX

INDEX

INDEX

INDEX

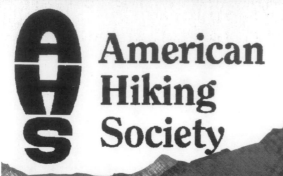
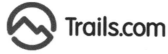
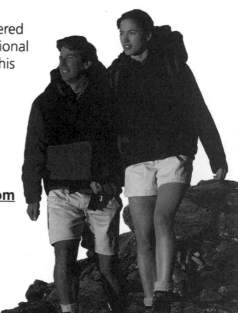